The Mental Health
Consequences of Torture

The Plenum Series on Stress and Coping

Series Editor:
Donald Meichenbaum, *University of Waterloo, Waterloo, Ontario, Canada*

A Continuation Order Plan is available for this series. A continuation order will bring delivery of each new volume immediately upon publication. Volumes are billed only upon actual shipment. For further information please contact the publisher.

The Mental Health Consequences of Torture

Edited by

Ellen Gerrity

National Institute of Mental Health
Bethesda, Maryland

Terence M. Keane

Boston University School of Medicine
Boston, Massachusetts

and

Farris Tuma

National Institute of Mental Health
Bethesda, Maryland

Kluwer Academic / Plenum Publishers
New York, Boston, Dordrecht, London, Moscow

Library of Congress Cataloging-in-Publication Data

The mental health consequences of torture/edited by Ellen T. Gerrity, Terence M. Keane, and Farris Tuma
    p. ; cm — (Plenum series on stress and coping)
    Includes bibliographical references and index.
    ISBN 0-306-46422-5
    1. Torture victims—Mental health.   2. Torture victims—Rehabilitation.   3. Torture—Psychological aspects.   4. Post-traumatic stress disorder—Treatment.   I. Gerrity, Ellen T.   II. Keane, Terence Martin.   III. Tuma, Farris.   IV. Series.
    [DNLM: 1. Stress Disorders, Post-Traumatic—psychology.   2. Torture—psychology.   3. Crime Victims—rehabilitation.   4. Mental Health Services.   5. Stress Disorders, Post-Traumatic—rehabilitation.   6. Violence—psychology.   WM 170 M549 2001]

RC451.4.T67 M46 2001
616.85′21—dc21

00-059276

ISBN: 0-306-46422-5

2001 Kluwer Academic / Plenum Publishers, New York
233 Spring Street, New York, N.Y. 10013

http://www.wkap.nl/

10   9   8   7   6   5   4   3   2   1

A C.I.P. record for this book is available from the Library of Congress

Printed in the United States of America

Contributors

Metin Basoglu, Section on Traumatic Studies, Institute of Psychiatry, King's College, London University SES 8AF London, England

Brian Engdahl, Veterans Administration Medical Center, Minneapolis, Minnesota 55417

John A. Fairbank, Department of Psychiatry, Duke University Medical Center, Durham, North Carolina 27710

Matthew J. Friedman, Dartmouth University, and the National Center for Post-Traumatic Stress Disorder, White River Junction, Vermont 05009

Merle Friedman, Psych-Action, Senderwood, Bedfordview, Gauteng 2007, South Africa

Ellen Gerrity, National Institute of Mental Health, Neuroscience Center Building, Bethesda, Maryland 20892

Malcolm Gordon, National Institute of Mental Health, Neuroscience Center Building, Bethesda, Maryland 20892

James M. Jaranson, Department of Psychiatry, University of Minnesota, St. Paul, Minnesota 55108-1300

Boaz Kahana, Department of Psychology, Cleveland State University, Cleveland, Ohio 44115

Eva Kahana, Department of Sociology, Case Western Reserve University, Cleveland, Ohio 44106

Marianne Kastrup, Rehabilitation and Research Center for Torture Victims, Borgergade 13/P.O. Box 2107, DK-1014 Copenhagen, Denmark

Terence M. Keane, Department of Psychiatry, Boston University School of Medicine, Boston, Massachusetts 02130

Dean G. Kilpatrick, National Crime Victims Research and Treatment Center, Department of Psychiatry and Behavioral Sciences, Medical University of South Carolina, Charleston, South Carolina 29425

J. David Kinzie, Department of Psychiatry, Oregon Health Sciences University, Portland, Oregon 97201

Mary P. Koss, Arizona Prevention Center, University of Arizona College of Medicine, Tucson, Arizona 85719

Kathryn M. Magruder, Department of Psychiatry and Behavioral Sciences, Medical University of South Carolina, Charleston, South Carolina 29425

Anthony J. Marsella, Department of Psychology, University of Hawaii, Honolulu, Hawaii 96821

Richard Mollica, Harvard Program in Refugee Trauma, Department of Psychiatry, Harvard University, Cambridge, Massachusetts 02138

Sister Dianna Ortiz, Guatemalan Human Rights Commission, Washington, D.C. 20017

Robert S. Pynoos, UCLA Trauma Psychiatry Service, Department of Psychiatry, University of California at Los Angeles, Los Angeles, California 90095

Margaret E. Ross, Cambridge Business Development Center and International Criminal Defense Attorneys Association, Cambridge, Massachusetts 02139

Agnes Rupp, National Institute of Mental Health, Neuroscience Center Building, Bethesda, Maryland 20892

Derrick Silove, School of Psychiatry, Southwestern School, University of New South Wales, Sydney, Australia

Eliot Sorel, Department of Psychiatry and Behavioral Sciences, George Washington University, 2021 K Street, NW, Washington, D.C. 20006

Steven Southwick, Department of Psychiatry, Yale University School of Medicine, West Haven, Connecticut 06516

Farris Tuma, National Institute of Mental Health, Neuroscience Center Building, Bethesda, Maryland 20892

Foreword

Torture has no ideological, geographical, or other boundaries: survivors of torture are everywhere. While some argue that we as a nation can no longer afford to remain engaged with the world—especially the poor, the abused, refugees, and those seeking asylum—often those most in need of aid are right here in our midst and stand as a repudiation of that idea.

The practice of torture is one of the most serious human rights abuses of our time. Torture and other forms of severe ill treatment conducted by paramilitaries or government security forces (or condoned by other government officials) occur in 125 countries today, according to the 1999 report of Amnesty International. The same Amnesty International report cites 78 countries that incarcerate prisoners of conscience, 66 countries that allow detention without charge or trial, 47 countries where extrajudicial executions occur, and 37 countries where "disappearances" among citizens are common. In recent years, people in the United States and the international community have become increasingly aware of the need to prevent these human rights abuses and to punish the perpetrators forcefully when abuses take place. Yet too often we have failed to address the needs of survivors after their rights have been so severely violated. The mental health consequences of torture and the treatment of torture survivors must be a central focus of our efforts to promote human rights.

As part of its efforts to promote internationally recognized human rights, the United States can and must do more to stop torture abroad and to treat those in this country who suffer from its consequences. In 1994, the U.S. Senate ratified the Convention Against Torture and Other Forms of Cruel, Inhuman, or Degrading Treatment or Punishment. Although Congress has taken some modest steps to begin to implement parts of the convention, we have not yet taken action to provide sufficient rehabilitation services in the spirit of Article 14 of the convention. In 1981, the United Nations created the Voluntary Fund for Victims of Torture, which provides funding and support to rehabilitation centers worldwide. But since that time, the fund has dispensed only half of what was requested by centers worldwide, a paltry sum compared to the need.

My own agenda in the Senate has included a number of legislative initiatives designed to combat torture and to help rehabilitate its survivors. In the 103rd Congress, I sponsored the Comprehensive Torture Victims Relief Act, which became the basis for the Torture Victims Relief Act in the 105th Congress and was enacted on October 30, 1998, as Public Law 105–320. This law authorized $12.5 million over 2 years for assistance to torture victim treatment centers in the United

States and around the world. The funds were authorized through a U.S. contribution in the amount of $3 million per year to the U.N. Voluntary Fund for Torture Victims, the full amount of which was appropriated in 1999. On November 3, 1999, the Torture Victims Relief Reauthorization Act was enacted as Public Law 106–87, which extends and increases the authorizations of 1998 through fiscal year 2003. This law authorizes $10 million for domestic treatment centers, $10 million for the U.S. Agency for International Development, and $5 million to be distributed through the U.S. contribution to the U.N. fund. The act addresses the continuing need to provide treatment services to the millions of survivors of torture worldwide and the estimated hundreds of thousands of survivors in this country alone. Repressive governments frequently torture those who are defending human rights and democracy in their own country. Enactment of this legislation recognizes the debt we owe to these courageous people who have made such a sacrifice for cherished principles and was an important step forward in our efforts to provide needed relief for torture survivors.

Without adequately funded and effective programs of treatment and rehabilitation, torture survivors often endure tremendous mental and physical suffering and are unable to hold a job, study for a new profession, or acquire other skills needed for successful adjustment into society. We need look no further than today's headlines about Kosovo, East Timor, Iraq, or Bosnia to know that we will be dealing with the problems that torture survivors face for many years. That is why we need more research on the mental health consequences of exposure to torture, better information on the incidence and prevalence of torture in the U.S. refugee and asylee populations, and an expansion of domestic and international treatment programs. Direct treatment programs not only give medical and psychological care to those who have been traumatized by torture but also provide hope to those struggling for human rights. Further, they provide documentation on the practice of torture that cannot be effectively refuted by governments, and this can help to eradicate torture as a systematic practice.

While many thousands of men, women, and children who are torture survivors live in the United States today, there are far too few centers with the resources and capabilities to treat the unique and critical problems they face. As a senator from Minnesota, I am extraordinarily proud of the Center for Victims of Torture in Minneapolis, which since 1985 has been doing pioneering work to address the complex needs of survivors of torture. In addition to the Center for Victims of Torture, centers have been established in New York, San Francisco, Chicago, Los Angeles, Denver, Eugene (Oregon), Baltimore, and Dallas. Yet, these centers are woefully underfunded and their sizes are inadequate to meet the need. The serious personal, familial, and community consequences of torture demand that federal, state, and local governments work together more vigorously to expand existing services and to develop more intervention and treatment programs. In the wake of so many wars and other catastrophes in recent years that have prompted tremendous human migrations from one region or country to another on several continents, we must devote greater resources to meeting the diverse human needs of refugees, asylees, and displaced persons. We must recognize that the losses sustained by these individuals are not just material losses but psychological and emotional as well.

It has been more than 50 years since the Universal Declaration on Human Rights and its attendant enforcement mechanisms, including the U.N. Commission, placed a new premium on the rights of individuals. Since then, the basic work of standard-setting, adjudication, enforcement, and institution-building has gone on, with international covenants and treaties adopted, international and regional commissions and bodies established, and other key steps being taken by the United States, other nations, and international bodies like the United Nations.

But even with such progress, much more must be done. The United States, by its history, its position, and its values, is uniquely situated to play an important role by injecting a new emphasis on human rights into its foreign policy and by being prepared to support much more vigorously—politically, legally, and diplomatically— application of international human rights law through the domestic legal systems of states, in bilateral and multilateral state relations, and through ad hoc legal bodies and permanent international organizations. A minimum guarantee of basic human dignity with a commitment to the continually expanding promotion and application of human rights standards is clearly in America's best tradition.

At the same time, we must continue to support those who suffer from the consequences of human rights abuses, especially those who experience the unspeakable betrayal of torture, by providing the necessary resources for better research, services, and treatment and by providing the necessary legal protections. We have a responsibility to bear witness to these atrocities, to do what we can to end them, and to help those who have survived and want nothing more than to regain their lives and their faith in humanity.

PAUL DAVID WELLSTONE
UNITED STATES SENATOR
WASHINGTON, DC

Prologue

This volume testifies to the strength of the human spirit even as it examines with an unflinching eye the horrific acts and consequences of torture and other causes of violent trauma. The text attends particularly to the psychological scars that torture and trauma inflict on victims and observers. First-person accounts that have been described with searing vividness both by famous writers and by anonymous voices afford us glimpses of both evil and triumph. Hope persists that the tragic, unadorned accounts of those who have survived will serve to raise awareness on the part of peoples throughout the world and ultimately prevent future incidents of torture and malicious violence. Yet if we are truly to develop the capacity to begin to heal the wounded, educate the innocent, and prevent future atrocities, a more systematic understanding of torture and its consequences is imperative.

The scientific challenge of understanding and stopping the practice of torture and violent trauma is global in scale; contributions of the research community are necessary, but these will be effective only to the extent that they encourage the participation of people from all walks of life. The National Institute of Mental Health (NIMH) is a component of the U.S. National Institutes of Health. The mission of NIMH is to reduce the burden of mental disorders through research on mind, brain, and behavior. NIMH's expertise and convening power equip it well to play a role in the search for knowledge that will provide improved treatments for the profound psychological sequelae of torture and violence. We are pleased to have had the opportunity to cosponsor the seminal 1997 conference on mental health research and services for survivors of torture and to have participated in the development of this volume, a product of the conference.

A strong consensus among peoples throughout the world holds that research involving humans is a sacred trust, one that demands respect for the dignity and welfare of research participants and the highest level of ethical accountability on the part of researchers. In no instance are these demands more critical than when research—whether clinical, observational, descriptive, or any other approach—involves the participation of individuals whose lives have been shattered through the malice of others. The demand for particular sensitivity and respect extends to any research-derived intervention strategies for posttraumatic stress disorder (PTSD) and other consequences of violent trauma. Among the potential obstacles to research and treatment alike is the possibility that medical professionals may have played a role in perpetrating torture or in resuscitating victims, so that subsequent interactions with medical professionals may be extremely stressful for survivors. People who were victimized may harbor realistic concerns that by recounting or publicizing their experiences, they may place themselves or their families at risk for yet further assault. Also, researchers and clinicians must be exquisitely aware of the danger of retraumatizing victims through well-intentioned questions or treatment strategies.

The mental health research community has made considerable progress in recent years in refining clinical interventions for use in the context of PTSD. At the same time, we recognize that the general diagnosis of PTSD likely does not capture or reflect the full range of symptoms and aftereffects associated with the unique experience of purposeful physical or psychological torture.

From a research perspective, one promising avenue for understanding PTSD and related conditions—and, in turn, improving our clinical treatments—lies in research that is beginning to pinpoint the way in which the human brain is altered by torture and violent trauma. We have learned much in recent years about how our brains and bodies respond to danger. Based on the fundamental need for survival, the brain assigns special significance to experiences and memories of the most dangerous, life-threatening events. Researchers have labeled an important component of the resulting traces "emotional memories" and have determined that they are processed through a particular part of the brain, the amygdala, that coordinates responses to threat, danger, or pain. In an "ordinary" dangerous situation, the amygdala's processing of a particular emotional memory plays a critical role in activating the "fight-or-flight" response, marked by an increase in heart rate, as well as a surge in stress hormones, a change in pain thresholds, and other automatic responses that permit an organism to respond appropriately to danger. We must understand, however, how in the situation of torture, our neural circuitry is altered by an uncontrollable, inescapable, and often repeated set of experiences for which the brain was never prepared by evolution. An unnatural environmental force, the experience of torture, is fully capable of fundamentally changing the function and, indeed, the actual structure of the brain. Although one should not be surprised that existing treatments are frustratingly inadequate in helping many survivors of torture, we should be heartened that accumulating knowledge about brain and behavior offers the promise for more specific, effective approaches to intervention and rehabilitation. As this promise comes to fruition, we must not fail to conduct the clinical trials and health service systems research that will ensure that effective treatments are identified and implemented.

We hope that this volume will find a place in needed clinical education and training programs for health care providers who are called on to work with victims. And, as research progresses, our intent is that the volume, which is a product of collaboration among multiple federal agencies and individuals from around the world, will heighten global attention to the unconscionable frequency of systematic torture in diverse settings and steel the resolve of people throughout the world to banish torture from human experience.

Steven E. Hyman, M.D.
Director, National Institute of Mental Health
Bethesda, Maryland

Preface

Torture, as defined by the World Medical Association, is "the deliberate, systematic, or wanton infliction of physical or mental suffering by one or more persons acting alone or on the orders of any authority, to force another person to yield information, to make a confession, or for any other reason."[1] Accurate numbers are difficult to obtain, but it is estimated that among refugees alone, the number of individuals who have experienced torture ranges from 5% to 35% of the world's 14 million refugees. When internally displaced persons are added to this number, as well as asylees, it can be roughly estimated that the world situation now includes at least 40 million forced migrants, many of whom have faced torture and related trauma in their lives. A report from Amnesty International in 1999 stated that systematic use of torture or similar ill treatment was ongoing in 120 of the world's 204 countries. The experience of torture results in the development of a wide range of psychological, behavioral, medical, and economic problems, including severe physical injuries and disabilities; psychiatric disorders, such as posttraumatic stress disorder, depression, and anxiety disorders; and a variety of serious psychological and emotional symptoms. The use of torture represents a worldwide problem that needs to be addressed by policymakers, researchers, clinicians, and the survivors themselves.

In mid-1997, the National Institute of Mental Health (NIMH), a research institute with the National Institutes of Health (NIH) and the U.S. Public Health Service,[2] assembled a panel of international experts to address the topic of the mental health consequences of torture and related violence and trauma. The mission of the group, the NIMH Working Group on the Mental Health Consequences of Torture and Related Violence and Trauma, was to produce a report on the status of scientific knowledge on this topic and to include research recommendations with implications for treatment, services, and policy development for survi-

---

[1] Amnesty International. (1985). The Declaration of Tokyo (World Medical Association). In Amnesty International Secretariat (Ed.), *Ethical codes and declarations relevant to the health professions* (2nd ed.). London: Author, pp. 9–10.

[2] As part of its mission to improve the diagnosis, treatment, and prevention of mental disorders and promote mental health, NIMH conducts and supports a broad spectrum of biological, psychological, and social research on mental disorders and mental health. A portion of NIMH's mission is focused on supporting research and research training concerning various aspects of violence and traumatic stress. This book was developed by the members of the NIMH Working Group on the Mental Health Consequences of Torture and Related Violence and Trauma and may not necessarily reflect the views of NIMH, NIH, or the U.S. Department of Health and Human Services.

vors of torture. Early in the process, the group members recognized that a comprehensive report on this topic would necessarily include systematic reviews of closely related traumatic stress research areas, such as studies of war veterans, Holocaust survivors, rape and domestic violence survivors, former prisoners of war, refugees, and assault survivors, in addition to the literature focused on the mental health consequences of torture. From the beginning, torture survivors were involved directly and indirectly in the process of reviewing the relevant literature to ensure that their experiences and perspectives were part of the ongoing dialogue and review.

The establishment of the Working Group was stimulated by representatives of South Africa who attended a multidisciplinary, multiagency research conference on survivors of torture in April 1997, which was cosponsored by the National Institute of Mental Health, the U.S. Office for Refugee Resettlement, the Center for Mental Health Services (of the Substance Abuse and Mental Health Services Agency), and U.S. Senator Paul Wellstone. The South African delegates asked Steven E. Hyman, M.D., the Director of NIMH, for assistance in obtaining scientific information on the mental health consequences of torture, which they felt would be a major contribution to the field in general and to South Africa in particular as it began its healing process through the Truth and Reconciliation Commission. In response to this request, the 24-member NIMH Working Group on the Mental Health Consequences of Torture and Related Violence and Trauma was established. In keeping with the timeline established by the South African delegates, the Working Group completed the report and delivered it to South Africa in March 1998. This book is based on the report of the Working Group.

The study of the mental health consequences of torture is one that involves many people from many fields and disciplines throughout the world. To fully comprehend the horror of torture inflicted on human beings by other human beings and to understand how this experience affects a person psychologically requires the expertise not only of mental health professionals but also of other health care providers and social science researchers, policymakers and legislators, lawyers and advocates, and the survivors themselves. Through successful collaboration and mutual support, an understanding of the psychological effects of torture can be developed and applied toward effective treatments and support for those in need. The goal of this book is to contribute to this comprehensive effort by making available relevant scientific information about research, treatment, policy, and services as they relate to trauma and victimization for individuals and countries throughout the world.

This book is dedicated to those who experience the horror of torture—past, present, and future—and to those who work to end it.

ELLEN GERRITY
TERENCE M. KEANE
FARRIS TUMA

Acknowledgments

This book is the culmination of efforts by many people over many years, and it is appropriate that recognition, respect, and the utmost gratitude be extended to those who have participated directly and indirectly in its creation.

The leadership of the National Institute of Mental Health (NIMH)—most notably, Dr. Steven Hyman, Director; Dr. Rex Cowdry, former Acting Director; Dr. Darrel Regier, Associate Director for Epidemiology and Health Policy; Dr. Richard Nakamura, Deputy Director of NIMH; and Dr. Ellen Stover, Director of the Division of Mental Disorders, Behavioral Research, and AIDS—contributed their wisdom, time, resources, and encouragement at each step in the development of this book. Even more important, the long-standing history of NIMH's support for research on the effects of severe trauma provided the foundation of knowledge on which this book is based.

Senator Paul Wellstone (D-Minnesota) and his staff (Colin McGinnis, Charlotte Oldham-Moore, and Martin Gensler) continue to be instrumental in keeping uppermost in the minds of the members of the U.S. Congress and the American people the needs of those who have suffered the consequences of torture, whether those needs can be met through improved research, treatment, legislation, or public policy.

The editorial support of Barbara Hart and Chrysa Cullather of Publications Professionals, and of Eliot Werner and his staff at Kluwer Academic/Plenum Publishers, is gratefully acknowledged. The contributions of Catherine West, the NIMH graphic artist, during this entire project have been generous, creative, and inspiring, and are much appreciated.

We also want to acknowledge our families, friends, and loved ones, whose infinite support and encouragement has meant so much to us. Simply said, we could not have done this work without them, and we are deeply grateful.

Most important, we must acknowledge that this book would not be possible without the courage of those who have suffered the experience of torture and related violent and traumatic experiences. These individuals speak out about their experiences—whether it be through research participation, political activism, personal testimonies, treatment or support groups, or in their personal and private efforts to help others as they make their own journey in recovery—and it is the courage and generosity of these people that should be acknowledged and honored above all.

ELLEN GERRITY
TERENCE M. KEANE
FARRIS TUMA

Contents

PART I. THE IMPACT OF TORTURE

PART III. TORTURE AND THE TRAUMA OF WAR

Chapter 13. Homicide and Physical Assault 195

Dean G. Kilpatrick and Mary P. Koss

Chapter 14. Children, Adolescents, and Families Exposed to Torture and Related Trauma 211

Robert S. Pynoos, J. David Kinzie, and Malcolm Gordon

Chapter 15. Domestic Violence in Families Exposed to Torture and Related Violence and Trauma 227

Malcolm Gordon

PART V. CLINICAL ISSUES FOR SURVIVORS OF TORTURE

James M. Jaranson, J. David Kinzie, Merle Friedman, Sister Dianna Ortiz, Matthew J. Friedman, Steven Southwick, Marianne Kastrup, and Richard Mollica

Anthony J. Marsella

Kathryn M. Magruder, Richard Mollica, and Merle Friedman

I

The Impact of Torture

1

Introduction

ELLEN GERRITY, TERENCE M. KEANE,
and FARRIS TUMA

This book is a review of the scientific evidence about the mental health consequences of torture and related violence and trauma. As a broadly focused review, the book addresses such topics as the short- and long-term psychological, neurobiological, social, economic, and disability-related consequences of such trauma; models for studying these consequences; treatment and rehabilitation for survivors; and models for delivering mental health services. Research information related to public policy, legal issues, and caregiving is included. The perspective of the survivor of torture has been an integral part in the development of the information included throughout this book.

The key question addressed is how the experience of intentional psychological and physical torture affects individuals, families, and societies. Individual torture, large-scale massacres, religious or ethnic cleansings, death squads, the disappearance of loved ones, and random war-related violence can all have profound and enduring effects on the physical and mental health of people. The nature of these effects is addressed in this book through a review of relevant scientific information and a discussion of related policy, legal, and personal issues.

MENTAL HEALTH CONSEQUENCES OF VIOLENCE AND TRAUMATIC STRESS

A major problem of our time is the destructive role of violence and traumatic stress in the lives of millions of people throughout the world. Estimating the

ELLEN GERRITY • National Institute of Mental Health, Neuroscience Center Building, Bethesda, Maryland 20892.   TERENCE M. KEANE • Department of Psychiatry, Boston University School of Medicine, Boston, Massachusetts 02130.   FARRIS TUMA • National Institute of Mental Health, Neuroscience Center Building, Bethesda, Maryland 20892.

The Mental Health Consequences of Torture, edited by Ellen Gerrity, Terence M. Keane, and Farris Tuma. Kluwer Academic/Plenum Publishers, New York, 2001.

numbers (prevalence and incidence) of victims of violence and traumatic stress is a challenge, in large part because of the variations in the nature and definitions of these problems. Many life situations contribute to the scope of victimization, including poverty, political oppression, ethnopolitical warfare, torture, mass violence, violent crime, and family abuse, all of which occur without respect to geographical boundaries, social class, race, gender, or age. Because of the widespread and ongoing nature of such exposure, the consequences for people will continue to be a worldwide concern. Generally, the focus of research and treatment of those exposed to such violence and trauma is on individuals, but these kinds of experiences also affect the health and well-being of families, communities, societies, and entire nations. The legacy of these experiences often continues into subsequent generations, creating an enduring cycle of pain and suffering. Because of these widespread, profound, and enduring experiences, the prevalence of trauma-related disorders and disabilities may well exceed that of any other psychiatric disorder (de Girolamo & MacFarlane, 1996). Among the most enduring are the effects of torture.

BACKGROUND

In response to concerns regarding the mental health consequences of torture and related violence and trauma, especially among survivors of torture residing in the United States, the National Institute of Mental Health (NIMH), in collaboration with the Center for Mental Health Services, the Office of Refugee Resettlement, and Senator Paul Wellstone (D-Minnesota), sponsored an international conference on April 10–11, 1997, in Washington, D.C., to discuss mental health research and services for torture and trauma survivors. This conference, Survivors of Torture: Improving Our Understanding—A National Conference on Mental Health Research and Services for Refugees and Asylum-Seekers in the United States Who Are Survivors of Torture, brought together the representatives and converging interests of more than 100 research and service organizations, national and international agencies, human rights and advocacy groups, and survivors of torture. The participants included representatives of South Africa, who met with Steven E. Hyman, the Director of NIMH, and asked for help in compiling scientific information on the mental health consequences of torture. These participants felt such information would be a major contribution to South Africa and to the entire world, with a particular urgency for information about the psychological needs of the increasing number of torture and trauma survivors. In response to this request, NIMH established the Working Group on the Mental Health Consequences of Torture and Related Violence and Trauma. This panel, which was staffed with 24 international trauma and torture research experts, resulted in a report to the South Africa Truth and Reconciliation Committee and this book.

CONCEPTUAL AND DEFINITIONAL CONCERNS

To provide a foundation for this discussion of the mental health consequences of torture, a review of conceptual and methodological issues that permeate research and clinical practice may be helpful.

Focus on Torture

One fundamental question is why the primary focus for this book is on the torture experience itself, rather than on a general discussion of other forms of organized, interpersonal, or mass violence? As noted by several of the contributors to this volume, a reasonable argument could be made that the focus should be on the wider population of persons (survivors and perpetrators) who experience mass violence, other forms of severe trauma, stress in war, and other forms of social upheaval. However, ultimately, the focus on the mental health consequences of torture is inherently important for several reasons. Torture is one of the most extreme forms of human violence, and the consequences of torture represent a critically understudied area of scientific research. Because of the extreme and horrific nature of the torture experience, an understanding of how it affects human beings can contribute to better psychological and medical treatment and to overall improvements in the delivery of services to survivors. As a human action, torture horrifies and evokes a strong reaction among the public, governments, and policymakers. But it is the survivors themselves who can speak most directly to this experience, providing essential insights regarding necessary changes in policy and health care. While studies of other forms of trauma and violence have a great deal to offer an investigation of the effects of torture, the defining and unique characteristics of torture itself make the study of its effects one that enlarges and improves the field of trauma research.

Researchers and clinicians have begun to recognize that the destructive medical and psychological consequences associated with the experience of "torture and related violence and trauma" often extend beyond the survivor to include family members, the perpetrator, the treatment provider, and society (Basoglu, 1992; Kinzie & Boehnlein, 1993; McCann & Pearlman, 1990; Nightingale, 1990). In many instances, an individual may have multiple roles—refugee, survivor of torture, perpetrator of violence—and thus may have numerous and complex needs. It is not uncommon in contemporary civil wars for civilians to occupy such multiple roles concurrently or to move between the roles of combatant, victim, and survivor before, during, or after periods of victimization, persecution, and displacement. This complexity notwithstanding, the focus of this book is on survivors of torture and related trauma and not on perpetrators per se, with the recognition that the complex relationship between perpetrators and victims of human rights violations is also worthy of a full review.

Definitions: Torture and Related Violence and Trauma

Because of scientific, political, and national health policy concerns, a continuing debate is under way to examine the elements of a precise definition of torture. Specific issues are outlined below, but a number of relevant publications also address this controversial question (e.g., Basoglu, 1992; Jaranson, 1998; Marsella, Bornemann, Ekblad, & Orley, 1995; National Immigration Law Center, 1994).

Torture

The term "torture" has been defined in different ways by different organizations for different purposes. According to Jaranson (1995, 1998), the two most commonly used definitions of torture have been formulated by the World Medical Association and the United Nations. The World Medical Association's definition, frequently called the Declaration of Tokyo, was developed in 1975 and has been widely accepted among the medical community, where it governs professional standards and ethics. The Declaration of Tokyo defines torture as "the deliberate, systematic, or wanton infliction of physical or mental suffering by one or more persons acting alone or on the orders of any authority, to force another person to yield information, to make a confession, or for any other reason" (Amnesty International, 1985, pp. 9–10).

Alternatively, the definition of torture developed by the United Nations delineates the legal and political responsibilities of governments (Jaranson, 1995, 1998):

> For the purpose of this convention, the term "torture" means any act by which pain or suffering, whether physical or mental, is intentionally inflicted on a person for such purposes as obtaining from him or a third person, information or a confession, punishing him for an act he or a third person has committed or is suspected of having committed, or intimidating or coercing him or a third person for any reason based on discrimination of any kind, when such pain or suffering is inflicted by or at the instigation of or with the consent or acquiescence of a public official or other person acting in an official capacity. It does not include pain or suffering arising only from, inherent in, or incidental to lawful sanctions (United Nations, 1989, p. 17).

Jaranson (1998) describes the World Medical Association's version as the broader definition, one that does not require the perpetrator to be affiliated with a government or to act officially with governmental approval. Consequently, the actions described could be interpreted to include torture as part of domestic or ritualistic abuse as well as part of criminal activities. Conversely, the United Nations' definition limits torture to those acts perpetrated, directly or indirectly, by those in "an official capacity" and appears to exclude three groups: (a) torture perpetrated by unofficial rebels or terrorists who ignore national or international mandates, (b) random violence during war, and (c) punishment allowed by national laws, even if the punishment uses techniques similar to those of torturers. Jaranson concludes that some professionals in the torture rehabilitation field consider the United Nations' definition to be too restrictive and favor a definition of politically motivated torture that is broad enough to include all acts of "organized violence" (van Willigen, 1992).

In general usage, the term "torture" describes a situation of horrific pain and suffering being inflicted on someone, often in captivity. Torture, despite variations in cultural manifestations, is cruel and degrading abuse of human beings with the potential for serious lifelong suffering.

Throughout this volume, various legal or statutory definitions are used. However, it is also recognized that, for the purposes of this volume, the experience of torture may extend beyond statutory or legal definitions to include other characteristics, as documented in personal testimony or in clinical or medical settings.

Violence

Webster's II New Riverside University Dictionary (1995) defines violence as "physical force employed so as to violate, damage, or abuse; an act or instance of violent behavior or action; abusive or unjust use of power." In scientific, clinical, or general usage, the term "violence" has many definitions and applications. In this volume, the term "violence" refers to individual and group experiences (e.g., ethnopolitical warfare, crime, family abuse, political oppression, and torture) that combine the concepts of deliberate and wrongful use of force with the intention of violating, damaging, or abusing another.

Trauma

The term "trauma" has both a medical and a psychiatric definition. Medically, trauma refers to a serious or critical "bodily injury, wound, or shock" (Neufeldt, 1988). This definition is often associated with trauma medicine practiced in emergency rooms and is also a generally accepted layperson view of the term. However, in psychological terms, and in this volume, trauma assumes a different meaning, referring to a "painful emotional experience, or shock, often producing a lasting psychic effect" (Neufeldt, 1988).

Psychiatric Symptoms and Disability

The psychiatric definition of trauma has become inherently associated with the diagnosis of posttraumatic stress disorder (PTSD). PTSD is a formally recognized psychiatric disorder. According to the American Psychiatric Association, PTSD can result from "exposure to an extreme traumatic stressor involving direct personal experience of an event that involves actual or threatened death or serious injury, or other threat to one's physical integrity; or witnessing an event that involves death, injury, or a threat to the physical integrity of another person; or learning about unexpected or violent death, serious harm, or threat of death, injury, experienced by a family member or other close associate" (American Psychiatric Association, 1994, p. 424).

The diagnosis of PTSD varies according to onset patterns, including acute (symptoms last less than 3 months), chronic (symptoms last 3 months or longer), and delayed (at least 6 months pass between the traumatic event and the appearance of symptoms) onset patterns (American Psychiatric Association, 1994). For

PTSD to be diagnosed, the fourth edition of the *Diagnostic and Statistical Manual of Mental Disorders* (DSM-IV; American Psychiatric Association, 1994) requires a particular combination of symptoms, including some relating to a reexperiencing of the traumatic event, persistent avoidance of stimuli associated with the event, persistent symptoms of increased arousal, symptom duration of greater than 1 month, and significant clinical distress or impairment in various areas of functioning.

Most groups, including survivors of torture, mental health researchers, and therapists, agree that the PTSD diagnosis can be a useful tool for describing the suffering and symptoms of survivors of torture and trauma, for gauging the extent and severity of traumatic experiences, and for planning and delivering clinical interventions. At the same time, these experts generally agree that the PTSD diagnosis alone is wholly inadequate to describe what it means to be a survivor of such trauma. As noted in the next chapter of this book by Ortiz, "The consequences of torture are multidimensional and interconnected; no part of the survivor's life is untouched." And as a survivor recounted at the April 1997 NIMH conference, "We struggle to make sense of what happened to us, to our community, and to our world. We are survivors who struggle to reclaim our dignity and our trust in humanity and in ourselves."

Researchers and clinicians have also proposed a number of other trauma-related clinical syndromes, including survivor syndrome, torture syndrome, prisoner of war syndrome, concentration camp syndrome, vicarious traumatization syndrome, and gross stress reaction syndrome. Although these syndromes are not recognized as medical diagnoses in either the *International Classification of Diseases and Related Health Problems* (10th revision) (World Health Organization, 1992) or DSM-IV, they have often proven to be useful within clinical settings where therapists and other professionals strive to understand the broad spectrum of symptoms and disabilities associated with torture experiences.

ORGANIZATION OF THE BOOK

Torture is a horror designed by human beings, one that is difficult to describe or understand. The role of survivors is crucial in bridging the gap of communication and understanding between survivors and those who have not directly experienced torture, particularly those designated as their caregivers. For this reason, in chapter 2 the perspective of the survivor is introduced, and it is integrated throughout the book. The survivor perspective challenges researchers, clinicians, and others working with survivors of torture to carefully consider the changes in the world of the survivor, the many meanings of mental health and medical diagnoses, the sources of ongoing stress, the role of faith and support, and the purposes of therapy. The experiences of survivors provide a window to this unique perspective. The survivor perspective also highlights the extraordinary ability of some individuals to manage and function with strength and courage in the wake of almost unimaginable experiences.

While most of this book is a review of the empirical literature on a number of relevant topics, chapter 3 reviews the mental health research work that focuses directly on survivors of torture. Research has been conducted on the scope and effect of torture and the role of risk and protective factors. Outcome studies have focused on a variety of measures, including PTSD; other psychological disorders and outcomes; neurobiological findings; cognitive outcomes; physical health; and economic, disability, and social consequences. Recommendations for future research are included in this section and throughout the book.

Next, for readers who are less familiar with psychological research in the area of trauma, three approaches for conceptualizing the consequences of torture and related violence and trauma are reviewed. Psychosocial, neurobiological, and economic models for examining the etiology, course, treatment, and prevention of the consequences of traumatic stress, including torture and related violence and trauma, are discussed. First, chapter 4 outlines some of the major psychological and psychosocial models that have been used to examine and conceptually understand the consequences of traumatic stress. For example, because of the inherent relationship between trauma and torture, PTSD has emerged as the most frequently studied disorder associated with torture (Basoglu, 1992). However, other researchers have pointed out that responses to torture and trauma can include a broad spectrum of disorders, including depression, psychosis, anger and rage, paranoia, sleep disorders, substance abuse, anxiety, and dissociative disorders (e.g., Marsella, Friedman, Gerrity, & Scurfield, 1996; Turner & Gorst-Unsworth, 1993). In addition to these disorders, survivors may also experience hopelessness and existential despair in the aftermath of torture as they seek to construct some sort of meaning and coherence from this gross violation of their being. The Italian writer, Primo Levi, a survivor of the torture of the Nazi concentration camps, wrote, "The purpose of existence itself is challenged by the fact of torture" (Levi, 1979).

Next, chapter 5 briefly reviews the literature concerning trauma-related neurobiological research and presents several useful models coming from animal and human studies. Recently, medical researchers have identified a range of neurophysiological disorders associated with traumatic stress, including disorders of the hypothalamic–pituitary–adrenal axis, the prefrontal dopaminergic system, the locus coeruleus noradrenergic system, and the thyroid gland and hippocampus (Grillon, Southwick, & Charney, 1996).

Chapter 6 on economic models discusses the health effects of torture from the perspective of the cost to society and the economic burden of disease, disorder, and disability. Recently, many mental health-related scientific disciplines have been recognizing that the value and success of research and interventions targeting mental disorder and illness need to be judged not only on their ability to reduce and prevent symptoms of such conditions, but also on their ability to explain the relationship between disorder, disability, and functioning. This chapter briefly reviews current literature on individual and societal disability, including the economic effects of trauma. While it is unusual in psychological literature to discuss life and health in economic terms, this perspective is inherently valuable in developing comprehensive and humane public health policy.

The next major sections of this book review several relevant bodies of literature on violence and trauma (chapters 7 to 15). Relevance was judged based on the extent to which a research area focused on traumatic experiences that can involve similar patterns of exposure, psychobiological responses, or therapeutic treatments. The research topics or groups reviewed in these chapters are as follows: refugees and asylum-seekers; veterans of armed conflicts; former prisoners of war; and victims of Holocaust trauma, rape and sexual assault, homicide and physical assault, war-related trauma, domestic violence, and child trauma. Included is a review of the scientific literature related to exposure, effects, risk, and protective factors, and recommendations for future research.

A discussion of the complex and challenging assessment and intervention issues follows in chapter 16. Examining successful interventions at various levels (e.g., individual, communal, and societal) for survivors of other traumatic experiences has the potential to benefit torture survivors who are also at risk of developing a range of psychobiological, emotional, behavioral, and social difficulties following the torture experience. Measurement issues are discussed in chapter 17, emphasizing the numerous procedural and psychometric challenges in this area of study. This chapter gives a brief discussion of current instruments and approaches and ethical considerations for research and treatment.

Services for survivors of torture are delivered by many different kinds of providers in many different settings throughout the world. Chapter 18 focuses on mental health services delivery models relevant to the treatment of survivors of torture. By addressing the structure or organization of systems of care, including access, process, and outcomes, the material in this chapter explores ways in which existing systems can be made more sensitive and effective in providing mental health care for survivors of torture. Survivors of torture can be from many countries and are found in many different health care situations (e.g., as refugees in a new country, as individuals who stay in their home countries, or as individuals tortured in a foreign country who then return to a home country). Although it is impossible to describe a single system that would be responsive and practical in all situations, the general field of mental health services research has struggled with many similar issues, and relevant research findings are presented here.

The role of professional caregivers and the relationship between the caregiver and the survivor are important to the process of healing. Chapter 19 presents research and clinical findings and addresses the complex challenges of providing care when caregivers are confronted each day with often horrific human experiences, as well as the difficulties of developing appropriate treatment with limited resources.

How public policy and the law can influence the lives of survivors and those who care for them is reviewed in chapter 20, which presents research findings regarding public policy and legal approaches to addressing the needs of survivors, with a particular emphasis on the role of reparation and restorative justice for survivors.

Finally, chapter 21 summarizes selected research findings reported in this book to point to future directions for further work.

This book was developed in the spirit of collaboration and cooperation among survivors, clinicians, researchers, and policymakers in an effort to make scientific and other critical information more readily available to those who undertake to solve this complex and disturbing problem throughout the world.

REFERENCES

American Psychiatric Association. (1994). *Diagnostic and statistical manual of mental disorders* (4th ed.). Washington, DC: Author.

Amnesty International. (1985). The Declaration of Tokyo (World Medical Association). In Amnesty International Secretariat (Ed.), *Ethical codes and declarations relevant to the health professions* (2nd ed.). London: Author.

Basoglu, M. (Ed.). (1992). *Torture and its consequences: Current treatment approaches.* Cambridge: Cambridge University Press.

de Girolamo, G., & MacFarlane, A. (1996). The epidemiology of PTSD: A comprehensive review of the international literature. In A. J. Marsella, M. Friedman, E. Gerrity, & R. Scurfield (Eds.), *Ethnocultural aspects of post traumatic stress disorder: Issues, research, and clinical applications* (pp. 33–85). Washington, DC: American Psychological Association.

Grillon, C., Southwick, S., & Charney, D. (1996). The psychobiological basis of posttraumatic stress disorder. *Molecular Psychiatry, 1,* 278–297.

Jaranson, J. (1995). Government-sanctioned torture: Status of the rehabilitation movement. *Transcultural Psychiatric Research Review, 32,* 253–286.

Jaranson, J. (1998). The science and politics of rehabilitating torture survivors: An overview. In J. Jaranson & M. Popkin (Eds.), *Caring for victims of torture* (pp. 15–40). Washington, DC: American Psychiatric Press.

Kinzie, D., & Boehnlein, J. (1993). Psychotherapy of the victims of massive violence: Countertransference and ethical issues. *American Journal of Psychotherapy, 47,* 90–102.

Levi, P. (1979). *If this is a man: The truce.* New York: Harmondsworth Penguin.

Marsella, A. J., Bornemann, T., Ekblad, S., & Orley, J. (1995). *Amidst peril and pain: The mental health and psychosocial well-being of the world's refugees.* Washington, DC: American Psychological Association.

Marsella, A. J., Friedman, M. J., Gerrity, E. T., & Scurfield, R. M. (1996). *Ethnocultural aspects of posttraumatic stress disorder: Issues, research, and clinical applications.* Washington, DC: American Psychological Association.

McCann, L., & Pearlman, L. (1990). Vicarious traumatization: A framework for understanding the psychological effects of working with victims. *Journal of Traumatic Stress, 3,* 131–148.

National Immigration Law Center. (1994). *Guide to alien eligibility for federal programs* (3rd ed.). Los Angeles: Author.

Neufeldt, V. (Ed.). (1988). *Webster's new world dictionary of the English language* (3rd ed.). New York: Simon & Schuster.

Nightingale, E. (1990). The problem of torture and the response of the health professional. In J. Gurschow & K. Hannibal (Eds.), *Health services for the treatment of torture and trauma survivors* (pp. 8–9). Washington, DC: American Association for the Advancement of Science.

Turner, S. W., & Gorst-Unsworth, C. (1993). Psychological sequelae of torture. In J. P. Wilson & B. Raphael (Eds.), *International handbook of traumatic stress syndromes* (pp. 703–713). New York: Plenum Press.

United Nations. (1989). Convention against torture and other cruel, inhuman, and degrading treatment or punishment. In United Nations (Ed.), *Methods of combating torture* (p. 17). Geneva, Switzerland: United Nations Center for Human Rights.

van Willigen, L. (1992). Organization of care and rehabilitation services for victims of torture and other forms of organized violence: A review of current issues. In M. Basoglu (Ed.), *Torture and its consequences: Current treatment approaches* (pp. 277–298). Cambridge: Cambridge University Press.

Webster's II new riverside university dictionary. (1995). Boston: Houghton Mifflin.

World Health Organization. (1992). *International statistical classification of diseases and related health problems* (10th revision). Geneva, Switzerland: Author.

2

The Survivors' Perspective
Voices from the Center

SISTER DIANNA ORTIZ

In the pages that follow, survivors share delicate pieces of their painful ordeal. For many, this was the first time they had spoken to another person of their agonizing experience of torture. This sharing did not come easily. Yet these men and women were willing to take a risk so that others might better understand the world of torture survivors.

In recounting the horror of their experiences, they did so with grace, strength, and a profound conviction that the silence which too often surrounds torture must be broken. They did so in a spirit of solidarity with those who, like themselves, physically survived torture, and with those children, women, and men who died as a result of this political violence.

Although both males and females are subject to torture, the pronoun "she" is used throughout this section for ease of presentation. Unless otherwise noted, quoted material comes from torture survivors with their permission, whose anonymity, both name and country of origin, has been guaranteed.

Increasingly, attention is being paid to torture and its survivors. We come from many nations and diverse cultures, all plagued by the same man-made epidemic. And in spite of differences in class, ethnicity, gender, religion, and political belief, this soul-searing experience unites us as one. In these pages, survivors from Asia, Africa, North and South America, and Europe have joined to set forth in the simplest of language a story only we can tell—that of the survivors' world. To understand this world, it is necessary to know what the terms torture, trauma, victim, and survivor mean to us.

SISTER DIANNA ORTIZ • Guatemalan Human Rights Commission, Washington, D.C. 20017.

The Mental Health Consequences of Torture, edited by Ellen Gerrity, Terence M. Keane, and Farris Tuma. Kluwer Academic/Plenum Publishers, New York, 2001.

TORTURE AND RELATED TRAUMA

We find the definitions of torture employed by the United Nations and cited in the World Medical Association's Declaration of Tokyo to be too narrow in scope. Torture, we believe, is much more than "a deliberate, systematic, or wanton infliction of physical or mental suffering by one or more persons acting alone or on the orders of any authority to extract information or a confession from an individual" (Amnesty International, 1985, pp. 9–10). Instead, we see it as an act of terrorism aimed at instilling a paralyzing fear not only in individuals but also in the family, the community, and society. This collective terror, practiced by more than 121 governments and yet ignored by world leaders, is intended to intimidate, silence, and control entire societies.

Events currently relegated to the category of "extreme" or "related" trauma— such as the disappearance, for political reasons, of a family member or a forced flight into exile—should be considered a form of torture. Their effects are equally devastating and widespread and result in permanent damage to the survivors' lives. Those who have survived a large-scale massacre in their community, attempts at religious or ethnic cleansing, the assassination of a loved one, or random violence during a war are affected much like the survivor of torture. The distinctions others have made among these violations of human rights are at best erroneous and at worst tragic. One survivor notes, "To have been victimized by and survived any one of them places us in a common pool with all other survivors of political crimes. Our experiences share a common theme, both in terms of victimization and survival."

As a refugee recounts,

> What I suffer is not considered to be torture by experts on the issue. If it is not torture, what is it then? When I met with the Truth and Reconciliation Commission, I was asked what kind of torture I had been subjected to and was provided with a long list to choose from. The word "disappearance" was nowhere to be found. When I spoke of how my children had been disappeared and therefore how I had been amputated from them, they didn't understand what I was talking about. As a woman and as a mother, [let me tell you] how it feels to be a survivor of disappearance as a form of torture. I have felt the same pain, despair, survivor's guilt ... the same anger, the same inability to trust anybody, including myself ... the same feelings of disempowerment, flashbacks, nightmares, feelings of madness, betrayal, and wanting to die, even by my own hands. My pain is so great that, sometimes, in my horrible hours of madness I wish I had been physically tortured instead of my children having been disappeared and taken away from me. (Used with permission.)

Her pain, like that of too many others, is seen as less severe than that of a person who has been subjected to electrical shock or assaulted with foreign objects or who has suffered amputations caused by instruments such as knives, saws, or land mines. But survivors understand that torture is torture, suffering is suffering, pain is pain.

Regardless of whether the pain inflicted is physical or psychological, the motivation is political. In some cases, the people targeted for terror are leaders of the movement that the terrorists want to destroy. In other cases, those targeted are innocent civilians, and the abuses against them are meant to warn the broader community that no one is immune to torture. Thus, the seeds of fear and mistrust are planted and germinate, resulting in silence on the part of the people and yielding a harvest of total domination for the torturers.

VICTIM VERSUS SURVIVOR

We who have been subjected to torture and extreme trauma are often given the label of "victim." This label focuses attention on the atrocities we have suffered, the shattering of our lives, and the fear and uncertainty with which we must live. But there is strength in us too, a resilience attested to by our very survival. We have lived through something unspeakable. We may greet each new day with fear and uncertainty, but we also meet it with a strength that empowers us to reclaim our dignity, our hope, and our trust in humanity, and to adapt to a new life.

The term "victim," says one survivor, implies that the experience of torture leaves a person weak, defenseless, and in desperate need of sympathy. A typical response to victims is to "lavish them with pity" and to take control of their lives. To reject the label "victim" is to risk being labeled again, this time as a troublemaker in denial and as an annoyance. Thus, the survivor who rejects the victim label subjects herself to possible retraumatization. To call us victims is to validate the image our torturers tried to mold us into and leave us—weak, subjugated, helpless. We are not victims. We are survivors.

THE CHANGED WORLD OF THE TORTURED

Emerging from the situation in which we were tortured, survivors often feel, and are, misunderstood. People expect us to be who we were before the torture occurred. But an individual changes dramatically. The consequences of torture are multidimensional and interconnected; no part of the survivor's life is untouched.

To understand the survivors' world, one must have a clear picture of the moment-by-moment effects of the torture. At the moment of victimization, the individual begins to die a slow death, which very few others can comprehend. The perpetrators see her as less than human; they strip her of her dignity, her sense of control, and her link with humanity. She begins to question the horrible reality before her eyes. Shattered by the very face of evil, treasured values of community, trust, and hope are lost in an instant—in their place are alienation, betrayal, and despair.

A grim example offered by one survivor is attested to by many others. One of the torturers is assigned to play the role of the good guy, feigning kindness toward the prisoner until she begins to trust and confide in him. She sees him as the Good Samaritan who will protect and rescue her. But this pretense reveals itself as the mockery it is, nothing but lies, false hopes, and broken promises. Thus, she is betrayed and has betrayed herself with her belief and possibly others with her revelations. The only consolation left is that death will not betray her. But she is wrong—another betrayal awaits. Her torturers do not kill her. She remembers,

> I was put into a small cell with another female prisoner. She was so broken. She had no hope at all. She told me that I was going to beg [the torturers] to kill me. But they're not going to do that. They will tell you that if you cooperate, they won't hurt you, that they will set you free. Oh, they'll release you after you give them the information they want, but before they set you free, you become a piece of meat—everyone gets a piece of you, even the rats. They do things to you that you can't even imagine. And you beg them to kill you. But they don't. By killing you, they lose. By keeping you alive and then releasing you, they win. You become a product of their creation. You're sent out to the world as a reminder: "This can happen to you if you oppose us." I was so convinced that couldn't happen to me, but it did. Today in my country, I am a living advertisement of what can happen to someone who gets mixed up in politics. (Used with permission.)

A metamorphosis takes place: The survivor emerges from this trauma alienated from all humanity. Her trust in herself, in others, and in God (or in the possible benevolence of the universe) has been shattered. She may feel more akin to the dead than to the living. As one survivor remembers, "People around me were celebrating my miraculous return while I was mourning my death, the emergence of a new person into a world I no longer felt a part of, a world I no longer trusted."

On the physical level, survivors may suffer life-long disabilities: Many have had limbs amputated or have incurred serious head injuries during severe beatings. Many of us carry scars from being bitten; hanged by wrists, arms, or legs; burned by electrical devices or cigarettes; or cut or stabbed with knives or machetes. Some of us are forever marked internally as well. The remnants of bone fractures show up years later in X rays. Inevitably the question arises: "What did you do to your wrist (or jaw, or rib)?" For us, such marks are more than topics for conversation in a doctor's office. Each mark is a tattoo, a permanent physical reminder of what was done to us, a symbol that in many cases brings shame. A male survivor who had fingernails and toenails removed during torture explains:

> My nails don't grow like they used to. They grow like a fungus—they really are a gruesome sight. Sometimes complete strangers come up to me and ask if I have a contagious disease. Others simply stare at me as if I were an odd piece of art on display. I don't know which is worse, the stares or the humiliating questions. Some of my friends know that I am ashamed to be seen in public, and they try to ease my pain by telling me to ignore people. Sometimes they say jokingly, "Soon winter will come and you can wear gloves. Then no one will see your hands." I can hide my hands from the outside world. But am I not part of that world? I can still see my hands and my feet. Doesn't that matter? And when the weather changes, I start to feel a pain so deep that I sometimes scream.... It's as if they [the torturers] are tearing out my nails again. Oh God, it hurts. It's like they're ripping every nerve out of my body, so slowly, one by one. Forget! That's what my family and friends tell me. How can I forget? How can I forget what they did to me when every morning I wake up to this gruesome sight? (Used with permission.)

While survivors may not always experience identical reactions to the situations we have undergone, we do share at least some of the same symptoms. In many cases, we are told that our reactions are too extreme considering the severity of what other people have suffered. Again, we say, torture is torture, suffering is suffering, pain is pain.

A SHROUD OF GUILT

Many survivors are suffused with feelings of guilt: guilt for being a silent witness to the torture and the death of another, guilt at being forced to participate in the torture of another, guilt for surviving while others perished, guilt for being picked up in the first place, or guilt for not being able to talk about the experience in a way that could help others.

In a monthly meeting of a group of survivors, both men and women, one person notes, "We are told that these feelings of guilt are unrealistic. We have nothing to feel guilty for. 'You had no control over what happened.'" But another survivor asks, "If that's true, then why do people ask us questions that make us feel that we are responsible? 'Why didn't you try to escape? Why didn't you defend yourself and others? Why did you give them information that put other people in danger?'" And a third survivor adds, "Then they ask why we remain silent. If I had gone public with my story, they tell me, I might have saved people who were being tortured. But are these people really interested in hearing our reasons or are they saying that, unlike them, we were just too weak. Are they telling us if they were in a similar situation, they would have acted differently?"

Guilt-ridden, another survivor goes over and over in his mind what he should have done to save the woman he loved:

> We were to be married that morning. After the church ceremony we were going to have a small reception. Then we would take the train to the beach where we would spend our honeymoon. Everything was perfect. I was the happiest man in town. Early that morning, we had agreed that we would meet at the park and then walk to the church together for the ceremony. The park is where we met; that was our sacred place. When I arrived there, two men were shoving her into the back seat of a car. She cried out to me to help her. But I just stood there. My feet would not move.... I never saw her again. I should have done—something.... (Used with permission.)

Guilt is not a universal phenomenon among survivors, however. One survivor speaks for others when he states with utter conviction, "I have nothing to feel guilty about. I did nothing wrong. I was doing what I believed was the right thing to do— standing up for my rights and those of other students."

In some cultures, fate or karma is thought to determine what happens to people. In others, the individual is believed to control her own destiny. Survivors' guilt is likely to be more common in the second type than the first. Therefore, in those cultures where fate or divine will is thought to control events, survivors' guilt may not afflict those who have been tortured. Yet it appears that most survivors do experience some form of guilt, although some discuss it more openly than others.

A survivor from a culture giving credence to a form of control by fate reports,

> I was brought up in a religious family, a religion that represents a certain outlook on life and life's experiences. Grandfather would tell me that fate would determine my destiny.

I never fully grasped the meaning of those words. In my culture, one doesn't ask questions, especially a woman. When I became a little older, I enrolled in the university, and the world opened up before me, and I learned that the leaders of my country were becoming more and more repressive. I participated with other students in demonstrations and even spoke out. Then one day I was arrested and beaten. After I was released, I returned to my grandfather's home. He wept when he saw me and kept repeating that I was not responsible for what had happened. To this day, grandfather still believes that it was fate that decided that I would suffer. But I know it was much more than fate. It was my insatiable hunger to indulge myself with knowledge that led me to the streets and which ultimately resulted in my arrest and torture. (Used with permission.)

HUMILIATION: HOW COULD I LET THAT HAPPEN?

With torture and extreme trauma comes humiliation. Torture is a situation in which we are stripped of all dignity. Frequently, we witness others' loss of dignity as well. Humiliation and guilt thus become intertwined. A father remembers not only his own horror and humiliation but also that of his teenage daughter and 9-year-old son, all of whom were detained by the military. He was immediately separated from them and given a choice—he could either reveal the names of those he worked with and then be reunited with his children, or he could refuse to speak and they would be punished. With great reluctance, he chose his children and surrendered the names of his friends to his captors. Upon doing so, he was brought before his son and his daughter, who had been stripped of her clothes.

I was given another choice; I rape my daughter or the guard does it. I tried to reason with them, telling them that she was an innocent child. I pleaded with them not to humiliate her, not to hurt her, but instead to rape me, to do with me as they wanted. They laughed and repeated the two choices. I looked at my daughter hoping that she would tell me what to do—our eyes met and I knew then that I could not violate my own daughter, and that I could not save her from those wretched men. I lowered my eyes in shame to keep from seeing my daughter abused. One guard held my face up, forcing me to watch this horrible scene. I watched, motionless, as she was raped before me and her little brother. When they were through, they forced me to do what they had done to her. My own daughter, my son forced to watch it all. How could anyone do that. What kind of men are they? What kind of a father am I? (Used with permission.)

CONTAMINATION: EVIL DANCING WITHIN

Guilt and humiliation are often accompanied by a feeling of contamination. For many of us, this may lead to distancing ourselves from family members, friends, and others. One survivor recalls,

Once I was safe, I thought I was free of my torturers. I actually believed that I would never see them again, that I would never have to smell them or hear their voices. But what I soon realized was that they were within me; they literally had made their home inside my soul. So often I felt as if they were dancing within me, reminding me that they were a part of my life. I felt so dirty, so contaminated by evil. I know it sounds strange, but often times I feared that I would contaminate my family and my friends—so I distanced myself from everyone. None of them could understand why I spent so much time alone or why I bathed so frequently. I was afraid if I told them I was trying to wash my torturers off me—if I shared my true feelings—they would think I was crazy and lock me up. (Used with permission.)

MISDIAGNOSIS

Mental health professionals often diagnose survivors of torture and extreme trauma as suffering from various disorders such as anorexia nervosa and chronic depression. As survivors, we readily acknowledge that the trauma we have endured has altered our lives. Yet it is incomprehensible to us how anyone in the mental health field can offer diagnoses of us without a thorough understanding of the experiences that prompted that behavior. Take, for example, a survivor diagnosed as anorexic by a psychiatrist:

> Like so many of the women in my village, I was raped, night after night. But one soldier took pity on me and helped me to escape. That's when I came to live with my aunt. She was very concerned for my health. You see, I wasn't eating. Then my health began to deteriorate. I became weaker and weaker, thinner and thinner. My aunt, not knowing what to do to help me, took me to the clinic to see a psychiatrist. She asked me many questions about my life and about being raped. I was too ashamed to talk about my personal self, but I did tell her that I didn't have control of my life—people around me were always telling me what to do and were always trying to get me to eat. She spoke to me about girls my age who have similar problems with control issues. That's when she told me that I had an eating disorder known as anorexia. My problem with eating had nothing to do with control. My throat hurt when I swallowed food. Each time I tried, I started to choke. I couldn't breathe and then I would remember.... They, the soldiers, after raping me, would make me swallow their sperm—sometimes even their urine. This is the reason I couldn't eat, not because I had an eating disorder. (Used with permission.)

An even more common diagnosis of survivors is that we suffer from chronic depression. It is true that some of us do suffer from depression. "I have the illness of depression. I am very sad much [of the] time. I [am] feeling depressed—very miserable," admits one man who was in prison for 6 months and who lost his mother, small sister, and friends in the war.

Others of us experience a profound sadness and despair, which we do not name as depression. As another survivor recalls,

> When I told the doctor that my heart was very sad—that I had no energy and wanted to sleep all the time—he told me that I was suffering from something called depression. He handed me a piece of paper and said, "Read this, it will tell you more about what's wrong with you." Later the doctor asked me if I had any questions. I thought about telling him that I couldn't understand what he was saying, that I couldn't read English. But I was too embarrassed to say anything. I used to tell my friends that I had depression. And what is that, they wanted to know? It's something the American doctor told me I had, I told them. Now that I'm better, I know that I was not suffering from depression.

All I know is that my heart was very sad. Wouldn't your heart be sad if you saw your
neighbors killing each other? Wouldn't your heart be sad if you were forced to leave
your homeland, if you were separated from your wife and children? Wouldn't you be
sad? All I know is that my heart was ... and is still very sad. (Used with permission.)

The diagnoses given by mental health professionals should be made carefully
and expressed carefully as well. As survivors, we ask experts and laypersons alike to
remember that we have endured what few people can imagine, and this requires
amazing strength. When we take offense at being labeled "client," "patient," "depressed," "sick," or "suffering from posttraumatic stress syndrome," it is because we
want to be recognized as normal people, people who were tortured and who have
survived with tenacity, grace, and dignity. Apfel and Simon have written, "Most
survivors are not sick, and attempts to categorize them can recapitulate oppressive
situations in which they were classified, numbered, and (literally) stamped as inferior, subhuman creatures" (Apfel & Simon, 1996, p. 13). As Victor Frankl has said,
despair about the worthwhileness of life may be "a spiritual distress" but is by no
means "mental disease" (Frankl, 1963, p. 163).

Researchers also apply labels in ways that can be even more dehumanizing.
One man, a survivor of sexual abuse, recalls being asked to participate in a study
with other survivors on the effects of rape among married men.

We thought he was going to help us resolve a problem that was ruining our marriages.
After we gave him the information he wanted, he diagnosed each of us as "sexually
dysfunctional" and recommended that we get help. We were devastated when we left his
office. We had been raped again, but this time by someone who we thought was going to
help us. (Used with permission.)

This experience mirrors those of other survivors. Another survivor adds,

Like guinea pigs and laboratory mice, we are providers of data, objects of someone else's
curiosity, nothing more. I think to myself, I am an expert on torture and its effects, but
do scientists seek input from me or other survivors? (Used with permission.)

Men and women who work in this field, we want to believe, are concerned
about the well-being of survivors and would not retraumatize us intentionally. Likewise, we want to believe that the data they gather on the physical and psychological
aspects of torture will benefit survivors and their families. We want to believe that,
ultimately, the research will serve as a vehicle to end the practice of torture. But as
we survivors make a good-faith effort to understand the importance of research
and the ways of researchers, we ask them to remember that we are human beings
and deserve to be treated with respect. We also believe we have a great deal to
contribute to the study of torture. We look forward to the day, says one survivor,
"when we will be regarded more as their colleagues than as research subjects."

SUICIDE: TO LIVE OR NOT?

There is no denying that many survivors of torture and extreme trauma sometimes contemplate suicide. The need to alleviate physical pain, to quiet haunting

memories, or to cleanse one's self may well lead to intense feelings of wanting to disappear or wanting to die. Upon hearing this, family members, friends, and mental health professionals automatically associate this feeling with suicide and take it on themselves to protect the individual from herself. In some cases, this has entailed forcibly committing the survivor to a mental institution, where all her control is taken away, where she is again detained against her will, where she is at the mercy of strangers, and where she hears the screams and shouts of other patients—all of which retraumatize her and place her back in the situation of the torture. Forced institutionalization should be considered very carefully in the light of the torture survivor's past and avoided wherever possible.

The concern that a torture survivor may commit suicide is well founded. As a last resort, some do put their self-destructive thoughts and feelings into action. For example, a young girl in the midst of a terrible conflict was imprisoned and raped every day. After each rape, her rapists left token wounds on her body as marks of pride and ownership. She was eventually released, but all attempts to resume a "normal" life failed. So deep was her pain that she eventually took her own life, not out of weakness or defenselessness, as the nontortured so often assume, but because she so desperately wanted to forget that which could not be forgotten. Finally, she found the way to erase the signatures of ownership that covered her mind and body. This young girl found a way to free herself.

Most, if not all, of us would like to erase the memories of the brutalities committed against ourselves and others. But how does one obliterate that which cannot be forgotten? And if they are impossible to forget, how does one live with the memories? A teenager speaks of such a moment when he was a young boy:

> I cannot forget that one afternoon when my village was ambushed by rebels. I can still see a little boy scurrying like a rabbit into the dead bushes, only to be shot in the back. And I remember my mother, throwing herself on top of me and my 9-month-old sister to protect us. Droplets of what I thought were my mother's tears fell on me. And I felt safe. The next morning when everything was quiet, I tried to awaken my mother to tell her that we were safe. But she wouldn't move. I managed to free myself ... and what I saw is something I can never erase from my memory. My mother's body was covered with blood and my sister's face was an ugly blue and her mouth was open as if she were gasping for air. She had suffocated. I no longer have a family. I am alone in this big world. Sometimes I think about killing myself, then I wouldn't be alone, but my mother died to save my life. She wanted me to live. I live to remind them [rebels] that they didn't kill all of us. My mother, my sister, and my village live in me. (Used with permission.)

For this young boy, and for others of us, suicide would be granting our perpetrators the satisfaction of knowing that they were successful in destroying us completely. Instead, for us, survival is our ultimate act of defiance.

It is part of one religious belief system that when a person contemplates suicide, evil spirits are at work. In another, suicide is deemed an unforgivable sin. Yet another belief holds that when one commits suicide, her soul or spirit is perpetually in limbo. However, religious beliefs do not always dissuade survivors from embracing suicide as their last hope to end their suffering.

As companions on this dreadful journey, we do not judge the actions of our sisters and brothers. To us, the act of suicide, whether attempted or carried out, is but a reminder of the appalling effects of torture and extreme trauma on the survivor and the survivor's family and society.

FAITH: TO BELIEVE OR NOT

During and after trauma, some survivors search for the answer to a question that is ultimately neither answerable nor dismissible: How could God allow people to be subjected to such heinous forms of violence? In the depths of our anguish, the faith of a lifetime is sorely tested and, in some cases, devastated. We begin to doubt God's compassion, God's very existence. That which once gave meaning and direction to our lives lies in ruins.

A newly ordained clergyman speaks of his first assignment—ministering to political prisoners. Appalled at the conditions under which they were forced to live, he challenged the authorities by initiating a series of demonstrations demanding prison reform. After several months, he and others were accused of conspiring to overthrow the government and were imprisoned.

> They put me into a frigid, damp, dark room with no windows, no lighting, and I was forced to undress. The dampness and cold were tolerable, but the torment of waiting was unbearable.... It was a Gethsemane moment, a time of waiting, not knowing what would happen from one minute to the next. I don't remember how long I was kept in solitary confinement; it could have been hours, days, weeks. Being deprived of food, water, light, and contact with other human beings nearly turned me into a madman. I saw myself as a forgotten pea in a pod, disintegrating. I screamed, screamed, screamed. Every scream was a scream for God. Where were you God? Why had you forsaken me? How could God torment someone like me, who had dedicated his life to Him? What was most frightening was that I had completely forgotten about my fellow prisoners; I was thinking only of myself, my own survival. Relief came when one of the guards took me into a brightly lit room crowded with unclothed prisoners who seemed oblivious to their nakedness. But then the guard, with a gun aimed at another prisoner's head, said, "Man of God" (that was the name they gave me), "dance, dance, dance ... or he dies." I danced like a wild man, flapping my arms to the silent music, which ended with a gun shot and a loud THUMP as the prisoner fell to the floor ... and I kept dancing on and on and on. In a flash, my faith in God and in mankind had been completely shattered. (Used with permission.)

Yet in the face of similarly shattering events, some survivors emerge with their faith unscathed, perhaps even strengthened by what they have experienced. A medical worker writes about her faith's greatest test.

> One afternoon, a wounded man appeared at the parish clinic. He was covered with blood and was asking for medical attention. I was told to send him away immediately, that if I were to help him, I would be seen as sympathetic to the opposition. When I looked into his eyes, he was just a child. At that moment, I was looking into the eyes of Christ. How could I send him away? It was my duty; this was a medical clinic, and I am a Christian. The following day, the local police arrested me. They accused me of being a guerrilla sympathizer, charging me with terrorism. After they had beaten me, slapped and kicked me, they grabbed me by the hair and shoved my head into a barrel of something that smelled like urine. I couldn't breathe. I thought I was going to die. And I

prayed aloud to God, pleading with Him to help me, not to let me die. My captors told me that God had forsaken me. But I knew better. God would never abandon me or any others in need. Three days later I was released. God had heard my prayer. He did not let me die in the hands of my enemy. (Used with permission.)

"I no longer take my life for granted," says another survivor.

With my experience has come a deeper understanding of the fragility of humanity and the evil that dwells in the world. If I can survive torture, I'm confident that I can survive anything that life can dish out to me, with or without God, Allah, Buddha, or anyone else. (Used with permission.)

RESILIENCE OF SURVIVORS

In the introduction to his book, *The Aftermath: Living With the Holocaust,* Aaron Hass contends that

The mental health community, writers, and artists have focused their attention on the pathological inheritance of the Holocaust, but they rarely acknowledged or credited the strengths residing in survivors, which not only have enabled them to pick up the shattered pieces of their lives but also in many cases have resulted in more than adequate postwar functioning. One reason for this failure to note the positive adjustment of many survivors may be the fear of permitting the denial of the trauma's severity. We may feel forced to emphasize survivors' subsequent pain in order not to minimize the reality of previous losses and the pitiless brutality to which they were subjected. Nevertheless, to understand the survivor, to understand the obstinacy of the human spirit not to be permanently squashed, we must also appreciate the successes of those who emerged (Hass, 1995). (Used with permission.)

Like Hass, we believe that considerably more attention must be given to our resilience and less to what others may consider to be our weakness, our pathological behavior.

TRANSITIONAL SURVIVAL SKILLS

Family members, friends, and mental health professionals do not always understand the behaviors torture survivors exhibit. "The magnitude of this inhumanity [of torture]," one survivor notes, "overpowers the mind's ability to comprehend how anyone could wantonly harm another human being to that extent. Still more, how can those who have never experienced it even begin to comprehend what happens to a person who has been subjected to such evil?" Survivors have long noted the tendency of family members and mental health professionals to interpret certain of our behaviors as self-destructive, when in fact they are strategies for staying alive. We may try to cope with the aftermath of our trauma by searching for ways to numb the pain, whether it be with alcohol, drugs, prostitution, continual sleep, or "normalizing" our lives—that is, denying that anything of consequence has happened.

Through the clinical lens, such actions may be considered pathological behavioral disorders. If maintained indefinitely, these transitional survival skills are, in many cases, detrimental. Nonetheless, in the short run, these activities keep us alive. As normal people emerging from an abnormal situation—the situation of torture—we survivors fashion these lifesaving behaviors out of ingenuity, creativity, and survival. Intolerance for this type of conduct on the part of mental health professionals may ultimately be more destructive to the survivor than the behaviors themselves. Hearing the behaviors that have allowed us to survive described as deviant or pathological only reinforces our sense that we are misunderstood, alone, crazy, and incapable of helping ourselves on the road back to recovery. During the torture, all our control was taken from us. We truly were helpless, abandoned, and humiliated. We could trust no one. In the aftermath of this experience, we tend to make the most progress in therapy when we feel we have someone committed to working with us who understands and respects us and allows us some latitude and control over the course of our recovery.

RECLAIMING CONTROL

Consider the choice of a female survivor who turned to prostitution as a way to reclaim what was taken from her during her 28 days of captivity. Her perpetrators had used and abused her body at their pleasure. Throughout her imprisonment and after her release, the question that haunted her was how she could have permitted others to control her so completely:

> I know that to most people, my need to reclaim my sense of control could be interpreted as an obsession, as if I had a vendetta against men and against myself.... But it was much more than that; it was a matter of life and death. [Prostitution] kept me alive, and empowered me to confront my past and face the future. I knew the risks that I was taking. I was careful in the selection of my customers. I took every precaution to protect myself, my health, and that of others.... I had to prove to myself and to others that I was in control of myself, not my torturers, not my customers. (Used with permission.)

In this case, prostitution proved to be a transitional survival skill, one that represented a positive and life-affirming choice.

NORMALIZING LIFE THROUGH DENIAL

The process of normalizing one's life through denial is another example of a transitional survival skill. Denial represents a refusal to believe that such a terrible ordeal occurred at all, or that if it did occur, its psychological aftermath has not had any great impact on the individual, the family, or the community.

The practice of genocidal rape, among women and men, gives evidence of both forms of denial as well as an additional transitional survival skill: the simple refusal to discuss what happened. In some countries, rape has been used as a weapon of war, intended to terrorize entire populations and to leave behind shame and terrible social stigma. Women of all ages have been systematically raped, not only by strangers but also by men who were their neighbors. Military forces, in some instances, have used rape to reward their troops.

Some women whose rape resulted in impregnation by their perpetrators were held in concentration camps until it was too late for them to abort. A woman who found herself carrying the offspring of one of her perpetrators speaks.

> They kept us in their custody until it was too late for us to have an abortion. I was filled with so much shame, so much hate.... There was a very young girl who had been separated from her mother. She was well liked by the soldiers, maybe because she was young and pretty. We tried to protect her, but we couldn't. She became pregnant like the rest of us. Then one day she tried to remove the fetus that was growing inside her. She died with that fetus in her own pool of blood. (Used with permission.)

Afraid and filled with shame, women are released, their cultural identity no longer intact, carrying the offspring of their rapists and "giving birth to a new generation that no one wants," as one woman put it—least of all the women who were forced to conceive. Afraid and overwhelmed with shame, some women refuse to let their husbands or immediate families know what happened. Some leave the newborn in the care of orphanages; some, shortly after giving birth, leave the hospital when no one is looking, leaving the child behind. Others may keep these infants, only to be faced with a daily reminder of both their perpetrators and the war.

The woman continues,

> We were filled with so much shame. Many of us were afraid to tell our husbands, our mothers, and fathers about what happened. We were afraid they would blame us and expel us from the family. Some women killed themselves after they were released. Some of us, like me, carried it [the fetus] for the full term. When I gave birth, when no one was looking, I left the hospital. I walked out of the hospital as if nothing had happened. I couldn't raise it. My husband was away at war when I was taken to the camps and raped.... He'll never have to know. Besides, he wouldn't believe me. (Used with permission.)

Genocidal rape is not limited to women. One man testifies,

> Only women are raped, not men. That's what I used to believe. All of that changed when I was gang-raped by soldiers. As a child I was taught to believe that men, unlike women, were strong. Man could protect himself from all danger. Then when a man gets married, he becomes the man of the house, the protector of the family unit. How can I tell my wife that I cannot give her children because I was both raped and castrated? How can I tell my father, my mother, your son who you raised to be a man was not man enough to protect himself from being raped. Because I was weak, you will never have grandchildren. (Used with permission.)

The collective torture that has terrorized and traumatized an entire population may be denied, not only by individuals and their families, but by communities as well. "People don't want to see, to hear, to be reminded of what happened in my village, my country. But I remember. I was one of the thousands of young women raped. No one wants to talk about it. So I live like everyone around me, as though nothing happened," says a survivor of genocidal rape.

It is said that this "normalization process" delays the inevitable confrontation with the traumatic experience that has made the individual a victim/survivor and that has altered her entire worldview and understanding of herself (Bar-On, 1996, p. 168). As a long-term solution, of course, denial is unlikely to be a successful method of coping. But as a transitional survival skill, it may be an effective, life-affirming strategy.

THERAPY

Another transitional survival skill in which survivors find some form of relief is psychotherapy. Some survivors may begin this process shortly after having been tortured, whereas others may wait until months or years later. However, in many cases, cultural, political, economic, or all of these factors may serve as barriers. In some societies, therapy is not a viable option. As one survivor points out, her cultural beliefs hold that "talking to outsiders about traumatic experiences or emotional problems is just not done. In doing so, one risks being stigmatized as either weak or crazy." In other instances, the factors that hamper recovery may include a lack of therapeutic or medical resources, or both, where survivors reside or a lack of financial assistance to families with a member who needs to be in an extended therapeutic setting. Finally, in many countries, there is the public belief that the practice and effects of torture are limited to other, "less civilized" locales. Thus, no government monies are allocated for the treatment of survivors.

It is with both great fear and extreme caution that survivors seek assistance from mental health professionals. A genesis moment of rebuilding trust occurs when we risk allowing others to see, to hear, and to know of the horrors of our torture. One survivor who had a positive initial experience in therapy was able to begin confronting his past:

> My life was in turmoil. I couldn't sleep or eat. Since I didn't have a work permit, I couldn't get a job. No one would hire an "illegal alien" like me. I was alone in my pain. No one to turn to, no one to wipe away my tears. So I relied on drugs to cope with my problems, to forget the day that the soldiers executed my entire family. The memories might fade momentarily, but they would always return. There was so much rage inside me. People were afraid of me; I was even afraid of myself. Then I met a woman who told me about a place that offered counseling for people like me. The woman and man who talked with me were very kind. I felt a little safe, but still I didn't trust them. I was afraid that these people who said they wanted to help me would turn me over to immigration.... Then I would be deported. Their many questions made me feel like I was being interrogated, but still I wanted to trust them, because they knew of the persecution of my people. For the first time, I started to talk with others about the execution of my family. (Used with permission.)

The positive experience of another survivor offers a further example of how therapy can be helpful. Her therapist, knowledgeable about the survivors' world, understood when and how to offer support. She also understood that survivors must be in control of their own decisions and their own lives. Recall the case of the survivor mentioned above who used prostitution as a transitional survival skill. During therapy sessions, she and her therapist would discuss how to deal with her pervasive sense of loss of control:

> When I shared with my therapist how prostitution allowed me to reclaim my control, I expected her to tell me that what I was doing was morally wrong. Surprisingly, she never judged me. She trusted me and the decisions I was making; she trusted my common sense. We talked about the risk factors, such as AIDS, both for me and for others. But, again, she trusted me to know what I was doing. Her understanding helped me put my life back together. The memories of my imprisonment and rapes are still with me, but they no longer control and paralyze me as they did in the past. Today, I have regained control of my life and live what I believe to be a productive life. I am married to a man who loves me for who I am. I am the mother of three children, and I am a lawyer. I have reclaimed that which was taken from me. (Used with permission.)

Equally positive was the experience of another survivor:

> Ten years later, I was still being reminded of the brutal acts that had been committed by the army. Enmeshed in a world where you cannot forget the past is hell and sometimes one thinks that he is going crazy. I remember going to the corner store to buy milk when I saw a policeman. He was whistling, smoking a cigarette.... I panicked and ran home and hid inside a closet. I stayed in that closet for 2 days, afraid that they would return to torture me again. When I started to talk to the therapist about having flashbacks and nightmares, he didn't seem at all shocked and told me that it was not uncommon to have these reactions. These were normal reactions. I was a new person after that. (Used with permission.)

However positive the therapy experience may be, no one ever fully recovers from the trauma of political violence. Remnants of that trauma will always be with us. Nonetheless, efforts to heal, whether they be individual or with the support of others, are not futile. Many survivors believe that recovery on some level is possible in every case and that mental health professionals can play a significant role in this process. Unless the therapeutic process is rooted in the empowerment of the survivor, however, it is doomed before it begins. If mental health professionals are to grasp the importance of this aspect, they must have a clear understanding not only of the psychology of torture and its consequences but also of the survivors' world. In the absence of this understanding, therapy may prove to be detrimental to the survivor.

As a refugee woman who was urged to see a therapist recalls,

> I was told that I would feel better talking to someone who could help me. The therapy session was an absolute disaster. The therapist yawned and looked at her watch as I was trying to tell her about what had happened. As I continued to talk, I noticed that she kept raising her eyebrows; there was a clock behind me. She was looking at the clock! When it struck four, she told me that was all for today. (Used with permission.)

It had taken so much courage for this woman to begin to talk about her experience. Unfortunately, this encounter closed the door to the possibility of therapy from that day on.

Survivors' sense of profound isolation may be confronted effectively in a therapeutic setting, but only when the clinician understands the distinctive nature of the therapist–survivor interaction. As illustrated above, therapists have a special role to play, but they must play it carefully. As any survivor can tell you, there are times when we are unable to see the roads available to us in our recovery. Torture survivors often work best with a therapist who does not chart the way for the survivor but maps out possible routes, leaving to the survivor the decision of how best to proceed. In this way the therapist acts as a compass; the therapist does not determine the action but points the way to various alternatives. The survivor, meanwhile, feels empowered and in control of the course of action, which is essential after suffering the tyranny of the torturers in a situation where every form of control was denied.

Some survivors tell how the arts—such as writing poetry, playing a musical instrument, or dancing—have been vehicles for restoring a sense of autonomy and hope. One survivor was able to begin this artistic process when his psychologist proposed an alternative form of therapy that finally permitted him to express himself.

> Art as therapy was unfamiliar to me, but it made perfect sense. I used to be an artist. I was arrested in my studio and that was the last time I picked up a paintbrush. During one of our sessions, he [the therapist] had a sketch pad, drawing pencils, and watercolors on the table. I picked up a pencil and started to draw my feelings, to draw what I remembered of my imprisonment and torture. One day I hope to have an exhibition of my work … to illustrate to people the violent world in which we live. (Used with permission.)

For therapy to be successful, mental health professionals must also honor the cultural beliefs of survivors. Failure in this area jeopardizes the effectiveness of the therapy and at the same time may suggest to the survivor that her culture is inferior. One survivor recounts such an experience:

> The doctor didn't speak my language and so they had to use a translator. When I described how they [torturers] put ants inside my eyes and then taped them shut, the psychologist acted like he didn't believe me. He kept telling the translator to have me repeat what I had said. After the third time, I said no more. Then he told me that he was going to take me to see a real doctor who would prescribe medicine for my eye infection. When I told the translator to tell the psychologist that I was applying a paste that my people had used for centuries to cure infections, it seemed that didn't matter. First, he didn't seem to believe what I said, then he didn't think my medicine was as good as his. I told them I wouldn't come back unless I could talk to someone who could understand me. (Used with permission.)

On his next visit, the survivor met with a therapist who not only spoke his language but understood the culture as well. At this point, he began to make progress.

Although individual therapy has proven to be a useful tool for many survivors, others find group therapy to be of greater value. It is not uncommon for each survivor to feel as if she is the only person who has suffered horrible atrocities. In group therapy, one woman explains,

> I developed an understanding of the purpose of torture, about people who torture others. Most importantly, I learned that the torture inflicted on me was not a direct attack on me. I learned that torture is universal. People from all walks of life are subject

to torture. Trauma can cause you to become absorbed in yourself; you sometimes forget that other people are being persecuted. It's less painful to talk to other people who have had similar experiences—we recognize each other's pain. (Used with permission.)

Then there are those of us who do not wish to talk about our problems in a group setting. In some cases, survivors are mistrustful of people from their country:

During the war, you didn't know who to trust. The people that you thought were your friends turned out to be informants. I play soccer with my countrymen and even have a couple of beers with them, but I would never confide in them. How can I be certain that they are not informers for the government? (Used with permission.)

Talk therapy is not the only form of treatment that has proved useful. Some survivors use traditional medicines, such as natural remedies prepared by "folk" healers. Others favor techniques such as body work, massage, aroma and sound therapy, special breathing and relaxation exercises, or the ancient spiritual tradition of shamanism (Larson, 1997, p. 21). Still others are open to accepting psychotropic medications, which are often recommended by health professionals and may lessen depression-like symptoms and insomnia. In any case, it is the survivor's right to choose which, if any, of these approaches she will use.

Most, if not all, survivors of torture need time to grieve and to heal physical injuries, to confront the horrors of the past and to understand the immense impact of what was done to us, to adapt to a new country, and to rebuild trust in ourselves and in others. Transitional survival skills carry us through one terror-filled night to the next. Inadequate or destructive as they may seem to others, they do keep us alive. From a position of slowly increasing strength, many of us can then begin to redirect our energies to helping other survivors, raising public awareness about the practice of torture, confronting our perpetrators, or simply learning to live life anew and with some sense of hope.

EFFECTS OF TORTURE ON THE FAMILY

The trauma that has engulfed us reaches out to our families as well—those of us who have families. A mother who offered her legal services to an organization whose leaders were considered communist by the government says,

I was the mother of three teenage daughters—that was before they took two of them from me. My oldest daughter never came home from school. I searched everywhere, military bases, police stations, morgues, and government offices, demanding to know where my daughter was. Local authorities said that she was apparently a rebellious teenager who had run off with a boy. Then the phone calls started.... The caller told me to stop asking questions or the same thing would happen to my other daughters. But my search for my daughter continued. With the help of a lawyer friend, I presented a writ of habeas corpus to the Court. They would not process my complaint. Then our lawyer friend started to receive death threats and left, asking for asylum in another country. Then the call came—the same caller said they had purchased a coffin for one of my daughters. That night, my second oldest daughter did not come home. And in the morning we found her body left in front of our door. Her face was swollen, covered with blood. All her teeth had been removed. Her chest was covered with bite marks. She had been raped, her neck broken. My daughter, she died with her eyes open. And I am to blame. I want to know who took my daughters away from me. I want those criminals punished. But my husband tells me if I start asking questions, the same thing could happen to our youngest daughter. He tells me that he will leave me and take my last daughter with him. She's all I have left.... I don't want to lose her; she's all I have left. I must protect her, so I must be silent. (Used with permission.)

Another mother, whose daughter was wounded in an attack, recalls her feelings:

My daughter wouldn't let anyone call us until she could get out of the hospital the next day and call us herself.... I felt as much anger as grief. Had someone else called, I think I would have been terrified and perhaps tried to go down immediately. I felt helpless and tried to talk her into leaving the country as soon as possible. I felt horror and anger intensely when she showed me her scars, especially the one over her heart. I remember her own anger when we met her at the airport and I was very worried about her state of mind.... She warned me repeatedly to lock the door when I left the house. (Used with permission.)

Parents often experience feelings of powerlessness when they are unable to protect their children from danger. In some cases, unconsciously, they become overprotective and try taking control of the survivor's life, which may result in friction or resentment. In other instances, the family feigns that nothing happened, never talking about the incident and resuming a "normal life," into which the survivor is expected to fit.

Generally, families will experience emotions that parallel those experienced by survivors, guilt and rage among them. It is important to remember that children of survivors undergo many of the same emotions as their parents. As the effects of torture permeate the family, the question of healing arises for its members as well as for the survivor. As the survivor explores possible techniques to achieve some level of recovery, family members may join in that exploration. Either on their own or with the assistance of a third party, the family members and the survivor must establish a situation whereby they can attempt to break through the isolation that separates them so that they can share their feelings with each other. In their own, perhaps different, ways, each very likely needs a measure of support from the other members of the family, from the community, and from the mental health profession. The reactions of family members may cover a wide range; however, what is clear is that torture affects not only the survivor but also the family members—persons who may have no preparation for how to react, how to deal with the survivor, or how to respond to their own emotions.

THE CULTURE OF DENIAL

All too often, the world survivors reenter resembles the one that our torturers promised us. They told us, implicitly or explicitly, that we were worthless, that no one cared, that we could not be believed. As we tell our stories, we often meet with a lack of understanding or outright indifference. This suggests to many survivors an unwillingness to face the reality of torture in the world today. Unfortunately, these reactions are not limited to the anonymous masses of the general public. They extend to our own governments. And when governments are involved, political concerns are added to the lack of comprehension, the indifference, and the denial that characterize the general populace.

On the road to recovery, many survivors, as a way of rebuilding their lives, begin to ask for information regarding the perpetrators of their ordeal and for justice. But instead of receiving help from our governments, we are often retraumatized: Governments either ignore us or, because we may be politically "inconvenient," actively discredit or slander us.

Our own cases aside, when governments justify, ignore, or secretly foment and support genocidal rape, massacres of innocent civilians, and illegal detention and torture, survivors are outraged. When the government in question happens to be the survivor's own, the survivor is retraumatized. Metaphorically, she is an abused child, still in the abusive family, watching the abuse of a sibling. She is not safe.

The case of one survivor illustrates this dynamic. She escaped from her perpetrators after torture in a foreign country where she was a missionary. The torture was overseen by a man from her own country, apparently an advisor to the security forces that had abducted her. When she returned to her country of origin, seeking refuge and justice, she asked for information regarding the identity of her countryman, whom her torturers had referred to as their boss.

In response, she was vilified by her government's officials, who attempted to establish that she was an instrument of the subversion, fabricating stories to secure a cutoff of military aid to the foreign army. When this tactic failed, attempts were made to characterize her as a lesbian who had never been abducted but had sneaked out for sex. When this approach proved futile, her government tried to track down a nonexistent record of psychological treatment before the abduction in an attempt to establish that she was mentally unstable and therefore not credible. Years later, her government finally admitted it had financially supported the army that had tortured her, even after aid was officially cut off in light of that army's repeated human rights abuses; that it indeed had advisors from a number of its own agencies working within the country's military; and that it had taught torture at its own army's school to thousands of foreign military officers—in fact, to the man who was defense minister at the time of the missionary's torture. In seeking justice, the survivor was again placed in the torture chamber in a sense: she was again falsely accused, vilified, and abused—and again, by an entity she formerly trusted: her own government.

Many governments, giving priority to their own political agendas, make sure that torturers do not suffer punishment; neither do those who give them their orders. It is we survivors who become the criminals. As Martinez and Fabri, staff members of the Marjorie Kovler Center for the Treatment of Survivors of Torture, have written,

> Torture survivors, like rape victims, are in a precarious legal position that compromises the rights of the victim. They must prove that the event occurred, that they are innocent of some yet unidentified wrongdoing, and that they are of deserving character.

The legal system is experienced not as an advocate for victims but as an adversary. This experience complements the tactic of torturers of telling the victim, overtly or by inference, that no one will listen to them or care about what happened to them. This is a way of increasing the likelihood of later silence. The torturer's tactics are reexperienced and reinforced when the survivors are in a situation in which their stories are not believed. (Martinez & Fabri, 1992, p. 47) (Used with permission.)

A refugee woman who sought political asylum in a host country tells of her encounter with an immigration judge:

His voice was loud, like that of my torturers. He said that everyone in the courtroom knew that I was not telling the full truth ... that I was here to make money, just to make a better life. "Isn't that right? Look at me when I talk to you," he shouted at me. Eye contact with your elders is a sign of disrespect in my culture, but the judge thought since I was not looking at him that I was not being truthful. He was so very angry with me and said that he did not have time to listen to my lies. Without hearing my testimony, the judge decided to deport me. I started to cry and he handed me a tissue and told me to stop crying, to stop feeling sorry for myself, and he stormed out of the courtroom.... And my lawyer said nothing to defend me. I was so hurt. I didn't know why I was being treated in this manner. Afterwards, I had many bad dreams and then I tried to kill myself. (Used with permission.)

Even those who do not survive may be blamed, as in the case of four churchwomen raped and murdered in a foreign country. Their behavior was impugned by high officials of their own government who were attempting to cover up the role of the military in the killings. The military, of course, was backed by the murdered women's own government.

To take another example, in September 1997, a former police officer testified before the country's truth commission about the beating death of a human rights worker. "He was acting stubborn and too big for his boots," the policeman said. He described how the prisoner, "sleep-deprived and naked, sat down during the interrogation, disobeying orders to remain standing. That prompted a scuffle in which [his] head hit a wall leading to the fatal brain injury" (Associated Press, 1997, p. A29). The policeman was saying that this man died, not because of torture, not because his torturers beat him to death, but because he sat down when he knew he was supposed to remain standing. Who was the cause of this man's death? None other than the victim himself, or so the torturers would have us believe.

Even when their testimonies are believed, survivors risk retraumatization. The mere recounting of their experience can plunge them into flashbacks, lead to recurring nightmares, and land them in a vulnerable psychological state. When survivors and their families are asked to give testimony in a courtroom setting or in front of truth commissions or war tribunals, those who have issued the invitation have a moral responsibility. This responsibility is greater than simply listening to survivors recount the atrocities they have suffered and witnessed. During and after the testimony, survivors are highly vulnerable. The responsibility that those who would hear the testimony must accept is to ensure that survivors, first of all, are physically safe—safe from reprisals by those against whom they give testimony. Beyond their physical protection, those who arrange testimonial hearings have the responsibility to ensure the survivors' psychological safety. In many instances, survivors not only recount what happened but begin to relive the torture once again; they are no longer on the witness stand but back in that awful setting, hearing the voices of their torturers and the screams of those being tortured, experiencing the smell of death, feeling the blows all over again.

Arrangements must be made to minimize the effects of this trauma. We survivors must be permitted to present our evidence in the manner we choose. Most specifically, we must not be rushed in our presentations, we should be allowed ample "break times," and, if possible, we should be permitted to have a person of our own choosing present with us. Finally, survivors who testify must know that there is a sturdy support network at their disposal. That network, which should include members of the survivor's family and community as well as mental health and legal professionals, should not wait passively for a phone call from the witness. Instead, members of the network, fully conversant with the survivor's world, should initiate contact from time to time to assure themselves of the survivor's well-being.

Torture, which Jean-Paul Sartre called the plague of our era, is an epidemic infecting people from every walk of life in more than 121 countries (Amnesty International, 1997). This act of terrorism poisons nations, destroys communities, and shatters its victims. Many of us ask why there is so little outrage toward what is so clearly a crime against all humanity. Whether the horror is physical or psychological makes no difference. Survivors wonder why there is little evidence of a public moral stance against this form of terrorism from national, economic, and religious leaders or those who are specialists in this field. "The Holocaust will be understood," Jacobo Timerman rightly reminds us, "not so much for the number of victims as for the magnitude of the silence, and what obsesses me most is the repetition of silence rather than the possibility of another Holocaust" (Timerman, 1981, p. 141).

RESEARCH RECOMMENDATIONS FROM THE SURVIVORS' PERSPECTIVE

From the perspective of survivors, the focus of current research tends to overemphasize the importance of the survivor and underemphasize those agents and organizations responsible for torture in the first place. In the case of survivor-oriented research, insufficient attention is paid to the survivor as an active participant in the project. As echoed by many survivors, those who have survived torture or any form of political violence tend to be treated as research objects, reactors rather than actors in the process.

Torture, initiated at the level of government, is followed by government-imposed secrecy and impunity for those involved in it. Research into the issue of how to eliminate the practice of torture as well as how to improve the healing process thus requires research into how to reduce or end secrecy and impunity in government.

On the issue of the healing process itself, controlled studies are needed in a number of areas:

- The effectiveness of "alternative" approaches, such as "folk" or traditional medicine; shamanism; sound, dance, and art therapy; and so forth.
- The use of family- and community-based therapy, as opposed to survivor-based therapy.
- The development and evaluation of community-based programs in torture and its survival.
- The short- and long-term effects of torture on society (e.g., attitudes of indifference, denial, and complicity).
- North- and South-based therapeutic approaches conducted in both the North and the South.

This kind of survivor-focused research will contribute to our understanding of what survivors need as they attempt to rebuild their lives and hope for the future.

REFERENCES

Amnesty International. (1985). The Declaration of Tokyo (World Medical Association). In Amnesty International Secretariat (Ed.), *Ethical codes and declarations relevant to the health professions* (2nd ed.). London: Author.

Amnesty International. (1997). *Amnesty International report 1997.* London: Author.

Apfel, R. J., & Simon, B. (1996). Introduction. In R. Apfel & B. Simon (Eds.), *Minefields in their hearts: The mental health of children in war and communal violence* (pp. 1–17). New Haven, CT: Yale University Press.

Associated Press. (1997, September 12). Biko defied police, officer says. *The Washington Post,* p. A29.

Bar-On, D. (1996). Attempting to overcome the intergenerational transmission of trauma: Dialogue between descendants of victims and of perpetrators. In R. Apfel & B. Simon (Eds.), *Minefields in their hearts: The mental health of children in war and communal violence* (pp. 165–188). New Haven, CT: Yale University Press.

Frankl, V. E. (1963). *Man's search for meaning: An introduction to logotherapy.* New York: Pocket Books.

Hass, A. (1995). *The aftermath: Living with the Holocaust.* New York: Cambridge University Press.

Larson, M. A. (1997). *Journeys in healing: Care with survivors of torture and organized violence in the U.S. and Canada: An exploratory study of U.S. and Canadian treatment programs.* Unpublished master's thesis, The University of North Carolina at Chapel Hill, Department of Health Behavior and Health Education, Chapel Hill.

Martinez, A., & Fabri, M. (1992). The Kovler Center: The dilemma of revictimization. *Torture, 2*(2), 47–48.

Timerman, J. (1981). *Prisoner without a name, cell without a number.* New York: Vintage Books.

3

Torture and Mental Health
A Research Overview

METIN BASOGLU, JAMES M. JARANSON, RICHARD
MOLLICA, and MARIANNE KASTRUP

Over the last two decades, much work has been done on various forms of extreme
trauma, particularly after the recognition in the early 1980s of posttraumatic stress
disorder (PTSD) as a diagnostic entity. Since then, significant progress has been
made in the diagnosis, assessment, and treatment of trauma survivors. Such progress,
however, has not been paralleled by work specifically on the trauma of torture
despite the widespread evidence of torture in the world and its mental health
implications.

Traumatic events of human design such as rape, domestic or marital violence,
child abuse, physical assault, combat and other forms of war violence, prisoner-of-war
or concentration camp experience, kidnapping, hostage-taking, and terrorist acts,
among others, share important common elements with torture. Despite the apparent differences between these traumatic events, their psychological consequences
are remarkably similar, which suggests potential commonalities in the way these
events are mediated in the central nervous system (Basoglu, 1992a). Furthermore,
recent evidence from a controlled treatment study (Marks, Lovell, Noshirvani,
Livanou, & Thrasher, 1998) suggests that psychological symptoms related to different types of traumatic events, whether accidents, natural disasters, or traumas

METIN BASOGLU • Section on Traumatic Studies, Institute of Psychiatry, King's College, London University SES 8AF London, England.   **JAMES M. JARANSON** • Department of Psychiatry, University of Minnesota, St. Paul, Minnesota 55108-1300.   **RICHARD MOLLICA** • Harvard
Program in Refugee Trauma, Department of Psychiatry, Harvard University, Cambridge, Massachusetts 02138.   **MARIANNE KASTRUP** • Rehabilitation and Research Center for Torture
Victims, Borgergade 13/P.O. Box 2107, DK-1014 Copenhagen, Denmark.

The Mental Health Consequences of Torture, edited by Ellen Gerrity, Terence M. Keane, and Farris
Tuma. Kluwer Academic/Plenum Publishers, New York, 2001.

of human design, respond similarly to particular forms of treatment (Livanou, 1998). Current knowledge on assessment, diagnosis, and treatment of trauma survivors could therefore be useful in working with survivors of torture. Similarly, the study of torture can contribute to our understanding of the mechanisms of traumatization, as there are striking parallels between experimental models of anxiety and depression and what human beings experience under torture (Basoglu & Mineka, 1992). A review of current knowledge on both torture and other extreme traumas could be beneficial for all these related fields.

PREVALENCE OF TORTURE

The term "torture" is often used in a moral or sentimental sense to designate any form of ill treatment with or without any purpose (Peters, 1985). Scientific study of this problem requires a more precise definition. The definition of torture used for the purposes of this chapter is that provided by the 1986 United Nations Declaration of Human Rights (United Nations, 1987). This definition is described elsewhere in the introduction to this book.

There are few studies of the prevalence of torture in the world on which to base reliable estimates. Epidemiological studies are difficult, if not impossible, because of the politically sensitive nature of the issue. The only data available are those published by human rights organizations such as Amnesty International. Although Amnesty International figures probably represent a fraction of all human rights abuses in the world, they nevertheless give some idea about the extent of the problem. The 1999 *Amnesty International Report* lists more than 121 countries known for some form of human rights violation in the previous year (Amnesty International, 1999).

An analysis (Basoglu, 1993) of the 1992 *Amnesty International Report* demonstrated the nature and global distribution of human rights violations. In 1991, systematic torture was reported in 93 of the 204 countries included in the *Amnesty International Report*. Reports of torture were more common from regions affected by political unrest, including mass demonstrations, riots, outbreaks of violence, killings, coup attempts, civil war, separatist or guerilla groups, armed tribal conflict, rebellions, and conflicts with various social and political opposition. The problem was not confined to these regions, however, as systematic torture or ill treatment was also reported in 25% of the western European and North American countries. The 1999 *Amnesty International Report* shows an increase in the number of countries involved in such atrocities.

Little is known about the prevalence of torture among various at-risk populations. Between 5% and 35% of the world's 14 million refugees (700,000 to 4.9 million refugees) are estimated to have had at least one experience of torture (Baker, 1992). These figures do not reflect the current extent of the problem after the recent developments in Eastern Europe, the former Yugoslavia, the Middle East, and other parts of the world torn by political turmoil, nationalistic movements, and regional wars. Similarly, some studies of nonpolitical prisoners suggest that the prevalence of torture in some prison populations may be as high as 85% (Paker, Paker, & Yuksel, 1992).

PHYSICAL EFFECTS OF TORTURE

Because they vary according to the form of torture used, classifying the physical sequelae of torture is difficult. The physical sequelae following the most commonly used forms of torture are reviewed in detail by Skylv (1992) and will be briefly discussed here. Various forms of torture often give rise to both structural injury in the body and disturbed function (Skylv, 1992). Torture survivors are often subjected to multiple forms of torture that result in overlapping injuries. The physical sequelae in tortured refugees characteristically concern the musculoskeletal system (Rasmussen, 1990). These injuries often arise from blunt blows to the body, repeated blows to certain parts of the body such as in falanga (beating of the soles of the feet); hanging by the wrists or the arms; being tied around the body, neck, or extremities; electrical torture; torture involving cuts, burns, or corrosion with acid; torture involving the teeth such as drilling, extraction, or violent blows; prolonged immobilization in forced positions; and sexual assault. An increased risk of infectious disease, malignancies, cerebrovascular accidents, and heart disease has also been reported in survivors of torture or prolonged arbitrary detention (Goldman & Goldston, 1985).

A review of the literature (Goldfeld, Mollica, Pesavento, & Faraone, 1988) found that among the physical sequelae of torture reported were the following:

- Hearing loss from "telephono" (beating on the ears with cupped hands)
- Distinctive scarring in the skin from electrical torture; burning with cigarettes, molten rubber, corrosive liquids, or tight ropes; or beating with blunt instruments
- Occult fractures, lumbosacral spine injuries, dislocation of vertebrae, or paraplegia as a result of beating or being hung by one extremity
- Aseptic necrosis of a toe, chronic venous incompetence of the legs, and pain on walking secondary to falanga
- Mutilation of genitalia, pregnancy, venereal disease, infertility, and miscarriage as a result of rape and torture of women
- Sexual dysfunction and testicular atrophy from genital torture in men

The authors noted that the studies of the physical effects of torture did not consistently present historical descriptive data or physical findings that could elucidate the etiology of the clinical symptoms and their connection to torture. Furthermore, the length of time between torture and evaluation was not consistently noted.

Because torture survivors are often subjected to multiple forms of torture giving rise to overlapping injuries, it may be difficult, particularly in the long term, to trace the symptoms and signs to particular forms of torture (Skylv, 1992). This makes it difficult to provide evidence for physical torture. However, some studies

(Lok, Tunca, Kumanlioglu, Kapkin, & Dirik, 1991) using bone scintigraphy have been able to detect increased activity in bones as a result of beating or falanga, even months after the torture.

PSYCHOLOGICAL EFFECTS OF TORTURE

In the last two decades numerous studies of the psychological effects of torture have been performed. Recent reviews (Basoglu, 1993; Goldfeld et al., 1988; Somnier, Vesti, Kastrup, & Genefke, 1992) have drawn attention to the methodological problems in these studies. These problems include insufficient description of the interview procedures, assessment instruments, diagnostic criteria, and medical diagnoses. Inadequate reporting of neurological and neuropsychological findings has made it difficult to rule out head trauma as a possible etiological factor. The length of time between the torture and assessment was often not reported. Few studies examined the relationship between the symptoms and the diagnosis of PTSD. Often it was not clear how factors such as gender, age, education, cultural traits, and personality factors related to posttorture symptoms.

A significant shortcoming of most of these studies is their uncontrolled design. Many focus only on refugees, and the additional effects of refugee trauma were not controlled for. Similarly, studies of nonrefugee survivors have not controlled for other nontorture, potentially traumatic life events. Torture is only one of the many traumatic stressors in an environment characterized by political repression (Basoglu, 1993; van Willigen, 1992), and such stressors are associated with increased psychiatric morbidity (Venzlaff, 1964).

A REVIEW OF STUDIES ON TORTURE

In this chapter, we will focus on the controlled studies after a brief review of the uncontrolled studies. The purpose of this review is to determine whether sufficient scientific evidence exists to show that torture has long-term psychological effects independent of other associated nontorture stressors, including refugee trauma.

Uncontrolled Studies

The psychological problems most commonly reported by torture survivors in uncontrolled studies (Allodi & Cowgill, 1982; Berger, 1980; Cathcart, Berger, & Knazan, 1979; Domovitch, Berger, Waver, Etlin, & Marshall, 1984; Lunde, 1982; Rasmussen & Lunde, 1980; Wallach & Rasmussen, 1983; Warmenhoven, van Slooten, Lachinsky, de Hoog, & Smeulers, 1981) were reviewed by Goldfeld et al. (1988) and included (a) psychological symptoms (anxiety, depression, irritability or aggressiveness, emotional lability, self-isolation or social withdrawal), (b) cognitive symptoms (confusion or disorientation, impaired memory and concentration, impaired reading ability), and (c) neurovegetative symptoms (lack of energy, insomnia, nightmares, sexual dysfunction). These findings were supported by the results of later studies (Abildgaard et al., 1984; Bauer, Priebe, Haring, & Adamczak, 1993; Cunningham & Cunningham, 1997; Hougen, Kelstrup, Petersen, & Rasmussen, 1988; Kjaersgaard & Genefke, 1977; Lunde, Rasmussen, Lindholm, & Wagner, 1980; Petersen et al., 1985; Petersen & Jacobsen, 1985; Rasmussen, Dam, & Nielsen, 1977; Somnier & Genefke, 1986). Other findings reported in studies of torture survivors include abnormal sleep patterns (Astrom, Lunde, Ortmann, & Boysen, 1989), somatization (Mollica, Wyshak, & Lavelle, 1987), and personality changes (Ortmann & Lunde, 1988; Somnier & Genefke, 1986).

Traumatic brain injury is one factor that appears to be associated with psychiatric comorbidity in survivors of mass violence and torture. Some studies of Holocaust survivors (Astrom, 1968; Eitenger, 1961; Hermann & Thygesen, 1954; Thygesen, Hermann, & Willanger, 1970) have reported neuropsychiatric symptoms (described as the "KZ" or "concentration camp" syndrome) that were thought to be related to traumatic brain injury. Brain injury is also suggested as a significant risk factor in survivors of torture (Goldfeld et al., 1988). Some studies reported an association between neuropsychiatric symptoms and head trauma (Petersen & Jacobsen, 1985; Rasmussen, 1990). There have also been case reports of neuropsychiatric findings in torture survivors including neurological symptoms and cerebral atrophy (Jensen et al., 1982; Somnier et al., 1982). Another study using computerized tomography of the brain (Somnier, Jensen, Pedersen, Bruhn, Salinas, & Genefke, unpublished data, cited in Somnier et al., 1992), however, found no evidence of cerebral atrophy. Furthermore, no evidence of progressive cognitive impairment was found in other studies of torture survivors (Somnier & Genefke, 1986). A more recent study of 55 torture survivors (Basoglu, Paker, Paker, Ozmen, Marks, et al., 1994), which investigated the relationship between various torture events and long-term psychological status, found no correlations between reports of head trauma (e.g., beating or blows on the head) and psychological symptoms. The evidence on this issue is thus conflicting, and further studies using modern methods of neuropsychiatric and neuropsychological investigation are required to clarify the role of head trauma in developing posttorture symptoms.

In a more recent review of the literature (Somnier et al., 1992), the most commonly reported symptoms in torture survivors were anxiety; cognitive, memory, and attention problems; mood disturbance; sleeping difficulty; sexual dysfunctions; personality changes; lack of energy; and behavioral disturbances. These problems were also common in nonrefugee survivors of torture (Abildgaard et al., 1984; Foster, 1987; Jadresic, 1990; Kordon et al., 1988; Lunde et al., 1980; Lunde & Ortmann, 1990; Pagaduan-Lopez, 1987; Wallach & Rasmussen, 1983).

Other studies involved mixed samples of tortured and nontortured refugees. In a study of 993 displaced Cambodians living in a Thai border camp (Mollica et al., 1993), the prevalence of depression was as high as 82%, and 15% of the study participants had symptoms that were consistent with western criteria for PTSD. In a study of asylum-seekers in Australia (Silove, Sinnerbrink, Field, Manicavasagar, & Steel, 1997), the rate of PTSD was 36.8% (47% among those who were exposed to various traumatic events, including torture). High rates of PTSD and depression were also reported in other studies of Cambodian refugees (Kinzie & Boehnlein, 1989; Kinzie, Sack, Angell, & Manson, 1986; see also chapter 7 in this volume).

Controlled Studies

A Danish study (Hougen et al., 1988) of 14 tortured refugees and 14 control participants who were neither imprisoned nor tortured found more psychological problems in torture survivors compared with the control subjects. However, there were design problems in the study. The number of participants was very small, and the matching of controls was not adequate. Also, possible effects of nontorture stressors were not controlled for in comparing the two groups, and the symptoms were not assessed in sufficient detail. In addition, refugee status was found to be related to better psychological health, and the control group included refugees.

Another study of 105 Latin American refugees in Denmark (Thorvaldsen, 1986, as cited in Somnier et al., 1992) found more symptoms of headaches, fatigue, sleep disturbance, nightmares, and concentration difficulty among 44 tortured refugees than among those in the control group. The between-group differences were significant, despite the fact that some of the controls had been imprisoned and ill-treated—but not tortured—in their countries.

In a prospective controlled study of Spanish torture survivors (Petersen & Jacobsen, 1985), torture survivors had more symptoms of depression, anxiety, emotional lability, sleep disturbance, nightmares, and memory and concentration difficulties than did the nontortured controls. This study, however, did not use established diagnostic criteria and standardized measures of anxiety, depression, and posttraumatic stress symptoms. The small sample size ($n=10$) and inadequate controls in matching participants further weakened the study's findings.

Another study involved 246 inmates of a prison in Turkey (Paker et al., 1992), 208 of whom were tortured for nonpolitical reasons. The sample had some homogeneity with respect to nontorture stressors. Tortured and nontortured inmates were not matched, but multiple regression analyses were used to control for some of the confounding variables. The revised third edition of the *Diagnostic and Statistical Manual of Mental Disorders* (DSM-III-R; American Psychiatric Association, 1987) criteria for PTSD were used in assessing psychological status. Torture survivors had significantly more PTSD and higher scores on measures of general psychopathology than did the nontortured prisoners. The length of time since the last torture experience, however, was not taken into account. Furthermore, the specific effects of torture were confounded by other stressors during imprisonment and elsewhere.

A more recent study in Turkey (Basoglu, Paker, Paker, Ozman, Marks, et al., 1994) used semistructured interviews based on DSM-III-R and other standardized assessor- and self-rated instruments to compare 55 tortured political activists with 55 nontortured political activists and 55 nontortured individuals who had no history of political activity or involvement. All groups were matched for age, sex, and marital and sociocultural status. The first two groups were also matched for political ideology and extent of political involvement.

The study involved nonrefugee survivors of torture, thereby avoiding the confound of refugee status. The DSM-III-R Severity of Psychosocial Stressors Scale for adults was used to measure nontorture stressful life events before, during, and after detention or imprisonment. The groups were similar in all matching variables, as well as in other variables such as ethnic status, past psychiatric history, family history of psychiatric illness, history of alcohol and drug abuse, and lifetime exposure to nontorture stressful life events. Severity of torture was quantified by using an Exposure to Torture Scale, which yielded two objective (the number of forms of torture that individuals were exposed to and the total number of exposures to all forms of torture) and two subjective (the sum of perceived distress ratings with respect to each torture event reported and a global rating of overall stressfulness of torture) measures of torture severity. The study design and measures thus allowed both between- and within-group analyses to examine the effects of torture while controlling for other confounding variables such as nontorture stressors.

The torture survivors had significantly more lifetime and current PTSD than did the controls (33% vs. 11% and 18% vs. 4%, respectively). Compared with controls, torture survivors also had higher anxiety and depression, although these scores in both groups were within the normal range. Among the factors related to long-term psychological status were the secondary effect of captivity and torture on family, family history of psychiatric illness, and postcaptivity psychosocial stressors (Basoglu, Paker, Paker, Ozmen, and Sahin, 1994). However, age at trauma, gender, and marital and socioeconomic status did not predict posttorture psychological functioning.

Among the diagnostic categories assessed by using the Structured Clinical Interview for DSM-III-R (SCID), the most common psychiatric condition was PTSD. Overall, no evidence of a syndrome different from PTSD was found (Basoglu, 1992b). The most common symptoms were (in descending order of frequency) as follows:

- Memory and concentration impairment
- Nightmares
- Distress in response to reminders of trauma
- Recollections of trauma
- Startle reactions
- Psychogenic amnesia
- Reexperiencing of the trauma
- Sleep disturbance
- Irritability
- Avoidance of reminders of trauma
- Physiological arousal
- Restricted expectations for the future
- Detachment from others
- Hypervigilance
- Restricted affect
- Diminished interest in activities
- Avoidance of trauma thoughts

A principal-components analysis of all anxiety and depression measures and PTSD symptom ratings yielded seven components: (a) depression and anxiety, (b) social withdrawal and estrangement, (c) autonomic reactivity and avoidance of trauma stimuli, (d) problems of impulse control, (e) reexperiencing phenomena, (f) emotional numbing and amnesia, and (g) nightmares or memory and concentration impairment (bipolar). PTSD and depression, which are often overlapping features in trauma survivors, were independent in this study group, a finding that supported the validity of PTSD as a diagnostic entity in the study group.

Although the study clearly demonstrated the effects of torture, considering the severity of torture endured by the survivors (a mean of 291 exposures to a mean of 23 different forms of torture), the prevalence of PTSD and major depressive illness was lower than expected. In an attempt to explain this finding, the investigators pointed to the possible protective role of a strong belief system, commitment to a cause, prior knowledge and expectations of torture, and possible prior immunization to traumatic stress (Basoglu, Paker, Paker, Ozmen, & Sahin, 1994). The majority of the survivors were highly committed political activists who reported prior expectations of and psychological preparedness for torture. Many survivors also reported having used elaborate coping strategies during torture, a factor that has been hypothesized to play a role in the development of traumatic stress symptoms (Basoglu & Mineka, 1992).

Of all the measures of torture severity, only perceived distress during torture related to PTSD (Basoglu & Paker, 1995). Frequency of torture did not predict posttraumatic stress responses, suggesting that for some individuals, once torture reaches a certain individual "threshold," repeated torture does not have an additional effect. A differential relationship was found between stressors and symptoms: Perceived severity of torture predicted PTSD, but not depression, whereas postcaptivity lack of social support related to depression, but not to PTSD. Postcaptivity nontorture stressors, however, related to both PTSD and anxiety and depression. These findings suggest that both torture and posttorture psychosocial stressors are associated with traumatic stress symptoms in torture survivors.

The study also examined some of the cognitive factors that may have protected the survivors against the traumatic effects of torture (Basoglu et al., 1996). The three groups were compared in their appraisal of self, others, and state authority. There were no remarkable differences between tortured and nontortured political activists, and both groups differed from nonactivist controls in having a more negative appraisal of state authority. The study concluded that a pretrauma lack of belief in a "benevolent state" may be important in predicting posttorture reactions.

The earlier study by Basoglu, Paker, Paker, Ozmen, Marks, et al. (1994), while pointing to the possible protective role of "psychological preparedness for trauma," could not test this hypothesis because of insufficient variability in the sample; most of the study participants were highly committed political activists. A later study (Basoglu et al., 1997) was carried out to compare the previous sample of 55 tortured political activists with 34 torture survivors who had no history of political activity, commitment to a political cause, or expectations of arrest and torture and thus were presumed to be less "psychologically prepared." Compared with the political activists, the nonactivists were subjected to relatively less severe torture but had significantly more current PTSD (58% vs. 18%) and current major depression (24% vs. 4%) and higher levels of psychopathology on most clinical measures. Of all the predictor variables examined, less psychological preparation for trauma was the strongest predictor of greater perceived distress during torture and more severe psychological problems. These findings support the role of a possible "immunization" effect created by psychological preparation that may reduce the effects of traumatic stress. The study also showed that unpredictability and uncontrollability of stressors appeared to exacerbate the effect of torture. Higher education was also a significant predictor of better psychological health.

In a 1997 study of 61 torture survivors in Turkey (Basoglu, Aker, Kaptanoglu, Livanou, & Erol, n.d.), which included both political activists and nonactivists, the lifetime prevalence of PTSD was substantially higher (63%) than that found in the 1994 study. The authors observed that the higher rate may have been caused by the inclusion of nonactivists in the sample. To examine the cognitive and behavioral components of psychological preparedness for trauma, this study attempted to operationalize some of the cognitive constructs (e.g., beliefs about a just world, personal safety, and trust in others) that are thought to play a role in posttraumatic stress responses (Foa, Zinbarg, & Rothbaum, 1992; Janoff-Bulman, 1992) and examine their relationship with PTSD in survivors of torture. Preliminary results from this study suggested that loss of faith and trust in others was a mediating variable in traumatization. Survivors who had stronger feelings of injustice arising from the impunity enjoyed by the perpetrators of human rights violations had more severe psychological problems. On closer examination, both loss of control and fear of further persecution were critical to the survivor's reaction to the impunity of perpetrators.

Another recent study (Maercker & Schutzwohl, 1997) investigated the long-term effects of political imprisonment in the former German Democratic Republic and compared 146 former political prisoners with 75 controls matched for age and sex. Psychological status was assessed using a semistructured diagnostic interview based on DSM-III-R. In comparison with controls, the former political prisoners had significantly higher rates of lifetime (59.6%) and current (30.1%) PTSD, claustrophobia, social phobia, and substance abuse, as well as higher scores on measures of anxiety, depression, general psychopathology, and dissociative symptoms. The prevalence of PTSD in this sample was thus higher than that found in the Basoglu, Paker, Paker, Ozmen, Marks, et al. (1994) study. Maercker and Schutzwohl (1997) also suggested that this difference might be explained by the fact that their sample included both political activists and nonactivists, whereas the sample in the Basoglu, Paker, Paker, Ozmen, Marks, et al. (1994) study consisted mainly of political activists. Analysis of data from this later study showed a similar high rate of lifetime PTSD (63%) when the activist and nonactivist groups were combined.

A recent controlled study (Shrestha et al., 1998) of 526 Bhutanese refugee survivors of torture in Nepal matched on age and sex with 526 nontortured refugees is the largest study of tortured refugees that has used matched controls to date. Participants in the study group were randomly selected from among the Bhutanese refugee community in the United Nations refugee camps in the Terai in eastern Nepal. The DSM-III-R criteria for PTSD and the Hopkins Symptom Checklist were used as the main outcome measures. Compared with the control group, the torture survivors had more PTSD symptoms, higher anxiety and depression scores, and more musculoskeletal and respiratory system complaints. The authors concluded that torture may increase the risk for mental health problems among refugees displaced within the developing world and that PTSD symptoms appear to be part of a universal reaction to torture. They also pointed to the need for an increase in services for tortured refugees.

A study in the United States of 62 Vietnamese expolitical detainees and 22 controls (Mollica et al., 1998) included participants who had registered for social services with the Vietnamese Civic Association on arriving in the Boston area from abroad. The control group of 22 males from the Vietnamese community had spent less than 1 year in a Vietnamese prison or reeducation camp and were not from the expolitical detainee resettlement program. Although the study did not use matched controls, between-group differences in psychological status were examined by using regression analyses that controlled for differences in sample characteristics. Compared with the controls, the expolitical detainees showed significantly higher scores on depression and PTSD symptoms, but the difference in the prevalence rates of PTSD (77.3% vs. 88.2%, respectively) and major depression (36.4% vs. 56.9%, respectively) between the two groups did not reach statistical significance. A series of linear regression analyses using various sample characteristics and a measure of cumulative trauma severity (number of torture events reported) showed that severity of torture was the most significant predictor of depression and PTSD symptoms (particularly of arousal symptoms). The authors suggested that a small sample size may have accounted for the lack of statistically significant differences in the prevalence of psychiatric diagnoses. The fact that some of the control subjects had prior incarceration (mean 0.1 year) and torture experiences (mean 3.1 torture events) may also have minimized the between-group differences in posttrauma psychological status.

A controlled study (Holtz, 1998) that was carried out in India involved 35 tortured refugee Tibetan nuns and lay students and 35 nontortured refugee nuns and students matched for sex, age, lay status, and years in exile. In addition to ratings of anxiety and depression, the study used measures of preexile, flight, and postexile stressors; pretrauma and posttrauma political commitment; prior knowledge of and preparedness for torture; and social support in exile. Unfortunately, PTSD was not assessed because of a lack of agreement among the researchers on a culturally valid translation of PTSD criteria. Relative to the controls, the torture survivors had significantly higher scores on measures of anxiety, but the two groups did not differ on ratings of depression. However, a lack of prior knowledge of and psychological preparedness for torture was found to be a significant predictor of posttorture anxiety symptoms. Other predictors included male sex, longer duration of torture, exposure to solitary confinement, feelings of hopelessness in prison, and recent arrival in India. The author suggested that the survivors' Tibetan Buddhist training as nuns may have contributed to their preparedness for or resilience to the traumatic effect of torture.

EVIDENCE FOR A TORTURE-SPECIFIC SYNDROME

The claims for evidence for a "torture syndrome" were based on two earlier studies (Abildgaard et al., 1984; Allodi & Cowgill, 1982). A study of 22 Greek torture survivors (Abildgaard et al., 1984) distinguished four groups of symptoms that appeared to constitute a chronic organic psychosyndrome (COP): (a) impaired memory and concentration; (b) sleep disturbance and nightmares; (c) psycholability, anxiety, and depression; and (d) vegetative symptoms, including gastrointestinal symptoms, cardiopulmonary symptoms, and sudden attacks of sweating without demonstrable organic cause. Eight survivors who had three or more of these symptoms were diagnosed as having COP. This study had several weaknesses: (a) a retrospective and uncontrolled design, (b) a fairly small sample size, (c) a failure to rule out the possible effects of head trauma, and (d) a failure to validate the three-symptom criterion. The syndrome was not related to age, sex, neurological signs, frequency of head trauma, or history of loss of consciousness during torture or following head trauma. On the other hand, it was related to longer duration of torture, suggesting that COP might have reflected greater severity of illness caused by more severe trauma. Also, the symptoms did not appear to be different from PTSD.

The other study (Allodi & Cowgill, 1982) involved 41 survivors who had been tortured a few months to 6 years before the assessment. The symptoms reported in this study were no different from those of other studies reviewed earlier. The study was also uncontrolled and involved only asylum-seekers. In addition, it was not clear how the symptoms related to PTSD criteria.

None of the other studies reviewed here examined whether the symptoms of torture survivors cluster in a coherent fashion so as to constitute a syndrome. Indeed, these studies appear to have merely listed the symptoms observed in torture survivors (Turner & Gorst-Unsworth, 1993). Evidence for a torture-specific syndrome would require (a) evidence of a causal connection between the torture and subsequent symptoms; (b) a meaningful grouping of symptoms, validated across samples and cultures; and (c) a comparison of symptoms with established diagnoses such as PTSD (Basoglu, 1997). Recent studies (Basoglu, Paker, Paker, Ozmen, Marks, et al., 1994; Maercker & Schutzwohl, 1997; Mollica et al., 1998; Shrestha et al., 1998) that addressed some of these requirements have not provided evidence for a torture syndrome different from PTSD.

SOCIAL AND ECONOMIC CONSEQUENCES OF TORTURE

Relatively little is known about the social and economic consequences of torture. After release, torture survivors may stay in their own country, escape to a nearby refugee camp, or travel to interim resettlement countries before final resettlement. Some do all of these in succession, although most survivors stay in their native countries where they were tortured (Somnier et al., 1992). The social and economic costs of torture are, therefore, important issues for the countries where torture systematically occurs, as well as for host countries that provide asylum to large numbers of tortured refugees.

Several factors may account for the social and economic consequences of torture and associated life events. Loss of social or occupational status or educational opportunities as a result of prolonged imprisonment, as well as problems in finding employment after release, may contribute to social and economic difficulties. These problems may also be compounded by the physical and psychological effects of torture. Physical disability may arise from permanent bodily injury (Skylv, 1992) or head trauma leading to cognitive impairment. Psychological problems, including PTSD and depression, may cause significant social disability and undermine the chances of finding employment. Irritability and rage reactions may impair interpersonal relationships. Marital and family problems may occur because of the inability to feel intimacy or to reestablish trust. Memory and concentration difficulties may reduce the capacity for learning and impair work performance. Symptoms of impulsivity and irritability may lead to problems with the law.

Several lines of evidence suggest that a particular symptom of PTSD, that is, avoidance of trauma reminders, warrants special attention in understanding the causes of social and economic disability in torture survivors. Although the avoided situations or activities can be infinitely varied depending on the extent of stimulus generalization, they often included crowded places; police or army officers; social or political meetings; street demonstrations; police or army cars on the street; authority figures; people who share certain physical characteristics (e.g., facial features, moustache) with the torturers; television (e.g., news of violence); newspapers; public transportation; hospitals; medical examinations or investigations; close spaces; close physical contact with others; and activities such as walking on the street, being alone at home, sleeping in the dark, and sleeping alone (Basoglu & Aker, 1996; Basoglu, Paker, Paker, Ozmen, Marks, et al., 1994). General anxiety disorders research has shown that behavioral avoidance of feared situations is the primary cause of disability in work, social, and family functioning (Basoglu, Lax, Kasvikis, & Marks, 1988; Basoglu, Marks, Swinson, et al., 1994). Similarly, global clinical improvement is most closely associated with improvement in behavioral avoidance of feared situations (Basoglu, Marks, Kilic, Noshirvani, & O'Sullivan, 1994). In a recent study of a mixed group of trauma survivors (Marks et al., 1998), avoidance of trauma reminders was one of the most significant predictors of social disability and severity of illness (Livanou, 1998). No comparable studies are yet available with torture survivors, but some preliminary evidence suggests that this symptom is also an important determinant of social disability in torture survivors. In one of the studies reviewed above (Basoglu, Paker, Paker, Ozmen, Marks, et al., 1994), 33% of tortured political activists had significant avoidance of trauma reminders, despite their observed resilience to torture. The avoidance symptom occurred more often (53%) among nonactivist survivors of torture (Basoglu et al.,

1997). Furthermore, some case studies (Basoglu & Aker, 1996; Basoglu, 1998) suggest that interventions aimed at reducing avoidance behavior lead to a significant improvement in social disability. Further investigation of this symptom, therefore, is warranted in future studies of the social and economic consequences of torture.

Other commonly observed psychological problems in torture survivors need to be taken into account in estimating economic costs of torture, especially the tendency to develop somatic symptoms and preoccupation with bodily complaints (Basoglu, 1992b; Mollica et al., 1987; Somnier et al., 1992). Somatization is said to be more common in certain nonwestern cultures (Kleinman & Good, 1985), and it is unclear whether torture has a unique effect on this tendency. Torture survivors with somatic symptoms often seek costly medical examinations and treatments that may not be necessary. Currently, there are no estimates of the degree of medical services sought by torture survivors, whether in their country of origin or in a host country. An investigation of this issue appears worthwhile.

There have been relatively few systematic studies of the effects of torture on the survivor's family. This issue deserves special attention in light of the findings from a recent study (Basoglu, Paker, Paker, Ozmen, & Sahin, 1994) that showed that the presence of additional family stressors was a more significant predictor of PTSD than the actual trauma of torture itself. These stressors included events such as persecution or torture of family members as a result of the survivor's political involvement, loss of contact with the family because of long-term captivity or geographic distance, and breakdown in marital relationships as a result of prolonged imprisonment or later psychological problems.

A number of other factors associated with the torture survivor's experience have been shown to affect family functioning. Psychological problems may arise in the children of torture survivors as a result of witnessing the torture of parents, parental absence, or posttraumatic behavioral problems in parents. Common problems in survivors' children include anxiety, hypersensitivity to noise, insomnia, and nightmares (Cohn, Holzer, Koch, & Severin, 1980); withdrawal, depression, irritability, aggressiveness, generalized fear, excessive clinging, and dependence on parents (Acuna, 1989); and psychosomatic problems and deterioration in school performance (Weile, Wingender, Bach-Mortensen, & Busch, 1990). In addition, posttorture behavioral problems of the torture survivor, such as introversion, withdrawal, isolation, excessive stubbornness, and authoritarian attitudes aimed at regaining status and control in the family (Comite de Defensa de los Derechos del Pueblo, 1989), may cause further maladjustment in the family. Furthermore, the survivor's family may come under further strain by additional stressors, such as unemployment, poverty, and various social stigmas (e.g., being labeled terrorists) when the torture experience is linked to involvement in dissident political activity (Daly, 1980).

Flight into exile, asylum-seeking, and settlement in a new country are additional events that aggravate the social and economic consequences of political persecution and torture. Separation from family, loss of social and occupational status, deprivation of social support networks and physical needs, uncertainty about the future, problems settling in a new country and adapting to a new culture, and housing and economic problems are among the many issues faced by refugee survivors of torture (van Willigen, 1992; Witterholt & Jaranson, 1998). In addition, racism and antiimmigrant bias may be part of the survivor's resettlement experience in much of the western world (Baker, 1992), even for those who have already been granted permanent residency in a host country. Those who have escaped to a host country without proper documents may face the risk of being summarily deported back to their home country or placed in detention. A more detailed review of the social and economic consequences of refugee trauma can be found in chapter 7 in this volume.

DISCUSSION AND CONCLUSIONS

Evidence on the Psychological Effects of Torture

In this chapter we have attempted a rather stringent review of the evidence on the independent psychological effects of torture because trauma research in general is often plagued by confounding factors. These factors, such as length of time since the trauma, other stressful life events, previous psychiatric history, individual variables, and concomitant depression, make demonstrating a stressor–response relationship difficult. Reliable conclusions require controlled comparisons between torture survivors and nontortured individuals with careful matching on relevant variables and statistical techniques to control for the effects of confounding variables. The reliability of conclusions is not merely a scientific concern; valid and reliable information is a critical element of effective human rights activity against torture.

The findings from both uncontrolled and controlled studies indicate there is substantial evidence that in some individuals torture has psychological effects independent of other associated stressors. Recent studies (Basoglu, Paker, Paker, Ozmen, Marks, et al., 1994; Maercker & Schutzwohl, 1997; Mollica et al., 1998; Shrestha et al., 1998) using standardized measures and controls supported the results of earlier investigations. In the study by Basoglu, Paker, Paker, Ozmen, Marks, et al. (1994), the effects of torture could be demonstrated despite a potential referral bias (i.e., highly resilient and less severely traumatized political activists coming forward to take part in the study). Indeed, more representative samples of torture survivors might show higher levels of traumatization, as suggested by findings of higher rates of PTSD in subsequent studies also involving nonactivist torture survivors (Basoglu et al., 1997, n.d.).

Given the possible confounding factors, can the findings in the Basoglu et al. (1997) study be attributed to torture per se? Confounding variables such as previous psychiatric history, concomitant anxiety, depression, drug or alcohol abuse, and nontorture stressors were either balanced across groups or very uncommon among the torture survivors. Major depression, for example, which often overlaps with PTSD and confounds the clinical picture, was quite rare in the study group.

Furthermore, personality factors that often obscure the stressor–response relationship were somewhat different in this study because the study involved political activists, who seem to share some common experiences or personal characteristics that may be protective in torture situations. The PTSD symptoms observed in such individuals, therefore, may be more likely to reflect the specific effects of torture. Finally, certain PTSD symptoms such as nightmares, intrusive thoughts, reexperiencing phenomena, and avoidance of trauma-related cues were clearly related to the torture experience.

Torture in the Context of Refugee Trauma: Implications of Current Knowledge for Refugee Care

The relative importance of torture and trauma within the full context of the refugee experience is a focus of ongoing debate among mental health professionals working with refugees. Some workers emphasize the trauma of torture, whereas others regard torture as one of the many traumatic events experienced by refugees (van Willigen, 1992). Although there are no direct comparisons of refugee and nonrefugee torture survivors yet, there is some indirect information that may shed light on this issue.

The rates of psychological problems reported in studies of refugee survivors of torture (Somnier et al., 1992) appear to be higher than those found in studies of nonrefugee torture survivors. This effect may be a result of further traumatization by additional stressors involved in the refugee experience. This observation is supported by at least two lines of evidence concerning the mechanisms of traumatization in torture survivors. First, in the Basoglu, Paker, Paker, Ozmen, and Sahin (1994) study, posttorture psychosocial stressors contributed independently to traumatic stress reactions, which supports the notion of "sequential" traumatization. Second, postcaptivity lack of social support predicted depression. These findings suggest that additional stressors such as refugee trauma, which involve deprivation of social support networks, may contribute to traumatic stress responses.

There may, however, be different psychological problems associated with torture and other forms of refugee trauma. This theory is supported by the fact that perceived severity of torture appears to be related to PTSD, but not to depression. However, lack of posttorture psychosocial support was associated with depression, but not with PTSD. The connection between torture and "core" PTSD symptoms such as reexperiencing phenomena, heightened physiological arousal, and avoidance of reminders of trauma may reflect the conditioning effects of torture. Conversely, lack of social support may lead to depression by reducing the sense of control over subsequent stressors and precipitating helplessness and hopelessness (Basoglu & Mineka, 1992). This observation is supported by findings from another study (Mollica et al., 1998) involving Vietnamese refugees in the United States that showed that the severity of torture related to both PTSD and depression, whereas length of residence in a host country (United States) was associated only with depression.

These findings suggest that both torture and trauma associated with the refugee experience are important issues in refugee care. However, further research is required to clarify the unique role that each may play, as well as their interaction. Comparisons between studies may not be entirely valid given the methodological and sampling differences between studies of refugee and nonrefugee survivors of torture. For example, the Basoglu et al. (n.d.) study found that the prevalence of lifetime PTSD was higher (63%) for nonrefugee survivors of torture involving political activists and nonactivists compared with a previous study involving mainly political activists (33%) (Basoglu, Paker, Paker, Ozmen, & Sahin, 1994). Additionally, "psychological preparedness for trauma" (as appropriately defined and operationalized for particular samples) appears to be one of several important factors to be addressed in any comparison between different samples of torture survivors.

The finding that torture and subsequent psychosocial stressors such as refugee trauma may have differential psychological effects has important implications for treatment. For example, rehabilitation programs with a focus on providing social support for refugees may be helpful in preventing or alleviating depression but may not be effective in reducing disabling PTSD symptoms. Indeed, more than 80% of the nonrefugee torture survivors studied by Basoglu, Paker, Paker, Ozmen, & Sahin (1994) had strong social and psychological support from their community; nevertheless, many of them had chronic PTSD symptoms. Rehabilitation programs may therefore need to be complemented with specific psychological interventions that are known to be effective in reducing PTSD symptoms, especially because the nature and extent of PTSD symptoms may make it difficult for the survivor to access and use social support (Keane, Albano, & Blake, 1992).

Factors Related to Long-Term Psychological Status in Torture Survivors

Relatively little is known about the factors that determine psychological response to torture, and few attempts have been made to investigate this issue in a systematic fashion in studies of nonrefugee survivors of torture. Furthermore, prediction studies require the use of special statistical techniques (e.g., multiple regression analysis) to examine the unique or independent effects of predictor variables, and few studies have employed such methods of analysis. Recent controlled studies of nonrefugee survivors of torture (Basoglu et al., 1997; Basoglu & Paker, 1995; Basoglu, Paker, Paker, Ozmen, & Sahin, 1994) identified subjective severity of torture, posttorture psychosocial stressors, family history of psychiatric illness, postcaptivity social support, "psychological preparedness for trauma," and education as predictors of long-term psychological status. Current age, gender, age at trauma, socioeconomic status, marital status, and frequency of torture were not significant predictors of long-term psychological functioning. These findings, however, need to be replicated in other groups of torture survivors in different cultures and in refugee torture survivors.

Among all the predictor variables examined in the above studies, "psychological preparedness for trauma" as a protective factor appears to be the most significant predictor of posttrauma psychological status. This finding has been replicated by a recent study by Holtz (1998). Holtz's findings point to the importance of the study of resilience and other protective factors in torture survivors as well as in survivors of other types of trauma. The mechanisms by which "psychological preparedness for trauma" serves as a protective factor against traumatic stress are yet unclear. In the Basoglu et al. (1997) study, this measure was used to assess pretrauma political activity, commitment to a political cause, and expectation of arrest and torture. Thus, the critical ingredients in psychological preparedness may be (a) cognitive processes, such as a strong belief system (political, religious, or other), the ability to give a meaning to the traumatic experience, or predictability or controllability of traumatic stressors; (b) behavioral processes, such as prior immunization to traumatic stressors during political activity; or (c) a combination of both cognitive and behavioral processes. Future research needs to operationalize these processes and examine their relative contributions to protective factors and resilience against traumatic stress.

It is critical to note that the concept of "psychological preparedness" for trauma as a protective factor against traumatic stress should not be seen as implying a weakness, failure, or personality deficit in torture survivors who develop psychological problems as a result of torture. "Psychological preparedness," as defined in the Basoglu, Paker, Paker, Ozmen, Marks, et al. (1994) study, is a new concept defined as a measure of resilience relating to a specific stressor situation (i.e., torture), and not as a measure of a general personality trait (Basoglu et al., 1997). Nor does it imply complete immunity against the traumatic effects of torture; many highly trained or "prepared" individual torture survivors develop core PTSD symptoms, such as reexperiencing and avoiding trauma reminders (Basoglu, Paker, Paker, Ozmen, Marks, et al., 1994). Furthermore, trauma researchers agree that personality factors play a greater role in PTSD at relatively lower levels of trauma intensity, and their effect is minimized as stressor intensity increases beyond a certain threshold.

Some recent evidence (Basoglu et al., 1997, n.d.; Holtz, 1998) suggests that certain situational variables, such as loss of control during torture, are related to greater perceived distress and subsequent posttraumatic stress responses. Individuals with less psychological preparedness for torture are less likely to have developed coping strategies to use during the torture experience (e.g., in using strategies to avoid severe torture or lessen the pain or distress involved) and thus may experience greater distress during torture and develop posttraumatic stress symptoms. In addition, certain forms of torture that involve greater loss of control and unpredictability (e.g., asphyxiation, restriction of body movements during torture, sham executions, helplessness in the face of extreme humiliation) are associated with greater perceived distress. This observation is consistent with evidence from animal work showing that uncontrollable and unpredictable stressors play an important role in the development of anxiety and fear responses (Basoglu & Mineka, 1992). These findings not only shed some light on the mechanisms of traumatization in torture survivors, but may also have implications for effective treatment. If loss of control is a critical factor in developing traumatic stress symptoms, then effective treatment would need to involve strategies that focus on helping the torture survivor regain a sense of control. Future research on this issue should include controlled clinical trials to test the efficacy of treatments with a focus on sense of control.

Impunity for Perpetrators and Posttraumatic Stress Responses

A commonly held view among mental health professionals working with survivors of human rights abuses is that impunity for perpetrators contributes to social and psychological problems and impedes healing processes in survivors (Carmichael & McKay, 1996; Flores, 1991; Gordon, 1994; Lagos, 1994; Lagos & Kordon, 1996; Neumann & Monasterio, 1991; Nicoletti, 1991; Roht-Arriaza, 1995). Impunity for torturers is said to lead to an erosion of moral codes; an implied acceptance of violent behavior in the community; feelings of fear, helplessness, and insecurity in society; and "social alienation" manifested by feelings of failure and skepticism, frustration, and addictive and violent behavior (Lagos, 1994). It has also been suggested that impunity impedes the bereavement process; induces self-blame and guilt; enhances reexperiencing of trauma; generates feelings of helplessness, isolation, or resentment toward the social environment; and generates survivor's guilt and other traumatic stress reactions such as nightmares, insomnia, depression, and somatization (Lagos, 1994).

This view is supported by cognitive theories of trauma, which maintain that PTSD is mediated by violation of previously held assumptions of invulnerability and personal safety (Foa, Steketee, & Rothbaum, 1989; Janoff-Bulman, 1992), inability to find an acceptable explanation for the trauma (Lifton & Olson, 1976), and violation of beliefs that the world is a just and orderly place (Lerner & Miller, 1978). There is also some evidence from a study of torture survivors (Basoglu et al., 1996) to suggest that lack of belief in a "just" or "benevolent" state may serve as a protective factor against posttorture stress responses. No systematic studies have been conducted, however, to examine how survivors of torture appraise the sociopolitical process of impunity for perpetrators and how such cognitive processes relate to posttraumatic stress responses. Similarly, little is known about how sociopolitical action that aims to bring perpetrators to justice and provide compensation or redress for the atrocities that were committed affects the healing processes in torture survivors.

Some preliminary evidence from a pilot study of 61 torture survivors in Turkey (Basoglu et al., n.d.) indicates that appraisal of sociopolitical processes and associated emotions, particularly a sense of injustice arising from the impunity enjoyed by torturers, are related to posttraumatic stress responses and depression. This study has identified three distinct groups of torture survivors in terms of their cognitive and emotional response to impunity for torturers: (a) those who respond with anger or distress and feelings of vengeance; (b) those who respond with anger or distress but no feelings of vengeance; and (c) those who respond with demoralization, despair, and depression. Emotional response characterized by desire for vengeance (Group 1) was associated with lower socioeducational status and "less psychological preparedness for trauma." The survivors in Group 2 and Group 3 were highly psychologically prepared political activists and, compared with the survivors in Group

1, had more education; fewer feelings of vengeance; less endorsement of "an-eye-for-an-eye, a-tooth-for-a-tooth" type of punishment for torturers; a more structured and sophisticated cognitive schema in relation to sociopolitical processes; stronger political beliefs; and a greater ability to give meaning to the torture experience. Group 3 differed from Group 2 in having less faith and trust in others and more traumatic stress responses. Multiple regression analysis identified loss of trust and faith in others as the possible mediating variable related to traumatic stress responses.

These results suggest that cognitive and emotional responses to sociopolitical processes are quite varied in torture survivors, and generalizations may not be justified. Future research on this issue needs to explore such responses in other cultures and sociopolitical environments, individual factors related to these responses, and how appraisal of sociopolitical events relates to posttraumatic stress reactions. Also important as a research objective, particularly for countries such as South Africa where a "truth and reconciliation" process took place, is to investigate whether and how compensation and redress (monetary or otherwise) for survivors of human rights abuses affect the psychological functioning of survivors. Such research may shed light on which forms of compensation and redress are most helpful in the process of recovery from trauma, both individually and collectively.

The role of sociopolitical factors in determining response to psychological treatment programs for survivors should also be a focus of future research. We do not yet know whether cognitive processes relating to impunity for torturers impede psychological treatment efforts. Indeed, relatively little is known about the role of cognitive factors in the treatment of PTSD (Keane et al., 1992). A recent controlled cognitive–behavioral treatment trial of PTSD (Livanou, 1998; Marks et al., 1998) in a mixed group of trauma survivors showed that (a) pretreatment beliefs about the trauma, self, and the world did not relate to treatment outcome; (b) improvement in PTSD symptoms preceded change in beliefs; and (c) behavioral treatment not involving cognitive interventions achieved as much improvement in PTSD as did cognitive therapy. These findings suggest that the role of certain cognitive factors in the treatment of PTSD may be more or less relevant to different groups of survivors or different types of trauma. It should also be remembered that many torture survivors never develop psychological problems, and many recover from the effects of trauma, either spontaneously or with treatment (Basoglu & Aker, 1996), despite a culture of complete impunity for torturers in their country. In conclusion, generalizations on this issue may be counterproductive, as an exclusive focus on sociopolitical factors in survivor care may impede the development of effective psychological treatments for survivors.

Research into Mental Health Effects of Torture and Refugee Trauma: An Alternative Approach

Most research on the mental health effects of torture and refugee trauma is based on a priori definitions of survivor populations (e.g., torture survivors, internally displaced people, asylum-seekers, refugees) and the assumption that the mental health problems observed in study subjects are caused by the trauma that defined the study group in the first place. Such a priori distinctions between trauma survivors may be helpful in political or advocacy work or in humanitarian and relief activities but may not have much value in formulating a conceptual model that would be useful in understanding the mental health effects of various stressors and possible ways of treating them.

A potentially useful research model developed by the authors would take multiple factors into account, including (a) the varied and overlapping nature of the traumatic stressors experienced by survivors of political violence, torture, and refugee trauma; (b) situational variables during the traumatic event, such as perceived severity of trauma, unpredictability and uncontrollability of stressors, and coping strategies; (c) the interactions between torture trauma, subsequent traumatic events in a politically repressive environment, and other stressful life events; (d) the differential relationships between stressors and psychological symptoms; and (e) the possible associations between sociopolitical and cultural factors, cognitive processes, and psychological symptoms.

This model would require careful operationalization and measurement of traumatic stressors, situational variables, cognitive factors (e.g., appraisal of sociopolitical events, culturally related beliefs about the trauma, and beliefs about self and the world), and traumatic stress symptoms to test hypotheses concerning mechanisms of traumatization. It would also use carefully matched controls. Hypothesis testing concerning the stressor–response relationship would be based on both between- and within-group analyses. This model would enable "mapping" of traumatic stress symptoms onto related stressors while controlling for other variables that may confound the stressor–response relationship. Multivariate statistical techniques, multiple regression analyses, or path analysis would be used to elucidate the complex relationships between demographic variables, personality characteristics, personal history variables, traumatic stressors, situational variables during the traumatic event, posttrauma psychosocial stressor social support, and psychological symptoms. This model would also use longitudinal research designs to examine the relationships between these variables.

Regarding refugee populations, future research based on this model needs to explore the possibly differential mental health effects of torture and refugee trauma and to examine how various traumatic stressors associated with these events interact in producing the symptoms commonly observed in tortured refugees. Of particular interest is whether the psychological effect of these stressors is additive or interactive. These issues could be best examined by controlled studies using a 2 x 2 design that would allow comparisons between tortured refugees, nontortured refugees, nonrefugee torture survivors, and nonrefugee controls with no torture experience.

Implications for Survivor Care Policies

The research evidence reviewed here may have important implications for legal, public health, and medical care policies concerning torture survivors. Some of these implications are briefly reviewed below.

Immigration and asylum policies and procedures should be informed by the knowledge that a substantial proportion of refugees seeking asylum may have had at least one experience of torture and that torture may lead to disabling psychological problems that may last decades or even a lifetime.

The traumatic effect of torture has been shown to be mediated by the subjective appraisal of its severity and perhaps less so by its nature, frequency, or duration (Basoglu & Paker, 1995). The definition and severity of torture are often important issues in legal cases involving asylum applications and compensation claims. Decisions are often influenced by the assumption that there is a relationship between the severity of the trauma and the ensuing psychological disability. Asylum applicants, for example, can make a stronger case if they can evidence the severity of their torture. Such an assumption can lead to problems in decisions concerning two groups of survivors: those who have experienced severe torture with minimal or no psychological problems and those who have developed severe traumatic stress as a result of less severe trauma. The former group of torture survivors may have difficulty evidencing past torture, while the latter may not be able to provide a convincing account for the severity of their psychological disability. Thus, the experiences of both of these groups may be misunderstood for different reasons. Subjective appraisal of the torture experience should, therefore, be given due consideration to avoid errors in assessing such cases.

Policies about refugee care benefit from information about the mental health effects of torture and refugee trauma. Attention to mental health issues may be as important as providing legal, social, and economic aid for refugees. As noted earlier, social support may not be sufficient for the recovery process unless it is complemented with effective psychological treatment. Furthermore, the therapeutic value of social support may be limited unless the person is psychologically able to process it. Greater consideration must be given to the need for mental health services for tortured refugees; mental health professionals need to play a more central role in the policymaking aspects of refugee care.

Given the estimates of the prevalence of torture in the world and the mental health hazard posed by its potential for chronic and disabling psychological consequences, psychological treatments with demonstrated efficacy are urgently needed. In view of the realities of mental health care delivery in troubled parts of the world where help is most needed, treatments are likely to be most appropriate if they are brief and cost-effective and if they integrate a variety of self-help and traditional healing models. Survivor care policies need to place greater emphasis on developing such treatments through systematic research and on training mental health workers in effective treatment techniques.

Considering the relationship between fear or avoidance of trauma reminders and social disability in torture survivors, treatment interventions with a demonstrated potential for reducing avoidance behavior may deserve increased attention in rehabilitating survivors. Exposure treatment as part of a behavioral program appears to be a promising approach in this regard (see chapter 16 in this volume). Indeed, 12 controlled studies (Boudewyns & Hyer, 1990, 1996; Brom, Kleber, & Defares, 1989; Cooper & Clum, 1989; Foa, Rothbaum, Riggs, & Murdock, 1991;

Keane, Fairbank, Caddell, & Zimering, 1989; Marks et al., 1998; Peniston, 1986; Resick, Jordan, Gierelli, Hutter, & Marhoefer-Dvorak, 1988; Resick & Schnicke, 1992; Tarrier et al., 1998; Vaughan et al., 1994) have demonstrated the efficacy of exposure-based treatments in PTSD related to a wide range of traumas. Some preliminary evidence indicates that such treatments are also effective in reducing fear and avoidance of trauma reminders and enhancing sense of control, thereby minimizing social disability in traumatized survivors of torture (Basoglu, 1992b, 1998; Basoglu & Aker, 1996). Although such treatments are promising, care should be taken both in the training and delivery of such treatments.

Finally, relatively little scientific interest has been expressed in the study of torture, its psychological effects, and their treatment, despite the prevalence of torture and the mental health hazard posed by the experience. Many of the available resources for survivor care are often used for social, legal, and economic aid and for various rehabilitation programs, the efficacy of which has not yet been demonstrated. Scientific research with due regard for ethical issues is possible and essential for effective survivor care and is important information for developing policies (Basoglu, 1993; Basoglu & Marks, 1988). Such scientific inquiry regarding torture survivors has important implications for human rights, theory, assessment, classification, treatment of traumatic stress responses, and legal issues concerning torture survivors. The effects of torture on the individual have interacting social, political, cultural, economic, medical, psychological, and biological dimensions. An integrated approach (Basoglu, 1993; Mollica, 1992) with due emphasis on all dimensions is needed for more effective preventive measures against torture and for more effective care of survivors.

Future Research Recommendations

In this discussion, we have highlighted some of the important current research issues and the directions for future research. To summarize, future research needs to focus on various important issues that include biological and neurological mechanisms of traumatization, factors related to long-term psychological functioning, and effective treatments for survivors of torture. Given the preliminary evidence on the importance of protective factors in trauma, further research is needed to elucidate the behavioral and cognitive components of such concepts. Such evidence also suggests that future research should focus on such protective factors, including resilience. A better understanding of resilience factors could be helpful in developing more effective treatment programs for torture survivors.

We also need a better understanding of how various stressors such as torture, uprooting, refugee trauma, and loss of social support relate to PTSD symptoms, anxiety, depression, and other psychological problems in survivors of torture. Controlled comparison studies involving refugee and nonrefugee torture survivors are needed to address this issue. Such studies may be best facilitated by multisite collaborative efforts. Collaborative studies may also help develop standardized and validated assessment instruments for refugee and nonrefugee torture survivors.

Systematic research is needed to understand how impunity for perpetrators and compensation or redress for the acts committed affect the psychological functioning of survivors of political violence and torture. Such research would be useful in clarifying the psychological effects of "truth and reconciliation" processes, such as in South Africa, on survivors as well as on the community. This research could also provide valuable insights into how such processes should be conducted to avoid further traumatization and promote the psychological well-being of survivors and their communities. The lessons learned could be useful for other countries where similar attempts are being considered.

Additional emphasis is needed on research in developing effective treatments for torture survivors. Controlled treatment trials with adequate follow-up are urgently needed to identify the most effective treatments and the mechanisms by which they exert their therapeutic effect. Pharmacological agents and psychological treatments with demonstrated efficacy in treating PTSD in survivors of other types of trauma need to be subjected to controlled trials to test their efficacy in both refugee and nonrefugee torture survivors. Of particular interest would be the study of combined drug–psychotherapy interventions in reducing traumatic stress reactions.

Outcome evaluation in rehabilitation work with torture survivors should also receive greater emphasis. Given the scarce resources available for the care of torture survivors, the efficacy of current rehabilitation models needs to be evaluated, and their therapeutic ingredients need to be clarified.

Within western countries that serve as resettlement countries, research priorities can focus on the prevalence of past torture experience among refugee populations, the prevalence and nature of medical and psychosocial problems among torture survivors, and the recovery process. Such studies could also be undertaken in countries of origin where the political circumstances are relatively favorable for this type of research.

REFERENCES

Abildgaard, U., Daugaard, G., Marcussen, H., Jess, P., Petersen, H. D., & Wallach, M. (1984). Chronic organic psycho-syndrome in Greek torture victims. *Danish Medical Bulletin, 31*, 239–241.

Acuna, J. E. (1989). *Children of the storm.* Quezon City, Philippines: Children's Rehabilitation Center.

Allodi, F., & Cowgill, G. (1982). Ethical and psychiatric aspects of torture: A Canadian study. *Canadian Journal of Psychiatry, 27*, 98–102.

American Psychiatric Association. (1987). *Diagnostic and statistical manual of mental disorders.* (3rd ed., rev.). Washington, DC: Author.

Amnesty International. (1999). *Amnesty International report.* London: Author.

Astrom, C. (1968). *Norwegian concentration camp survivors.* Oslo, Norway: Oslo University Press.

Astrom, C., Lunde, I., Ortmann, J., & Boysen, G. (1989). Sleep disturbances in torture survivors. *Acta Neurologia Scandinavica, 79*, 150–154.

Baker, R. (1992). Psychosocial consequences for tortured refugees seeking asylum and refugee status in Europe. In M. Basoglu (Ed.), *Torture and its consequences: Current treatment approaches* (pp. 83–106). Cambridge: Cambridge University Press.

Basoglu, M. (1992a). Introduction. In M. Basoglu (Ed.), *Torture and its consequences: Current treatment approaches* (pp. 1–8). Cambridge: Cambridge University Press.

Basoglu, M. (1992b). Behavioural and cognitive approach in the treatment of torture-related psychological problems. In M. Basoglu (Ed.), *Torture and its consequences: Current treatment approaches* (pp. 402–429). Cambridge: Cambridge University Press.

Basoglu, M. (1993). Prevention of torture and care of survivors: An integrated approach. *Journal of the American Medical Association, 270*(5), 606–611.

Basoglu, M. (1995). The impact of torture experience on psychological adjustment: Approaches to research. In Y. Kasvikis (Ed.), *25 years of scientific progress in behavioural and cognitive therapies* (pp. 174–190). Athens, Greece: Ellinika Grammata.

Basoglu, M. (1997). Torture as a stressful life event: A review of the current status of knowledge. In T. W. Miller (Ed.), *Clinical disorders and stressful life events* (pp. 45–70). Madison, CT: International Universities Press.

Basoglu, M. (1998). Behavioral and cognitive treatment of survivors of torture. In J. M. Jaranson & M. K. Popkin (Eds.), *Caring for victims of torture* (pp. 131–148). Washington, DC: American Psychiatric Press.

Basoglu, M., & Aker, T. (1996). Cognitive–behavioural treatment of torture survivors: A case study. *Torture, 6*(3), 61–65.

Basoglu, M., Aker, T., Kaptanoglu, C., Livanou, M., & Erol, A. (n.d.). *Cognitive and emotional responses to impunity for torturers and traumatic stress responses in survivors of torture.* Unpublished manuscript.

Basoglu, M., Lax, T., Kasvikis, Y. G., & Marks, I. M. (1988). Predictors of improvement in obsessive-compulsive disorder. *Journal of Anxiety Disorders, 2,* 229–317.

Basoglu, M., & Marks, I. M. (1988). Torture: Research needed into how to help those who have been tortured. *British Medical Journal, 297,* 1423–1424.

Basoglu, M., Marks, I. M., Kilic, C., Noshirvani, H., & O'Sullivan, G. (1994). The relationship between panic, anticipatory anxiety, agoraphobia, and global improvement in panic disorder with agoraphobia treated with alprazolam and exposure. *British Journal of Psychiatry, 164,* 647–652.

Basoglu, M., Marks, I. M., Swinson, R. P., Noshirvani, H., O'Sullivan, G., & Kuch, K. (1994). Pretreatment predictors of treatment outcome in panic disorder agoraphobia treated with alprazolam and exposure. *Journal of Affective Disorders, 30,* 123–132.

Basoglu, M., & Mineka, S. (1992). The role of uncontrollability and unpredictability of stress in the development of post-torture stress symptoms. In M. Basoglu (Ed.), *Torture and its consequences: Current treatment approaches* (pp. 182–225). Cambridge: Cambridge University Press.

Basoglu, M., Mineka, S., Paker, M., Aker, T., Livanou, M., & Gok, S. (1997). Psychological preparedness for trauma as a protective factor in survivors of torture. *Psychological Medicine, 27,* 1421–1433.

Basoglu, M., & Paker, M. (1995). Severity of trauma as predictor of long-term psychological status in survivors of torture. *Journal of Anxiety Disorders, 9*(4), 339–350.

Basoglu, M., Paker, M., Ozmen, E., Tasdemir, O., Sahin, D., Ceyhanli, A., Incesu, C., & Sarimurat, N. (1996). Appraisal of self, social environment, and state authority as a possible mediator of post-traumatic stress disorder in tortured political activists. *Journal of Abnormal Psychology, 105*(2), 232–236.

Basoglu, M., Paker, M., Paker, O., Ozmen, E., Marks, I. M., Incesu, C., Sahin, D., & Sarimurat, N. (1994). Psychological effects of torture: A comparison of tortured with nontortured political activists in Turkey. *American Journal of Psychiatry, 151,* 76–81.

Basoglu, M., Paker, M., Paker, O., Ozmen, E., & Sahin, D. (1994). Factors related to long-term traumatic stress responses in survivors of torture. *Journal of the American Medical Association, 272*(5), 357–363.

Bauer, M., Priebe, S., Haring, B., & Adamczak, K. (1993). Long-term mental sequelae of political imprisonment in East Germany. *Journal of Nervous and Mental Disease, 181,* 257–262.

Berger, P. (1980). Documentation of physical sequelae. *Danish Medical Bulletin, 27*, 215–217.

Boudewyns, P., & Hyer, L. A. (1990). Physiological response to combat memories and preliminary treatment outcome in Vietnam veteran PTSD patients treated with direct therapeutic exposure. *Behavior Therapy, 21*, 63–87.

Boudewyns, P., & Hyer, L. (1996). Eye movement desensitization and reprocessing (EMDR) as treatment for post-traumatic stress disorder. *Clinical Psychology and Psychotherapy, 3*(3), 185–195.

Brom, D., Kleber, R. J., & Defares, P. B. (1989). Brief psychotherapy for posttraumatic stress disorders. *Journal of Consulting and Clinical Psychology, 57*(5), 607–612.

Carmichael, K., & McKay, F. (1996). The need for redress: Why seek a remedy—Reparation as rehabilitation. *Torture, 6*, 7–9.

Cathcart, L. M., Berger, P., & Knazan, B. (1979). Medical examination of torture victims applying for refugee status. *Canadian Medical Association Journal, 121*, 179–184.

Cohn, J., Holzer, K., Koch, L., & Severin, B. (1980). Children and torture: An investigation of Chilean immigrant children in Denmark. *Danish Medical Bulletin, 27*, 238–239.

Comite de Defensa de los Derechos del Pueblo. (1989). The effects of torture and political repression in a sample of Chilean families. *Social Science and Medicine, 28*, 735–740.

Cooper, N. A., & Clum, G. (1989). Imaginal flooding as a supplementary treatment for PTSD in combat veterans: A controlled study. *Behavior Therapy, 20*, 381–391.

Cunningham, M., & Cunningham, J. D. (1997). Patterns of symptomatology and patterns of torture and trauma experiences in resettled refugees. *Australian and New Zealand Journal of Psychiatry, 31*, 555–565.

Daly, R. J. (1980). Compensation and rehabilitation of victims of torture: An example of preventive psychiatry. *Danish Medical Bulletin, 27*, 245–248.

Domovitch, E., Berger, P. B., Waver, M. J., Etlin, D. D., & Marshall, J. C. (1984). Human torture: Description and sequelae of 104 cases. *Canadian Journal of Family Physicians, 30*, 827–830.

Eitenger, L. (1961). Pathology of the concentration camp syndrome. *Archives of General Psychiatry, 5*, 371–379.

Flores, O. (1991, November). *Social disadjustments caused by impunity*. Paper presented at the 3rd International Conference on Health, Political Repression, and Human Rights, Santiago, Chile.

Foa, E. B., Rothbaum, B. O., Riggs, D. S., & Murdock, T. B. (1991). Treatment of posttraumatic stress disorder in rape victims: A comparison between cognitive-behavioral procedures and counseling. *Journal of Consulting and Clinical Psychology, 59*(5), 715–723.

Foa, E. B., Steketee, G., & Rothbaum, B. O. (1989). Behavioral/cognitive conceptualizations of post-traumatic stress disorder. *Behavior Therapy, 20*, 155–176.

Foa, E. B., Zinbarg, R., & Rothbaum, B. O. (1992). Uncontrollability and unpredictability in post-traumatic stress disorder: An animal model. *Psychological Bulletin, 112*, 218–238.

Foster, D. (1987). *Detention and torture in South Africa: Psychological, legal, and historical aspects*. Cape Town, South Africa: Phillip.

Goldfeld, A. E., Mollica, R. F., Pesavento, B. H., & Faraone, S. V. (1988). The physical and psychological sequelae of torture: Symptomatology and diagnosis. *Journal of the American Medical Association, 259*, 2725–2729.

Goldman, H. H., & Goldston, S. W. (1985). *Preventing stress-related psychiatric disorders*. Department of Health and Human Services Publication No. (ADM) 85-1366. Washington, DC: U.S. Government Printing Office.

Gordon, N. (1994). Compensation suits as an instrument in the rehabilitation of tortured persons. *Torture, 4*, 111–114.

Hermann, K., & Thygesen, P. (1954). KZ syndromet: Hungerdystrofiens folgetilstand 8 ar efter. *Ugeskrift for Laeger, 116*, 825–836.

Holtz, T. H. (1998). Refugee versus torture trauma: A retrospective controlled cohort study of Tibetan refugees. *Journal of Nervous and Mental Disease, 186*, 24–34.

Hougen, H. P., Kelstrup, J., Petersen, H. D., & Rasmussen, O. V. (1988). Sequelae to torture: A controlled study of torture victims living in exile. *Forensic Science International, 36*, 153–160.

Jadresic, D. (1990). Medical, psychological, and social aspects of torture: Prevention and treatment. *Medicine and War, 6*, 197–203.

Janoff-Bulman, R. (1992). *Shattered assumptions*. New York: Free Press.

Jensen, T. S., Genefke, I. K., Hyldebrandt, N., Pedersen, H., Petersen, H. D., & Weile, B. (1982). Cerebral atrophy in young torture victims. *New England Journal of Medicine, 307*(21), 1341.

Keane, T. M., Albano, A. M., & Blake, D. D. (1992). Current trends in the treatment of post-traumatic stress symptoms. In M. Basoglu (Ed.), *Torture and its consequences: Current treatment approaches* (pp. 363–401). Cambridge: Cambridge University Press.

Keane, T. M., Fairbank, J. A., Caddell, J. M., & Zimering, R. T. (1989). Implosive (flooding) therapy reduces symptoms of PTSD in Vietnam combat veterans. *Behavior Therapy, 20*, 245–260.

Kinzie, J. D., & Boehnlein, J. K. (1989). Post-traumatic psychosis among Cambodian refugees. *Journal of Traumatic Stress, 2*, 75–91.

Kinzie, J. D., Sack, W. H., Angell, R. H., & Manson, S. (1986). The psychiatric effects of massive trauma on Cambodian children: I. The children. *Journal of the American Academy of Child Psychiatry, 25*(3), 370–376.

Kjaersgaard, A. R., & Genefke, I. K. (1977). Victims of torture in Uruguay and Argentina: Case studies. In *Evidence of torture: Studies by the Amnesty International Danish Medical Group* (pp. 20–26). London: Amnesty International.

Kleinman, A., & Good, B. J. (1985). *Culture and depression: Study in the anthropology and cross-cultural psychiatry of affective disorder*. Berkeley: University of California Press.

Kordon, D., Edelman, L. I., Nicoletti, E., Lagos, D. M., Bozzolo, R. C., & Kandel, E. (1988). Torture in Argentina. In Group of Psychological Assistance to Mothers of "Plaza de Mayo" (Ed.), *Psychological effects of political repression* (pp. 95–107). Buenos Aires, Argentina: Sudamericana/Planeta.

Lagos, D. (1994). Argentina: Psycho-social and clinical consequences of political repression and impunity in the medium term. *Torture, 4*(1), 13–15.

Lagos, D., & Kordon, D. (1996). Psychological effects of political repression and impunity in Argentina. *Torture, 6*, 54–56.

Lerner, M. J., & Miller, D. (1978). Just world research and the attribution process: Looking back and ahead. *Psychological Bulletin, 85*, 1030–1051.

Lifton, J. R., & Olson, O. (1976). Human meaning of total disaster. *Psychiatry, 39*, 1–18.

Livanou, M. (1998). *Beliefs about self and the world as predictors of outcome in the treatment of post-traumatic stress disorder*. Unpublished doctoral dissertation, University of London, England.

Lok, V., Tunca, M., Kumanlioglu, K., Kapkin, E., & Dirik, G. (1991). Bone scintigraphy as clue to previous torture. *Lancet, 337*, 846–847.

Lunde, I. (1982). Mental sequelae of torture (Psykiske folger has torturofet). *Manedsskrift for Praktisk Laegegerning, 60*, 476–488.

Lunde, I., & Ortmann, J. (1990). Prevalence and sequelae of sexual torture. *Lancet, 336*, 289–291.

Lunde, I., Rasmussen, O. V., Lindholm, J., & Wagner, G. (1980). Gonadal and sexual functions in tortured Greek men. *Danish Medical Bulletin, 27*, 243–245.

Maercker, A., & Schutzwohl, M. (1997). Long-term effects of political imprisonment: A group comparison study. *Social Psychiatry and Psychiatric Epidemiology, 32*, 435–442.

Marks, I. M., Lovell, K., Noshirvani, H., Livanou, M., & Thrasher, S. (1998). Treatment of posttraumatic stress disorder by exposure and/or cognitive restructuring: A controlled study. *Archives of General Psychiatry, 55*(4), 317–325.

Mollica, R. F. (1992). The prevention of torture and the clinical care of survivors: A field in need of science. In M. Basoglu (Ed.), *Torture and its consequences: Current treatment approaches* (pp. 23–37). Cambridge: Cambridge University Press.

Mollica, R. F., Donelan, K., Tor, S., Lavalle, J., Elias, C., Frankel, M., & Blendon, R. J. (1993). The effect of trauma and confinement on functional health and mental health status of Cambodians living in Thailand–Cambodia border camps. *Journal of the American Medical Association, 270*, 581–586.

Mollica, R. F., McInnes, K., Pham, T., Smith-Fawzi, M. C., Murphy, E., & Lin, L. (1998). The dose–effect relationship between torture and psychiatric symptoms in Vietnamese expolitical detainees and a comparison group. *Journal of Nervous and Mental Disease, 186*(9), 543–553.

Mollica, R. F., Wyshak, G., & Lavelle, J. (1987). The psychosocial impact of war trauma and torture on Southeast Asian refugees. *American Journal of Psychiatry, 144*, 1567–1572.

Neumann, E., & Monasterio, H. (1991, November). *Impunity: A symbiotic element of terror.* Paper presented at the 3rd International Conference on Health, Political Repression and Human Rights, Santiago, Chile.

Nicoletti, E. (1991, November). *Impunity and social responsibility.* Paper presented at the 3rd International Conference on Health, Political Repression and Human Rights, Santiago, Chile.

Ortmann, J., & Lunde, I. (1988, August). *Changed identity, low self-esteem, depression, and anxiety in 148 torture victims treated at the RCT: Relation to sexual torture.* Paper presented at the World Health Organization workshop on the health situation of refugees and victims of organized violence, Gothenburg, Sweden.

Pagaduan-Lopez, J. C. (1987). *Torture survivors: What can we do for them?* Manila, Philippines: Medical Action Group.

Paker, M., Paker, O., & Yuksel, S. (1992). Psychological effects of torture: An empirical study of tortured and non-tortured non-political prisoners. In M. Basoglu (Ed.), *Torture and its consequences: Current treatment approaches* (pp. 72–82). Cambridge: Cambridge University Press.

Peniston, E. G. (1986). EMG biofeedback-assisted desensitization treatment for Vietnam combat veterans with post traumatic stress disorder. *Clinical Biofeedback and Health, 9*(1), 35–41.

Peters, E. (1985). *Torture.* Oxford, England: Blackwell.

Petersen, H. D., Abildgaard, U., Daugaard, G., Jess, P., Marcussen, H., & Wallach, M. (1985). Psychological and physical long-term effects of torture: A follow-up examination of 22 Greek persons exposed to torture 1967–1974. *Scandinavian Journal of Social Medicine, 13*, 89–93.

Petersen, H. D., & Jacobsen, P. (1985). Psychical and physical symptoms after torture: A prospective controlled study. *Forensic Science International, 29*, 179–189.

Rasmussen, O. V. (1990). Medical aspects of torture. *Danish Medical Bulletin, 37*, 1–88.

Rasmussen, O. V., Dam, A. M., & Nielsen, I. L. (1977). Torture: A study of Chilean and Greek victims. In *Evidence of torture: Studies by the Amnesty International Danish Medical Group* (pp. 9–19). London: Amnesty International.

Rasmussen, O. V., & Lunde, I. (1980). Evaluation of investigation of 200 torture victims. *Danish Medical Bulletin, 27*, 241–243.

Resick, P. A., Jordan, C. G., Girelli, S. A., Hutter, C. K., & Marhoefer-Dvorak, S. (1988). A comparative outcome study of a behavioral group therapy for sexual assault victims. *Behavior Therapy, 19*, 385–401.

Resick, P. A., & Schnicke, M. K. (1992). Cognitive processing therapy for sexual assault victims. *Journal of Consulting and Clinical Psychology, 60*(5), 748–756.

Roht-Arriaza, N. (1995). Punishment, redress, and pardon: Theoretical and psychological approaches. In N. Roht-Arriaza (Ed.), *Impunity and human rights in international law and practice* (pp. 13–23). Oxford, England: Oxford University Press.

Shrestha, N. M., Sharma, B., Van Ommermen, M., Regmi, S., Makaju, R., Komproe, I., Shresta, G. B., & de Jong, J. (1998). Impact of torture on refugees displaced within the developing world: Symptomatology among Bhutanese refugees in Nepal. *Journal of the American Medical Association, 280*(5), 443–448.

Silove, D., Sinnerbrink, I., Field, A., Manicavasagar, V., & Steel, Z. (1997). Anxiety, depression, and PTSD in asylum-seekers: Associations with pre-migration trauma and post-migration stressors. *British Journal of Psychiatry, 170*, 351–357.

Skylv, G. (1992). The physical sequelae of torture. In M. Basoglu (Ed.), *Torture and its consequences: Current treatment approaches* (pp. 38–55). Cambridge: Cambridge University Press.

Somnier, F. E., & Genefke, I. K. (1986). Psychotherapy for victims of torture. *British Journal of Psychiatry, 149*, 323–329.

Somnier, F. E., Jensen, T. S., Pedersen, H., Bruhn, P., Salinas, P., & Genefke, I. K. (1982). Cerebral atrophy in young torture victims. *Acta Neurologia Scandinavica, 65*, 321–322.

Somnier, F., Vesti, P., Kastrup, M., & Genefke, I. K. (1992). Psycho-social consequences of torture: Current knowledge and evidence. In M. Basoglu (Ed.), *Torture and its consequences: Current treatment approaches* (pp. 56–71). Cambridge: Cambridge University Press.

Tarrier, N., Pilgrim, H., Sommerfield, C., Faragher, B., Reynolds, M., & Graham, E. (1998). A randomised trial of cognitive therapy and imaginal exposure in the treatment of chronic post-traumatic stress disorder. *Journal of Consulting and Clinical Psychology, 67*(1), 13–18.

Thygesen, P., Hermann, K., & Willanger, R. (1970). Concentration camp survivors in Denmark: Persecution, disease, disability, compensation. *Danish Medical Bulletin, 17*, 65–108.

Turner, S. W., & Gorst-Unsworth, C. (1993). Psychological sequelae of torture. In J. Wilson & B. Raphael (Eds.), *International handbook of traumatic stress syndromes*. New York: Plenum Press.

United Nations. (1987). *United Nations convention against torture and other cruel, inhuman, or degrading treatment or punishment*. GA Res. 39/46,39 GAOR Supp. (No. 51) at 197, U.N. Doc. A/39/51, opened for signature February 4, 1985, entered into force, June 26, 1987.

van Willigen, L. H. M. (1992). Organisation of care and rehabilitation services for victims of torture and other forms of organised violence: A review of current issues. In M. Basoglu (Ed.), *Torture and its consequences: Current treatment approaches* (pp. 277–298). Cambridge: Cambridge University Press.

Vaughan, K., Armstrong, M. S., Gold, R., O'Connor, H., Jenneke, W., & Tarrier, N. (1994). A trial of eye movement desensitization compared to image habituation training and applied muscle relaxation in post-traumatic stress disorder. *Journal of Behaviour Therapy and Experimental Psychiatry, 25*(4), 283–291.

Venzlaff, U. (1964). Mental disorders resulting from social persecution outside concentration camps. *International Journal of Social Psychiatry, 10*, 177–183.

Wallach, M., & Rasmussen, O. V. (1983). An investigation in their own country of Chilean nationals submitted to torture (Tortur i Chile 1980–1982: En undersogelese of torturede chilenere i deres hjemland). *Ugeskrift for Laeger, 145*, 2349–2352.

Warmenhoven, C., van Slooten, H., Lachinsky, N., de Hoog, M. I., & Smeulers, J. (1981). Medische gevolgen van martelingen: Een onderzoek bij uluchtelingen in Nederland [Medical consequences of torture]. *Nederlands Tijdschrift voor Geneeskunde, 125*, 104–108.

Weile, B., Wingender, L. B., Bach-Mortensen, N., & Busch, P. (1990). Behavioral problems in children of torture victims: A sequel to cultural maladaptation or to parental torture? *Journal of Developmental and Behavioral Pediatrics, 11*, 79–80.

Witterholt, S., & Jaranson, J. (1998). Caring for victims on site: Bosnian refugees in Croatia. In J. Jaranson & M. Popkin (Eds.), *Caring for victims of torture* (pp. 243–252). Washington, DC: American Psychiatric Press.

II

Conceptual Models for Understanding Torture

4

Psychosocial Models

JOHN A. FAIRBANK, MATTHEW J. FRIEDMAN, and METIN BASOGLU

In this chapter we discuss a selected number of psychosocial conceptual models—learning theory, information processing, social–cognitive models, social support, developmental models, and learned helplessness—that purport to explain some aspects of the etiology, course, and treatment of the human response to traumatic experiences. These specific psychological models were selected for review because empirical information is available regarding their explanatory power for survivors of torture and related violence and trauma.

LEARNING THEORY: CLASSICAL AND INSTRUMENTAL CONDITIONING

Early behavioral conceptual models of traumatic stress reactions were based largely on the two-factor learning theory of psychopathology originally proposed by Mowrer (Fairbank & Keane, 1982; Keane, 1998; Keane, Zimering, & Caddell, 1985; Kilpatrick, Resick, & Veronen, 1981; Kilpatrick, Veronen, & Best, 1985). As applied to traumatic stress reactions, two-factor conditioning models posit that fear and other aversive emotions are learned through association via mechanisms of classical conditioning (Fairbank & Nicholson, 1987). Such fear conditioning is the first factor in the acquisition of aversive emotions characteristic of many persons

JOHN A. FAIRBANK • Department of Psychiatry, Duke University Medical Center, Durham, North Carolina 27710.   MATTHEW J. FRIEDMAN • Dartmouth University, and the National Center for Post-Traumatic Stress Disorder, White River Junction, Vermont 05009.   METIN BASOGLU • Section on Traumatic Studies, Institute of Psychiatry, King's College, London University SES 8AF London, England.

The Mental Health Consequences of Torture, edited by Ellen Gerrity, Terence M. Keane, and Farris Tuma. Kluwer Academic/Plenum Publishers, New York, 2001.

who have survived catastrophic events. The second factor involves principles of instrumental conditioning in that some persons will learn to escape from or avoid cues that stimulate aversive emotions (Keane, 1998).

Through the process of fear conditioning, neutral cues associated with a traumatic (or otherwise aversive) event acquire the capacity subsequently to evoke a conditioned emotional (fearful) response in the absence of the aversive stimulus. First described by Pavlov and associates, this psychological mechanism is posited to preserve information about exposure to previous threats to promote future survival. A line of research demonstrating the presence of fear conditioning among individuals with posttraumatic stress disorder (PTSD) involves laboratory paradigms in which persons with PTSD are exposed to auditory or visual stimuli pertaining to their traumatic event (Blanchard, Kolb, Pallmeyer, & Gerardi, 1982; Malloy, Fairbank, & Keane, 1983; Pitman, Orr, Forgue, De Jong, & Claiborn, 1987). Most people who have PTSD will exhibit sudden dramatic elevations of cardiovascular or other sympathetic nervous system activity immediately after exposure to such trauma-related stimuli in a laboratory setting (Blanchard, Kolb, & Prins, 1991; Malloy et al., 1983; Orr, Pitman, Lasko, & Herz, 1993).

More recent conceptual models have emphasized the central role of cognitive factors in the development and maintenance of stress-related symptoms and illnesses (Brewin, Dalgleish, & Joseph, 1996; Chemtob, Roitblatt, Hamada, Carlson, & Twentyman, 1988; Creamer, Burgess, & Pattison, 1992; Foa, Steketee, & Rothbaum, 1989; Lang, 1977; Litz & Keane, 1989; Resick & Schnicke, 1993).

COGNITIVE–BEHAVIORAL THEORIES: INFORMATION PROCESSING

Information processing theory has been proposed as an explanation of the ways in which information associated with traumatic experiences is encoded and recalled in memory (Foa & Kozak, 1986; Foa, Rothbaum, & Molnar, 1995; Foa et al., 1989). Foa et al. (1989), for example, have offered a model based on the concept of a fear structure that they describe as a "network in memory that includes three types of information: (a) information about the feared stimulus situation; (b) information about verbal, physiological, and overt behavioral responses; and (c) interpretive information about the meaning of the stimulus and the response elements of the structure" (p. 166). Foa et al. (1995) have proposed that treatment must be based on activation and correction of information in fear structures, accomplished through exposure to traumatic stimuli and cognitive restructuring, respectively. The information processing model has yielded a productive, theoretically grounded approach to basic laboratory studies and clinical efficacy research.

A widely replicated laboratory finding is that persons with PTSD selectively attend to and process trauma-relevant information (McNally, 1995). Experiments using Stroop Test paradigms have repeatedly shown that words closely related to trauma produce more cognitive interference than negative words less closely related to trauma (Kaspi, McNally, & Amir, 1995; Vrana, Roodman, & Beckham, 1995). In studies of Vietnam veterans, interference for trauma words has been found to be significantly related to severity of PTSD symptoms but not to level of exposure to combat, per se (Cassiday, McNally, & Zeitlin, 1992; McNally, Kaspi, Riemann, & Zeitlin, 1990). Additional studies have shown that people with PTSD show biases favoring trauma-related material in tasks designed to tap explicit memory (e.g., recall, recognition) as well as implicit memory (e.g., word-stem completion, lexical decision) (e.g., Vrana et al., 1995; Zeitlin & McNally, 1991).

Evidence in the animal literature also shows that predictable and controllable stressors generally have a less deleterious effect than do unpredictable and uncontrollable stressors (for a review, see Basoglu & Mineka, 1992; Mineka & Hendersen, 1985). Moreover, prior exposure to controllable stressors, perhaps leading to a sense of mastery, can immunize against the deleterious effects of subsequent exposure to uncontrollable stressors (e.g., Moye, Hyson, Grau, & Maier, 1983; Williams & Maier, 1977). A recent study (Basoglu & Mineka, 1997) found evidence in support of these hypotheses in survivors of torture. This study compared 55 tortured political activists who had greater "psychological preparedness for trauma" (i.e., prior exposure to similar stressors, greater extent of political involvement, stronger commitment to a political cause, and prior knowledge and expectations of torture) with 34 tortured nonactivists who had less psychological preparedness for trauma. Despite less severe torture, the nonactivist group reported greater perceived distress during torture and had more PTSD and more severe psychological symptoms than did the activist group.

SOCIAL–COGNITIVE MODELS

A number of authors (Horowitz, 1986; Janoff-Bulman, 1985; McCann & Pearlman, 1990; Roth & Newman, 1993) have proposed social–cognitive models that emphasize that traumatic experiences challenge people's preexisting core beliefs and assumptions about themselves and others, fostering negative emotions and maladaptive belief structures that produce and maintain the array of signs, symptoms, and disorders characteristic of stress-related illnesses. Although empirical studies of the social–cognitive model are still rare, some supporting research evidence has been reported. For example, Dalgleish (1993) examined maladaptive belief structures in survivors of a disaster involving the sinking of a ferry and found that survivors with PTSD were more likely to believe that a range of negative events would occur in the future than survivors without a traumatic stress disorder. With the use of a semistructured interview procedure, Newman, Riggs, and Roth (1997) examined an array of cognitive (e.g., ideas and expectations that the world is malevolent) and emotional (e.g., emotional self-reproach) issues in individuals with and without traumatic stress disorders. These investigators found that the severity of PTSD symptoms and the level of interpersonal violence associated with the traumatic events were associated with deficits in the processing of cognitive and emotional material.

SOCIAL SUPPORT MODELS

A vast body of research on acute and chronic stress has demonstrated that social support affects and influences physical and mental health and the likelihood that individuals will experience stress-related illnesses (e.g., Cohen & Wills, 1985; Holahan & Moos, 1981; King, King, Fairbank, Keane, & Adams, 1998; Norris & Murrell, 1990). Research on the readjustment of trauma survivors has also shown the importance of the quality and quantity of social support to recovery from stressful life events and overall well-being (e.g., Egendorf, Kadushin, Laufer, Rothbart, & Sloan, 1981; Keane, Scott, Chavoya, Lamparski, & Fairbank, 1985; Solomon & Mikulincer, 1990).

Researchers have also long recognized that posttrauma outcomes may not be solely the product of a single precipitating event (e.g., Green, 1994; Resnick, Kilpatrick, & Lipovsky, 1991). Rather, what is observed as a stress reaction may be the consequence of a series of highly stressful events that extend back into an individual's personal history before a focal traumatic experience. Current findings suggest that adverse life events have a strong negative relationship with social support, in that stressful life events appear to deplete social resources, which, in turn, exacerbates stress-related illnesses. In some instances, stressful life events in and of themselves are the loss of important interpersonal support resources (e.g., the loss of a spouse through death) (King et al., 1998). More commonly, stressful life events deplete social resources by placing an excessive demand on them.

DEVELOPMENTAL MODELS

Developmental models emphasize that knowing a person's developmental stage is essential to understanding reactivity to trauma throughout the course of life (Cole & Putnam, 1992; Marmar, Foy, Kagan, & Pynoos, 1993; Pynoos, Steinberg, & Wraith, 1995). A basic assumption of most developmental models is that the ways in which the effects of trauma are manifested are likely to vary by individuals' neurobiological, cognitive, emotional, and psychological maturation at the time of exposure (Cole & Putnam, 1992). A comprehensive model proposed by Pynoos et al. (1995) underscores the complexity and dynamic qualities of the developmental perspective. Focusing on the reactions of children and adolescents to traumatic events, this model posits a role for "the intricate matrix of a changing child and environment, evolving familial and societal expectations, and an essential linkage between disrupted and normal development" (p. 72). Developmental approaches to understanding reactivity to trauma have begun to be tested empirically. For example, a longitudinal study of children exposed to a severe brush fire in Australia found that trauma–reactivity relationships were not static over time (McFarlane, 1988). Over the next decade, developmentally appropriate research designs (e.g., longitudinal studies) are likely to be used to explore how maturational processes are involved in survivors' adaptation to severe traumatic events.

LEARNED HELPLESSNESS

Survivors of abusive and violent interpersonal trauma often experience apathy, dysphoria, passivity, decrements in performance on basic tasks, and highly generalized beliefs about personal lack of control over future events (Goodman, Koss, & Russo, 1993). To better understand the etiology of these symptoms, several authors (Campbell, 1989; Flannery, 1987; Flannery & Harvey, 1991; Walker, 1978) have considered the role of "learned helplessness," a theory developed by Martin Seligman (Garber & Seligman, 1980; Seligman, 1975). The construct of learned helplessness was originally proposed to explain the effect of prior exposure to inescapable shock on some animals' subsequent passive behavior and failure to respond under different conditions in which escape from the aversive shock was possible. Research animals showed a range of behavioral outcomes, from profound performance decrements to marked positive adaptation, in studies using Seligman's (1975) paradigm. This animal model provides researchers with a promising direction for studying aspects of the course of behavioral adaptation following exposure to uncontrollable and inescapable trauma (Pare, 1996).

RECOMMENDATIONS FOR FUTURE RESEARCH

Testable hypotheses need to be derived from each of the models, which can then be evaluated with regard to the following:

- Risk for PTSD and other signs, symptoms, conditions, and disorders
- Prediction of symptom patterns, course, severity, and chronicity of the stress response
- Methodological approaches to early detection
- Theory-driven interventions
- Measurement of outcomes within a theoretical context (e.g., evaluation of symptom reduction as an outcome of predicted changes in cognitions, appraisal, social support, etc.)
- Tests of goodness-of-fit of theoretical constructs with clinical or psychobiological phenomena

The complexity of the human response to torture and related violent and traumatic events suggests the need for continued effort to develop, refine, and test integrated models of traumatic stress that take into account the complexity of person–environment–outcome interactions. Promising work in this direction includes the dual representation theory proposed by Brewin et al. (1996).

Psychosocial models of traumatic stress generally focus on psychopathology and functional impairments associated with exposure to extreme events. Models are needed that examine the strength and resilience of survivors and that help to shape a conceptual framework for recovery.

REFERENCES

Basoglu, M., & Mineka, S. (1992). The role of uncontrollability and unpredictability of stress in the development of post-torture stress symptoms. In M. Basoglu (Ed.), *Torture and its consequences: Current treatment approaches* (pp. 182–225). Cambridge: Cambridge University Press.

Basoglu, M., & Mineka, S. (1997). Psychological preparedness for trauma as a protective factor in survivors of torture. *Psychological Medicine, 27*, 1421–1433.

Blanchard, E. B., Kolb, L. C., Pallmeyer, T. P., & Gerardi, R. J. (1982). A psychophysiological study of posttraumatic stress disorder in Vietnam veterans. *Psychiatric Quarterly, 54*(4), 220–229.

Blanchard, E. B., Kolb, L. C., & Prins, A. (1991). Psychophysiological responses in the diagnosis of posttraumatic stress disorder in Vietnam veterans. *Journal of Nervous and Mental Disease, 179*(2), 99–103.

Brewin, C. R., Dalgleish, T., & Joseph, S. (1996). A dual representation theory of posttraumatic stress disorder. *Psychological Review, 103*(4), 670–686.

Campbell, J. C. (1989). A test of two explanatory models of women's responses to battering. *Nursing Research, 38*, 18–24.

Cassiday, K. L., McNally, R. J., & Zeitlin, S. B. (1992). Cognitive processing of trauma cues in rape victims with posttraumatic stress disorder. *Cognitive Therapy and Research, 16*, 283–295.

Chemtob, C., Roitblatt, H. L., Hamada, R. S., Carlson, J. G., & Twentyman, C. T. (1988). A cognitive action theory of post-traumatic stress disorder. *Journal of Anxiety Disorders, 2*, 253–275.

Cohen, S., & Wills, T. A. (1985). Stress, social support, and the buffering hypothesis. *Psychological Bulletin, 98*, 310–357.

Cole, P. M., & Putnam, F. W. (1992). Effect of incest on self and social functioning: A developmental psychopathology perspective. *Journal of Consulting and Clinical Psychology, 60*(2), 174–184.

Creamer, M., Burgess, P., & Pattison, P. (1992). Reaction to trauma: A cognitive processing model. *Journal of Abnormal Psychology, 101*, 452–459.

Dalgleish, T. (1993). *The judgment of risk in traumatised and non-traumatised disaster survivors.* Unpublished master's thesis, University of London, England.

Egendorf, A., Kadushin, C., Laufer, R. S., Rothbart, G., & Sloan, L. (1981). *Legacies of Vietnam: Comparative adjustment of veterans and their peers.* Washington, DC: U.S. Government Printing Office.

Fairbank, J. A., & Keane, T. M. (1982). Flooding for combat-related stress disorders: Assessment of anxiety reduction across traumatic memories. *Behavior Therapy, 13*, 499–510.

Fairbank, J. A., & Nicholson, R. A. (1987). Theoretical and empirical issues in the treatment of post-traumatic stress disorder in Vietnam veterans. *Journal of Clinical Psychology, 43*(1), 44–55.

Flannery, R. B. (1987). From victim to survivor: A stress management approach in the treatment of learned helplessness. In B. A. van der Kolk (Ed.), *Psychological trauma.* Washington, DC: American Psychiatric Press.

Flannery, R. B., & Harvey, M. R. (1991). Psychological trauma and learned helplessness: Seligman's paradigm reconsidered. *Psychotherapy, 28*(2), 374–378.

Foa, E. B., & Kozak, M. J. (1986). Emotional processing of fear: Exposure to corrective information. *Psychological Bulletin, 99*(1), 20–35.

Foa, E. B., Rothbaum, B. O., & Molnar, C. (1995). Cognitive-behavioral therapy of post-traumatic stress disorder. *Journal of Traumatic Stress, 8*(4), 675–690.

Foa, E. B., Steketee, G., & Rothbaum, B. O. (1989). Behavioral/cognitive conceptualizations of post-traumatic stress disorder. *Behavior Therapy, 20*, 155–176.

Garber, J., & Seligman, M. E. D. (Eds.). (1980). *Human helplessness: Theory and application.* New York: Academic Press.

Goodman, L. A., Koss, M. P., & Russo, N. F. (1993). Violence against women: Mental health effects: Part II. Conceptualizations of posttraumatic stress. *Applied and Preventive Psychology, 2*(3), 123–130.

Green, B. L. (1994). Psychosocial research in traumatic stress: An update. *Journal of Traumatic Stress, 7*, 341–362.

Holahan, C. J., & Moos, R. H. (1981). Social support and psychological distress: A longitudinal analysis. *Journal of Abnormal Psychology, 90*, 365–370.

Horowitz, M. J. (1986). *Stress response syndromes.* New York: Aronson.

Janoff-Bulman, R. (1985). The aftermath of victimization: Rebuilding shattered assumptions. In C. R. Figley (Ed.), *Trauma and its wake: The study and treatment of post-traumatic stress disorder* (pp. 15–35). New York: Brunner/Mazel.

Kaspi, S. P., McNally, R. J., & Amir, N. (1995). Cognitive processing of emotional information in posttraumatic stress disorder. *Cognitive Therapy and Research, 19*, 319–330.

Keane, T. M. (1998). Psychological and behavioral treatment of post-traumatic stress disorder. In P. Nathan & J. Gorman (Eds.), *A guide to treatments that work* (pp. 398–407). New York: Oxford University Press.

Keane, T. M., Scott, W. O., Chavoya, G. A., Lamparski, D. M., & Fairbank, J. A. (1985). Social support in Vietnam veterans with posttraumatic stress disorder: A comparative analysis. *Journal of Consulting and Clinical Psychology, 53*, 95–102.

Keane, T. M., Zimering, R. T., & Caddell, J. M. (1985). A behavioral formulation of posttraumatic stress disorder in Vietnam veterans. *Behavior Therapist, 8*, 9–12.

Kilpatrick, D. G., Resick, P. A., & Veronen, L. J. (1981). Effects of a rape experience: A longitudinal study. *Journal of Social Issues, 37*, 105–122.

Kilpatrick, D. G., Veronen, L. J., & Best, C. L. (1985). Factors predicting psychological distress among rape victims. In C. R. Figley (Ed.), *Trauma and its wake: The study and treatment of post-traumatic disorder* (pp. 113–141). New York: Brunner/Mazel.

King, L. A., King, D. W., Fairbank, J. A., Keane, T. M., & Adams, G. A. (1998). Resilience recovery factors in post-traumatic stress disorder among female and male Vietnam veterans: Hardiness, postwar social support, and additional stressful life events. *Journal of Personality and Social Psychology, 74*(2), 420–434.

Lang, P. J. (1977). Imagery in therapy: An information processing analysis of fear. *Behavior Therapy, 8*, 862–886.

Litz, B. T., & Keane, T. M. (1989). Information processing in anxiety disorders: Application to the understanding of posttraumatic stress disorder. *Clinical Psychology Review, 9*, 243–257.

Malloy, P. F., Fairbank, J. A., & Keane, T. M. (1983). Validation of a multimethod assessment of posttraumatic stress disorders in Vietnam veterans. *Journal of Consulting and Clinical Psychology, 51*(4), 488–494.

Marmar, C. R., Foy, D., Kagan, B., & Pynoos, R. S. (1993). An integrated approach for treating posttraumatic stress. In J. M. Oldham, M. B. Riba, & A. Tasman (Eds.), *Review of psychiatry* (Vol. 12). Washington, DC: American Psychiatric Press.

McCann, I. L., & Pearlman, L. A. (1990). *Psychological trauma and the adult survivor: Theory, therapy, and transformation.* New York: Brunner/Mazel.

McFarlane, A. C. (1988). Recent life events and psychiatric disorder in children: The interaction with preceding extreme adversity. *Journal of Child Psychology and Psychiatry, 5*, 677–690.

McNally, R. J. (1995). *Cognitive processing of trauma-relevant information in PTSD.* White River Junction, VT: The National Center for Post-Traumatic Stress Disorder, VA Medical and Regional Office Center.

McNally, R. J., Kaspi, S. P., Riemann, B. C., & Zeitlin, S. B. (1990). Selective processing of threat cues in posttraumatic stress disorder. *Journal of Abnormal Psychology, 99*, 398–402.

Mineka, S., & Hendersen, R. (1985). Controllability and predictability in acquired motivation. *Annual Review of Psychology, 36*, 495–529.

Moye, T., Hyson, R., Grau, J., & Maier, S. (1983). Immunization of opioid analgesia: Effects of prior escapable shock on subsequent shock-induced and morphine-induced antinociception. *Learning and Motivation, 4*, 238–251.

Newman, E., Riggs, D. S., & Roth, S. (1997). Thematic resolution, PTSD, and complex PTSD: The relationship between meaning and trauma-related diagnoses. *Journal of Traumatic Stress, 10*(2), 197–213.

Norris, F. H., & Murrell, S. A. (1990). Social support, life events, and stress as modifiers of adjustment to bereavement by older adults. *Psychology and Aging, 5,* 429–436.

Orr, S. P., Pitman, R. K., Lasko, N. B., & Herz, L. R. (1993). Psychophysiological assessment of posttraumatic stress disorder imagery in World War II and Korean combat veterans. *Journal of Abnormal Psychology, 102*(1), 152–159.

Pare, W. P. (1996). Enhanced retrieval of unpleasant memories influenced by shock controllability, shock, sequence, and rat strain. *Biological Psychiatry, 39,* 808–813.

Pitman, R. K., Orr, S. P., Forgue, D. F., De Jong, J. B., & Claiborn, J. M. (1987). Psychophysiologic assessment of posttraumatic stress disorder imagery in Vietnam combat veterans. *Archives of General Psychiatry, 44*(11), 970–975.

Pynoos, R. S., Steinberg, A. M., & Wraith, R. (1995). A developmental model of childhood traumatic stress. In D. Cicchetti & D. Cohen (Eds.), *Developmental psychopathology, Vol. 2: Risk, disorder, and adaptation* (pp. 72–95). New York: Wiley.

Resick, P. A., & Schnicke, M. K. (Eds.). (1993). *Cognitive processing therapy for rape victims.* Newbury Park, CA: Sage.

Resnick, H. S., Kilpatrick, D. G., & Lipovsky, J. A. (1991). Assessment of rape-related posttraumatic stress disorder: Stressor and symptom dimensions. *Psychological Assessment, 3,* 561–572.

Roth, S., & Newman, E. (1993). The process of coping with incest for adult survivors: Measurement and implications for treatment and research. *Journal of Interpersonal Violence, 8*(3), 363–377.

Seligman, M. E. D. (1975). *Helplessness: On depression, development and death.* San Francisco: Freeman.

Solomon, Z., & Mikulincer, M. (1990). Life events and combat-related posttraumatic stress disorder: The intervening role of locus of control and social support. *Military Psychology, 2,* 241–256.

Vrana, S. R., Roodman, A., & Beckham, J. C. (1995). Selective processing of trauma-relevant words in posttraumatic stress disorder. *Journal of Anxiety Disorders, 9,* 515–530.

Walker, L. E. (1978). Battered women and learned helplessness. *Victimology, 2,* 525–534.

Williams, J., & Maier, S. (1977). Transsituational immunization and therapy of learned helplessness in the rat. *Journal of Experimental Psychology: Animal Behaviour Processes, 3,* 240–252.

Zeitlin, S. B., & McNally, R. J. (1991). Implicit and explicit memory bias for threat in posttraumatic stress disorder. *Behaviour Research and Therapy, 29,* 451–457.

5

Neurobiological Models of Posttraumatic Stress Disorder

STEVEN SOUTHWICK and MATTHEW J. FRIEDMAN

Posttraumatic stress disorder (PTSD) is commonly understood as a psychological disorder that results from exposure to life-threatening situations. Symptoms of reexperiencing, avoidance, and increased arousal are frequently treated with psychologically based interventions, including individual and group psychotherapy, behavior therapy, and psychoeducation. In recent years, however, it has become increasingly clear that PTSD also can be understood from a biological perspective.

Multiple neurobiological systems become activated when an organism is threatened. Parallel activation of various brain regions and neurotransmitter systems allows the organism to assess and appropriately respond to potential dangers. This highly complex process contributes to the development of anxiety, fear, and the fight–flight response that allows the organism to protect itself by either fleeing from or actively confronting danger. Whereas this process generally serves a protective role in the short run, it appears that maladaptive responses to stress can ensue in individuals who develop PTSD (Charney, Deutch, & Krystal, 1993).

In this chapter, we will focus on two neurobiological systems that are critical for survival—the sympathetic nervous system and the hypothalamic–pituitary–adrenal axis (HPA). To date, most neurobiological research in PTSD has focused on these two systems. It is clear that numerous other neurobiological systems, such as the opiate, serotonin, and dopamine systems, also are involved in acute and chronic responses to stress, although far less is known about them as they relate to PTSD.

STEVEN SOUTHWICK • Department of Psychiatry, Yale University School of Medicine, West Haven, Connecticut 06516.   MATTHEW J. FRIEDMAN • Dartmouth University, and the National Center for Post-Traumatic Stress Disorder, White River Junction, Vermont 05009.

The Mental Health Consequences of Torture, edited by Ellen Gerrity, Terence M. Keane, and Farris Tuma. Kluwer Academic/Plenum Publishers, New York, 2001.

How these stress-related neurobiological systems interact with one another in complex ways is only partially understood (Southwick, Krystal, Johnson, & Charney, 1992). This chapter will also describe several neurobiological models of PTSD. These models grow out of animal and human studies and represent an attempt to understand the rapidly growing body of trauma-related neurobiological research.

SYMPATHETIC NERVOUS SYSTEM ALTERATIONS IN PTSD

The sympathetic nervous system plays a central role in the organism's fight–flight response by increasing blood flow to muscles and vital organs, dilating pupils, limiting blood loss, and mobilizing energy for use by large muscle groups. Epinephrine (adrenaline) and norepinephrine (noradrenaline), both catecholamines, are two key neurotransmitters that facilitate the above sympathetic nervous system functions (Cannon, 1914; Gagnon, 1977; Mountcastle, 1973). They also play an important role in the development of fear and in the organism's ability to selectively focus on, respond to, and then remember the feared stimulus (Aston-Jones, Valentino, & Van Bockstaele, 1994; Gold & McCarty, 1995; Liang, Juler, & McGaugh, 1990; McGaugh, 1989; Zigmond, Finlay, & Sved, 1995).

Since World War II, numerous psychophysiological studies have documented the heightened sympathetic nervous system arousal of combat veterans who suffer from PTSD (Orr, 1990; Prins, Kaloupek, & Keane, 1995). Psychophysiological studies typically measure biological parameters such as heart rate, blood pressure, and skin conductance and electromyographic activity of facial muscles at baseline and in response to various trauma-relevant stimuli and neutral stimuli and generic stressors. Trauma-relevant stimuli include auditory and visual reminders of traumas similar to the one experienced by the participant as well as script-driven imagery of the individual's own specific traumatic experience.

A review of this extensive literature shows that trauma victims with PTSD demonstrate greater psychophysiological reactivity (especially heart rate) to trauma-relevant stimuli than do comparison groups such as trauma victims without PTSD and nontraumatized healthy controls. Although some studies have reported a higher baseline resting heart rate in PTSD compared with control groups, most studies have found no differences (Orr, 1990; Prins et al., 1995). Further, response to generic stressors typically has been the same between PTSD and non-PTSD groups (McFall, Murburg, & Ko, 1990; Pitman et al., 1990). In summary, trauma victims with PTSD appear to have normal resting sympathetic nervous system activity (as reflected by heart rate and blood pressure) that becomes abnormally reactive in response to specific reminders of a personally experienced trauma but not in response to generic stressors (Murburg, 1994; Prins et al., 1995).

Biochemical correlates of this heightened sympathetic nervous system activity in veterans and civilians with PTSD include increased excretion of epinephrine and norepinephrine in urine collected over a 24-hour period (L. M. Davidson & Baum, 1986; DeBellis, Baum, Birmaher, & Ryan, 1997; Kosten, Mason, & Giller, 1987; Yehuda, Southwick, & Giller, 1992) and decreased numbers of alpha-2 adrenergic receptors on the surface of platelets (circulating blood elements) (Perry, 1994; Perry, Giller, & Southwick, 1987). For epinephrine and norepinephrine to have a physiological effect, they must first attach to adrenergic receptors. A decrease in the number of adrenergic receptors most likely results from chronic elevation of circulating epinephrine and norepinephrine. Thus, as a group, individuals with PTSD appear to have higher levels of epinephrine and norepinephrine than nontraumatized individuals even many years after a trauma.

This increase in epinephrine and norepinephrine may not be present during calm, resting states. However, it appears that PTSD subjects, as a group, respond to a variety of stressors with exaggerated increases in catecholamines compared with healthy controls (McFall et al., 1990; Murburg, 1994; Southwick, Bremner, Krystal, & Charney, 1994; Southwick et al., 1993; Southwick, Yehuda, & Morgan, 1995). For example, greater increases in epinephrine have been observed in veterans with war-related PTSD compared with controls during and after viewing a combat film but not in response to a film depicting an automobile accident (McFall et al., 1990). Exaggerated increases in catecholamines also have been noted in response to pharmacological provocation. To more directly assess adrenergic responsivity of both the peripheral and central nervous system, one study administered intravenous yohimbine to 20 Vietnam combat veterans with PTSD and 18 healthy controls (Southwick et al., 1993). Yohimbine is an alpha-2 adrenergic receptor antagonist that activates noradrenergic neurons by blocking the alpha-2-adrenergic autoreceptor, thereby increasing the release of endogenous norepinephrine. Yohimbine caused panic attacks in 70% and flashbacks in 40% of combat veterans with PTSD but had minimal effects in the control group. Subjects with PTSD also had significantly greater increases in heart rate and a greater than twofold increase in methoxyhydroxyphenylglycol (MHPG), a breakdown product of norepinephrine.

In a recent positron emission tomography (PET) study (Bremner, Innis, et al., 1997), the effect of yohimbine on the brain activity of 10 combat veterans with PTSD was compared with that of 10 healthy controls. A single bolus of [F-18]2-fluoro-2-deoxyglucose was administered to each subject following either yohimbine or placebo infusion. Subjects were then scanned, and PET images were reconstructed to determine brain-tissue activity. Yohimbine caused an exaggerated release of plasma MHPG and a relative decrease in brain metabolism. It was hypothesized that this relative decrease in brain metabolism may have resulted in a possible increase in signal-to-noise ratio and vigilance among combat veterans with PTSD as compared with normal controls. Taken together, the above catecholamine findings suggest that at least a subgroup of individuals with PTSD has increased responsivity of the sympathetic nervous system that is most evident when the individual is restressed (Murburg, 1994; Southwick et al., 1995).

THE HYPOTHALAMIC–PITUITARY–ADRENAL AXIS

Whereas the sympathetic nervous system prepares the organism to react to stressful stimuli, the HPA axis appears to serve a catabolic restorative role (Munck, Guyre, & Holbrook, 1984; Yehuda, 1997). When an organism is stressed, the hypothalamus releases corticotropin-releasing hormone (CRH), which then stimulates the release of adrenocorticotropic hormone (ACTH) from the pituitary gland. ACTH in turn stimulates the adrenal gland to release cortisol, which helps to terminate a variety of neurobiological reactions that have been set in motion by stressful stimuli.

Under normal circumstances, cortisol rises in response to stress. However, several recent studies have found that trauma victims who develop PTSD have lower initial cortisol responses to a traumatic event than trauma victims who do not develop PTSD (McFarlane, Atchison, & Yehuda, 1997; Resnick, Yehuda, & Acierno, 1997). Further, in studies of civilians and veterans with chronic PTSD, baseline plasma cortisol levels and 24-hour urine cortisol excretion have been reported as low compared with controls (Yehuda, Giller, Levengood, Southwick, & Siever, 1995). In combat veterans with chronic PTSD, these low plasma levels of cortisol have been reported throughout the day and night, especially in the very early morning and late evening (Yehuda, 1997).

Receptor-binding studies, however, have found an increased number of glucocorticoid receptors in subjects with PTSD compared with nontraumatized controls (Yehuda, 1997; Yehuda, Giller, et al., 1995). An increased number of receptors would enhance sensitivity by providing more binding sites for cortisol. Consistent with increased receptor number and sensitivity is the finding that subjects with PTSD hyperrespond to administration of dexamethasone, a synthetic glucocorticoid that acts like cortisol (Yehuda, 1997; Yehuda, Boisoneau, & Lowy, 1995; Yehuda, Giller, et al., 1995; Yehuda, Southwick, & Krystal, 1993). Normally, when dexamethasone is administered to healthy individuals, it stimulates glucocorticoid receptors that serve as part of a negative feedback mechanism. When stimulated, these receptors signal the hypothalamus and pituitary to decrease the release of CRH and ACTH, which in turn results in decreased stimulation of the adrenal gland and diminished release of endogenous cortisol. In several different populations of trauma survivors with PTSD, dexamethasone has an exaggerated effect with the result that endogenous cortisol release is reduced to a greater degree than in normal controls. This finding is consistent with an increased number of glucocorticoid receptors and increased negative feedback at the level of the hypothalamus and pituitary in traumatized individuals with PTSD compared with controls (Yehuda, Giller, et al., 1995). These findings in PTSD differ markedly from findings in studies of major depressive disorder (American Psychiatric Association Task Force on Laboratory Tests in Psychiatry, 1987).

Other important HPA axis findings in combat veterans with PTSD include elevated CRH levels in the cerebrospinal fluid (Bremner, Licinio et al., 1997), blunted ACTH response to CRH infusion (Smith, Davidson, & Ritchie, 1989), and increased ACTH response to metyrapone (Yehuda, 1997). In conjunction with plasma and 24-hour urine cortisol, glucocorticoid receptor, and dexamethasone suppression studies, these findings are consistent with the notion of enhanced negative feedback of the HPA axis and elevated CRH release in PTSD (Yehuda, 1997). It has been hypothesized that these alterations help to explain why individuals with PTSD hyperrespond to stress (Yehuda, 1997).

STRESS SENSITIZATION

Sensitization refers to a stressor-induced increase in behavioral or physiological responsiveness following exposure to subsequent stressors of the same or lesser magnitude (Post, 1992; Post, Weiss, & Smith, 1995; Sorg & Kalivas, 1995). When a neurobiological system becomes sensitized, its behavioral, physiological, and biochemical responses to a given stressor gradually increase. The time interval between the initial stressors appears to be an important factor in the development of sensitization. If sufficient time has passed between the initial stressor and subsequent stressors, a single stressful stimulus may be capable of initiating behavior sensitization. The capacity to respond more readily to future stressors may be adaptive with regard to survival (Post et al., 1995; Sorg & Kalivas, 1995). The organism is better prepared for future dangers. However, it appears that sensitization may also be maladaptive, leaving the organism in a hyperreactive state in which it overresponds to minor stressors. The organism may become hypervigilant and continue to act biologically as if a danger exists even when no real danger is currently present (Southwick et al., 1995).

Neurochemical and neuroanatomical systems mediating sensitization are only partially understood. Most extensively studied in the development and maintenance of stress-induced sensitization in mammals have been catecholamine systems (especially dopamine and norepinephrine). For example, limited shock exposure that does not increase norepinephrine utilization in control rats does increase norepinephrine release in animals previously exposed to the stressor (Anisman & Sklar, 1978; Irwin, Ahluwalia, & Anismar, 1986). Similarly, equivalent doses of yohimbine have been shown to cause significantly greater increases in anxiety, vigilance, intrusive traumatic memories, heart rate, and plasma MHPG in combat veterans with PTSD compared with healthy controls (Southwick et al., 1993). This finding is consistent with a behavioral sensitization model of PTSD.

A large body of evidence also suggests that the HPA axis can become sensitized in trauma victims with PTSD. Consistent with a sensitization model (Yehuda, 1997), most HPA axis studies in veterans and civilians with PTSD have found decreased plasma cortisol and decreased 24-hour urine cortisol, but larger numbers of plasma lymphocyte glucocorticoid receptors and increased suppression of cortisol by the synthetic glucocorticoid dexamethasone. A larger number of glucocorticoid receptors at the level of the hypothalamus and the pituitary may explain why cortisol and dexamethasone appear to have an exaggerated inhibitory effect on HPA axis function.

Although sensitization has not been shown clearly in clinical studies of traumatized subjects, it has been hypothesized that sensitization of sympathetic nervous system and HPA axis function may contribute to a number of PTSD symptoms including hypervigilance, irritability, poor concentration, insomnia, exaggerated startle, and, perhaps, intrusive memories (Charney et al., 1993; Yehuda, 1997). Whereas most neurobiological studies in traumatized humans have focused on the sympathetic nervous system and the HPA axis, preliminary evidence exists that other neurobiological systems, including the serotonin system (Arora, Fitcner, & O'Connor, 1993; Southwick et al., 1997), also may be sensitized in trauma survivors with PTSD. Exactly how various neurobiological stress systems interact during the acute and chronic phases of trauma and thereafter are not well understood. However, it is possible that sensitization (increased negative feedback) of the HPA axis results in decreased levels of cortisol and thus a diminished capacity to terminate the sympathetic nervous system's response to traumatic stress (Yehuda, 1997). Overall, a behavioral sensitization model appears to fit many of the findings reported to date in subjects with PTSD in which systems gradually become hyperresponsive to stress. Further, recent evidence suggests that sensitization may be associated with changes in gene expression (Post et al., 1995).

FEAR CONDITIONING

Numerous researchers have noted a remarkable similarity between the effects of fear conditioning in animals and the behavioral and physiological responses seen in combat veterans with severe war neuroses (Kardiner & Spiegel, 1947; Keane, Fairbank, & Caddell, 1985; Kolb, 1987). Fear conditioning involves the pairing of a fear-provoking aversive event (unconditioned stimulus, or US) with an explicit neutral stimulus (conditioned stimulus, or CS) that then serves as a specific reminder of the trauma or aversive event. For example, if a neutral light is paired with an aversive stimulus such as a shock, eventually the light by itself (in the absence of the shock) can elicit fear and fear-related physiologic responses. The light becomes an explicit conditioned stimulus (Grillon, Southwick, & Charney, 1996). Conditioning also can occur to contextual cues that were present during the pairing of the CS and US (Bolles & Fanselow, 1980; Foa, Zinbarg, & Rothbaum, 1992). Thus, the cage in which the shock was delivered can become a contextual cue with the capacity to evoke fear in the absence of either aversive unconditioned stimuli (e.g., shock) or explicit conditioned stimuli (e.g., light).

As an example, after surviving a life-threatening fire (US) in which others were killed, a combat veteran may no longer experience the smell of burning wood as a neutral stimulus that evokes feelings of peace and comfort. Instead, the smell now may serve as an explicit CS that is capable of evoking fear and fear-related behaviors. Other contextual stimuli that were present at the time of the fire, but that were not directly associated with the fire, also can acquire the capacity to evoke fear. Thus, if the fire occurred on a hot and muggy day, many years later hot and muggy days, even in locations thousands of miles away from the original fire, may leave the veteran feeling anxious and irritable (Southwick et al., 1994).

The neurobiological underpinnings of fear conditioning are not completely understood. However, it is clear that the amygdala plays a pivotal role in both unconditioned and conditioned fear (Aggleton, 1992; Blanchard & Blanchard, 1972). The amygdala is a structure in the limbic system that receives rich input from sensory regions of the cortex and from numerous subcortical regions. It also has extensive efferent, or outgoing, neuronal connections to autonomic, motor, and neuroendocrine systems. This rich array of neuronal input and output makes the amygdala ideally suited for its role in assessing and responding to emotionally significant stimuli such as those that indicate potential threat (Aggleton, 1992).

In animals, electric stimulation of the amygdala produces fear-related behaviors, whereas lesions of the amygdala have been shown to reduce fear and aggression as well as the overall ability to attach meaning to sensory information, a capacity that allows the organism to generate appropriate behavioral responses. In general, amygdala neuronal activity is increased with stimuli of high emotional significance, especially threat. It also has been demonstrated that a formerly neutral stimulus that has been conditioned to a fear-related stimulus (US) can, on its own, increase neuronal firing in the amygdala and that lesions of the amygdala attenuate fear-related behaviors seen in response to fear-conditioned stimuli (CS). Thus, the amygdala is highly responsive to both unconditioned and conditioned fear cues (Charney, Deutch, Southwick, & Krystal, 1995).

Separate neurobiological mechanisms appear to mediate explicit fear conditioning and contextual fear conditioning. Although much evidence suggests that the amygdala is involved in both types of conditioning (Aggleton, 1992; Blanchard & Blanchard, 1972; Davis, 1992), the hippocampus appears to play a critical role in contextual but not explicit fear conditioning (Phillips & LeDoux, 1992). The hippocampus is a limbic structure that plays a key role in processing spatial and contextual cues with an emphasis on the relationship of multiple stimuli (O'Keefe, 1993; O'Keefe & Nadel, 1978; Parkinson, Murray, & Mishkin, 1990). Lesions of the hippocampus attenuate fear responses to conditioned contextual stimuli but not conditioned explicit stimuli (O'Keefe & Nadel, 1978; Phillips & LeDoux, 1992). Thus, after hippocampal lesions, animals are no longer afraid of the cage (contextual stimuli) in which shock was delivered but are still afraid of the explicit stimulus (light) that was paired with the shock. Research evidence also suggests that various neurotransmitters, such as noradrenaline and acetylcholine, have differential roles in explicit and contextual conditioning (McAlonan, Wilkinson, Robbins, & Everitt, 1995; Selden, Everitt, Jarrard, & Robbins, 1991).

Fear conditioning can occur very rapidly (Blanchard, Yudko, Rodgers, & Blanchard, 1993; LeDoux, 1996). For example, in some cases, a neutral stimulus can become conditioned to fear after a single pairing with an unconditioned fear stimulus. This pairing allows the organism to avoid lengthy trial-and-error learning about situations that are potentially dangerous. Rapid conditioning of characteristics of the danger itself (explicit stimuli) and characteristics of the place in which the danger occurred (contextual stimuli) maximize future chances for survival (LeDoux, 1996).

Fear conditioning also can occur outside of conscious awareness (LeDoux, 1996; Ohman, 1992). Thus, the traumatized human may not be consciously aware that a formerly neutral stimulus has become frightening through its association with an unconditioned fear stimulus. This concept applies for both explicit and contextual stimuli. The result may be an individual who becomes anxious, irritable, or frightened for reasons that he or she does not understand. The earlier cited trauma victim, for example, may become anxious or frightened on hot, muggy days without having any conscious appreciation for the cause of these feelings.

Once established, fear conditioning can last for long periods of time. Theoretically, once a conditioned fear stimulus is no longer associated with an aversive outcome, the conditioned fear response should extinguish. However, recent evidence suggests that extinction is an active process that involves new learning. The old fear-conditioned learning has not really been extinguished or replaced (LeDoux, Farb, & Ruggiero, 1990). This finding has led to the suggestion that subcortical fear-related learning is essentially indelible in nature (Bouton, 1994; LeDoux, 1996). Even though the fear-conditioned response seems to have disappeared over time, it can return under the right circumstances.

ENHANCED MEMORY FOR AVERSIVE EVENTS

A large body of evidence suggests that arousing, fearful, or emotionally exciting events are remembered better and for longer periods of time than emotionally neutral events (McGaugh, 1989). Such arousing events reportedly can produce what Brown and Kulik (1977) have termed flashbulb memories that resemble a photographic print. It has been proposed that emotional arousal activates neurobiological systems that facilitate the encoding and consolidation of memory. Enhanced memory for arousing situations may have significance for survival. The organism that remembers arousing and dangerous situations may be less vulnerable to similar potentially dangerous situations in the future. Unfortunately, these memories (in the form of intrusive recollections and nightmares) also may repetitively haunt the trauma survivor long after the event (LeDoux, 1996; Reiser, 1991).

Animal and human studies strongly suggest that enhanced memory for emotionally arousing, stressful, and traumatic events may, in part, be mediated by catecholamines (adrenaline, noradrenaline). Gold and Van Buskirk (1975) reported that posttraining injections of epinephrine enhanced retention for an inhibitory avoidance task in rats with intact adrenal glands. Enhanced retention was dependent on both dose and time. Norepinephrine, particularly in the amygdala, is also involved in learning and memory. Intra-amygdala infusion of norepinephrine immediately after training for a variety of learning tasks enhanced retention (Liang et al., 1990).

It has been hypothesized that highly stressful traumatic events can cause overstimulation of endogenous stress-responsive neuromodulators such as epinephrine and norepinephrine and that these neuromodulators cause an overconsolidation of memory for the event. The resulting, deeply engraved traumatic memory would then be responsible for conditioned emotional responses and intrusive recollections typically seen in PTSD (Pitman, 1989). Further, when the traumatic event is relived through intrusive recollections, flashbacks, and nightmares, epinephrine and norepinephrine are again released, leading to an additional strengthening of the memory trace and an even greater likelihood of subsequent intrusive recollections. This positive-feedback loop could explain the progression from subclinical to clinical PTSD seen in patients with delayed-onset PTSD (Liang et al., 1990). Whereas evidence suggests that biochemical correlates of moderate- and high-arousal events facilitate encoding, it may be that extreme arousal may actually disrupt encoding, with the result that memory for some traumatic events becomes fragmented (Koss, Tromp, & Tharan, 1995).

An important recent human investigation addresses the relationship between catecholamine activation and acquisition of memory. Cahil, Prins, Weber, and McGaugh (1994) examined the effect of propranolol, a drug that blocks beta-adrenergic activation, on long-term memory for an emotionally arousing story in comparison with a closely matched emotionally neutral story among normal controls. In randomized double-blind fashion, participants received either propranolol or a placebo 1 hour before viewing a series of slides. Some of the slides depicted scenes that were considered to be neutral in nature (e.g., one of the neutral slides showed a mother and her son walking together), whereas others depicted scenes that were classified as stressful and emotional (e.g., the boy in a terrible automobile accident). In a surprise memory test 1 week after viewing the slides, participants were tested for their memory of the slides. Participants in the placebo-condition group had significantly better memory for the emotional slides than for the neutral slides. Conversely, subjects in the propranolol-condition group did not remember the emotional slides any better than the neutral slides. That is, propranolol did not affect memory for the neutral slides but did affect memory for the emotionally arousing slides, suggesting that beta-adrenergic activation is involved in the enhanced memory associated with arousing or emotional experiences. The results could not be explained by potential effects of propranolol on attention or sedation.

Support for the idea that catecholamine stimulation also can facilitate memory retrieval for arousing or emotional experiences comes from a study of 20 Vietnam combat veterans with PTSD who, in response to disinhibition of the noradrenergic system by yohimbine infusion, experienced vivid intrusive memories of traumatic combat experiences. Forty percent had a full-blown flashback (Southwick et al., 1993). These intrusive recollections were accompanied by evidence of increased catecholamine activity, including significant elevations of MHPG, heart rate, and blood pressure. The retrieval of traumatic memories with yohimbine infusion is consistent with animal studies demonstrating enhanced retrieval of aversive memories through adrenergic and noradrenergic stimulation (Conway, Anderson, & Larsen, 1994). Creating a biological context (i.e., yohimbine-induced increase in catecholamine activity) that resembles the biological state at the time of encoding (fear-induced increase in catecholamine activity) may have served to facilitate the retrieval of frightening memories.

OTHER CONSIDERATIONS

Other models, such as learned helplessness (a maladaptive behavioral depression resulting from inescapable stress), have also been offered as ways to understand the development of PTSD (Krystal, 1990; Rasmusson & Charney, 1997). In all models of PTSD, the role of premorbid and developmental factors must be considered. To what degree are sensitization, fear conditioning, learned helplessness, and enhanced memory for trauma affected by neurobiological factors that have been inherited or influenced by the course of development?

Clearly, heredity plays a key role in animal and human behavior, including defensive and fear-related behaviors (LeDoux, 1996). For example, it is well known that animals can be bred for a variety of behavioral traits, including responsivity (ranging from timid to courageous) to novel stimuli. In general, these traits remain relatively stable over time (Gray, 1987). Similarly, in humans, it is believed that temperament and the individual's characteristic response to stressful stimuli are, in part, genetically determined (Kagan & Snidman, 1991; Marks, 1987). It is possible that these inherited behavioral traits and their neurobiological underpinnings influence the chances of developing PTSD when confronted with a traumatic stressor. For example, inherited variations in sympathetic nervous system functioning, the capacity for a particular neurobiological system to become sensitized or conditioned, or both may be, in part, genetically determined. Empirical evidence for a heritable component of PTSD comes from family history data supporting a relationship between PTSD and other anxiety disorders (J. Davidson, Smith, & Kudler, 1989) and from twin-study data suggesting that approximately 13% to 34% of the variance for specific PTSD-symptom clusters is genetically transmitted (True et al., 1993).

Experiences during early development also have an important influence on later behavioral and neurobiological responses to stress. It has been proposed that trauma in childhood may differentially affect maturation of various brain regions by overstimulating areas involved in fear and alarm reactions (limbic, midbrain, and brain stem) and by retarding cortical development through neglect and sensory deprivation (Perry, Pollard, Blakely, Baker, & Vigilante, 1995). Development and responsivity of various stress-related neuroendocrine systems might also be affected. Such effects would likely influence a child's ability to regulate impulses, aggression, and emotions and to accurately process information. It also is possible that early trauma-related neurobiological alterations might predispose an individual to develop PTSD in the future (Pynoos, Steinberg, & Wraith, 1995). For example, combat veterans with histories of childhood abuse are more likely to develop combat-related PTSD than are soldiers without histories of abuse (Bremner, Southwick, Johnson, Yehuda, & Charney, 1993).

Animal studies have provided strong support for the notion that severe psychological stress can cause tissue damage to the nervous system. Functional and morphological changes within the hippocampus have been reported in traumatized rodents and primates (Sapolsky, 1994). These changes may be mediated by stress-induced elevations of glucocorticoids. In humans, several recent magnetic resonance imaging (MRI) studies have reported decreased hippocampal volume in traumatized civilian and combat veteran populations with PTSD compared with controls (Bremner et al., 1995; Bremner, Randall, et al., 1997; Gurvits et al., 1996; Stein, Hanna, Koverola, Torchia, & McClarty, 1997). Because the hippocampus plays an important role in memory and learning, researchers investigated whether stress-induced damage to the hippocampus could help to explain reexperiencing symptoms, reported deficits in explicit memory, and fragmented memory for details of the traumatic event among subjects with PTSD.

In addition to MRI studies that raise the possibility of structural brain abnormalities (i.e., reduced hippocampal volume) among PTSD subjects, brain imaging studies with PET suggest that PTSD may also be associated with functional brain alterations. Preliminary PET studies indicate that when PTSD subjects are exposed to reminders of their personal trauma (e.g., traumatic images or scripts), they exhibit increased regional cerebral blood flow to brain structures thought to process emotionally charged information, such as the amygdala and the anterior cingulate cortex (Rauch & Shin, 1997). These findings appear to be consistent with the above models of PTSD.

In this brief review, we have touched on some of the most consistent neurobiological findings in humans with PTSD. We also have described a number of models that may help to explain these findings. Clearly, the neurobiology of acute and chronic trauma, as well as PTSD, is extremely complex. Human research in this area is still in its infancy.

REFERENCES

Aggleton, J. (1992). *The amygdala: Neurobiological aspects of emotion, memory, and mental dysfunction.* New York: Wiley-Liss.

American Psychiatric Association Task Force on Laboratory Tests in Psychiatry. (1987). The dexamethasone suppression test: An overview of its current status in psychiatry. *American Journal of Psychiatry, 144,* 1253–1262.

Anisman, H., & Sklar, L. S. (1978). Catecholamine depletion upon reexposure to stress: Mediation of the escape deficits produced by inescapable shock. *Journal of Comprehensive Physiological Psychology, 93,* 610–625.

Arora, R. C., Fitcner, C. G., & O'Connor, F. (1993). Paroxetine binding in the blood platelets of posttraumatic stress disordered patients. *Life Science, 53,* 919–928.

Aston-Jones, G., Valentino, R., & Van Bockstaele, M. (1994). Locus coeruleus, stress, and PTSD: Neurobiological and clinical parallels. In M. Murburg (Ed.), *Catecholamine function in posttraumatic stress disorder: Emerging concepts.* Washington, DC: American Psychological Association Press.

Blanchard, D. C., & Blanchard, R. J. (1972). Innate and conditioned reactions to threat in rats with amygdaloid lesions. *Journal of Comparative Physiology and Psychology, 81,* 281–290.

Blanchard, R. J., Yudko, E. B., Rodgers, R. J., & Blanchard, D. C. (1993). Defense system psychopharmacology: An ethological approach to the pharmacology of fear and anxiety. *Behavioural Brain Research, 58,* 155–166.

Bolles, R. C., & Fanselow, M. S. (1980). A perceptual–defense–recuperative model of fear and pain. *Behavior and Brain Sciences, 3,* 291–323.

Bouton, M. E. (1994). Conditioning, remembering, and forgetting. *Journal of Experimental Psychology: Animal Behavior Processes, 20,* 219–231.

Bremner, J. D., Innis, R. B., Salomon, R. M., Staib, L., Ng, C. K., Miller, H. L., Bronen, R. A., Duncan, J., Krystal, J. H., Rich, D., Malison, R., Price, L. H., Dey, H., Soufer, R., & Charney, D. S. (1997). PET measurement of cerebral metabolic correlates of yohimbine administration in combat related posttraumatic stress disorder. *Archives of General Psychiatry, 54,* 246–254.

Bremner, J. D., Licinio, J., Darnell, A., Krystal, J., Owens, M., Southwick, S., Nemeroff, C., & Charney, D. (1997). Elevated CSF corticotropin-releasing factor concentrations in posttraumatic stress disorder. *American Journal of Psychiatry, 154,* 624–629.

Bremner, J. D., Randall, P., Scott, T. M., Bronen, R. A., Seibyl, J. P., Southwick, S. M., Delaney, R. C., McCarthy, G., Charney, D. S., & Innis, R. B. (1995). MRI-based measurement of hippocampal volume in patients with combat-related posttraumatic stress disorder. *American Journal of Psychiatry, 152,* 973–981.

Bremner, J. D., Randall, P., Vermetten, E., Staib, L., Bronen, R. A., Capelli, S., Mazure, C. M., McCarthy, G., Innis, R. B., & Charney, D. S. (1997). MRI-based measurement of hippocampal volume in posttraumatic stress disorder related to childhood physical and sexual abuse: A preliminary report. *Biological Psychiatry, 41,* 23–32.

Bremner, J. D., Southwick, S. M., Johnson, D. R., Yehuda, R., & Charney, D. S. (1993). Childhood physical abuse and combat-related posttraumatic stress disorder in Vietnam veterans. *American Journal of Psychiatry, 150,* 235–239.

Brown, R., & Kulik, J. (1977). Flashbulb memories. *Cognition, 5,* 73–99.

Cahill, L., Prins, B., Weber, M., & McGaugh, J. L. (1994). Adrenergic activation and memory for emotional events. *Nature, 371,* 702–704.

Cannon, W. B. (1914). Emergency function of adrenal medulla in pain and the major emotions. *American Journal of Physiology, 3,* 356–372.

Charney, D. S., Deutch, A., & Krystal, J. (1993). Psychobiological mechanisms of posttraumatic stress disorder. *Archives of General Psychiatry, 50,* 294–305.

Charney, D. S., Deutch, A. Y., Southwick, S. M., & Krystal, J. H. (1995). Neural circuits and mechanisms of post-traumatic stress disorder. In M. J. Friedman, D. S. Charney, & A. Y. Deutch (Eds.), *Neurobiological and clinical consequences of stress: From normal adaptation to post-traumatic stress disorder* (pp. 271–290). Philadelphia: Lippincott–Raven.

Conway, M. A., Anderson, S. J., & Larsen, S. F. (1994). The formation of flashbulb memories. *Memory and Cognition, 22,* 326–343.

Davidson, J., Smith, R., & Kudler, H. (1989). Familial psychiatric illness in chronic posttraumatic stress disorder. *Comprehensive Psychiatry, 30,* 339–345.

Davidson, L. M., & Baum, A. (1986). Chronic stress and posttraumatic stress disorder. *Journal of Consulting and Clinical Psychology, 54,* 303–308.

Davis, M. (1992). The role of the amygdala in conditioned fear. In J. Aggleton (Ed.), *The amygdala: Neurobiological aspects of emotion, memory and mental dysfunction* (pp. 255–306). New York: Wiley-Liss.

De Bellis, M. D., Baum, A. S., Birmaher, B., & Ryan, N. D. (1997). Urinary catecholamine excretion in childhood overanxious and posttraumatic stress disorder. *Annals of the New York Academy of Sciences, 821,* 451–455.

Foa, E. B., Zinbarg, R., & Rothbaum, B. O. (1992). Uncontrollability and unpredictability in posttraumatic stress disorder: An animal model. *Psychological Bulletin, 112,* 218–238.

Gagnon, W. F. (1977). *The nervous system.* Los Altos, CA: Lange.

Gold, P. E., & McCarty, R. C. (1995). Stress regulation of memory processes: Role of peripheral catecholamines and glucose. In M. J. Friedman, D. S. Charney, & A. Y. Deutch (Eds.), *Neurobiological and clinical consequences of stress: From normal adaptation to post-traumatic stress disorder* (pp. 151–162). Philadelphia: Lippincott-Raven.

Gold, P. E., & van Buskirk, R. B. (1975). Facilitation of time-dependent memory processes with posttrial epinephrine injections. *Behavioral Biology, 13,* 145–153.

Gray, J. A. (1987). *The psychology of fear and stress* (Vol. 2). New York: Cambridge University Press.

Grillon, C., Southwick, S. M., & Charney, D. S. (1996). The psychobiological basis of posttraumatic stress disorder. *Molecular Psychiatry, 1,* 278–297.

Gurvits, T. G., Shenton, M. R., Hokama, H., Ohta, H., Lasko, N. B., Gilberson, M. W., Orr, S. P., Kikinis, R., Lolesz, F. A., McCarley, R. W., & Pitman, R. K. (1996). Magnetic resonance imaging study of hippocampal volume in chronic combat-related posttraumatic stress disorder. *Biological Psychiatry, 40,* 192–199.

Irwin, J., Ahluwalia, P., & Anismar, H. (1986). Sensitization of norepinephrine activity following acute and chronic foot-shock. *Brain Research, 379,* 98–103.

Kagan, J., & Snidman, N. (1991). Infant predictors of inhibited and uninhibited profiles. *Psychological Science, 2,* 40–43.

Kardiner A., & Spiegel, H. (1947). *The traumatic neuroses of war.* New York: Hoeber.

Keane, T. M., Fairbank, J. P., & Caddell, J. M. (1985). A behavioral approach to assessing and treating post traumatic stress disorder in Vietnam veterans. In C. R. Figley (Ed.), *Trauma and its wake: The study and treatment of post-traumatic stress disorder* (pp. 257–294). New York: Brunner/Mazel.

Kolb, L. C. (1987). A neuropsychological hypothesis explaining post traumatic stress disorders. *American Journal of Psychiatry, 144,* 989–995.

Koss, M. P., Tromp, S., & Tharan, M. (1995). Traumatic memories: Empirical foundations, forensic and clinical implications. *Clinical Psychology: Science and Practice, 2,* 111–132.

Kosten, T. R., Mason, J. W., & Giller, E. L. (1987). Sustained urinary norepinephrine and epinephrine elevation in post-traumatic stress disorder. *Psychoneuroendocrinology, 12,* 13–20.

Krystal, J. H. (1990). Animal models for posttraumatic stress disorder. In E. L. Giller (Ed.), *Biological assessment and treatment of posttraumatic stress disorder, progress in psychiatry* (pp. 3–64), Washington, DC: American Psychiatric Press.

LeDoux, J. E. (1996). *The emotional brain: The mysterious underpinnings of emotional life.* New York: Simon & Schuster.

LeDoux, J. E., Farb, C. F., & Ruggiero, D. A. (1990). Topographic organization of neurons in the acoustic thalamus that project to the amygdala. *Journal of Neuroscience, 10,* 1043–1054.

Liang, K. C., Juler, R., & McGaugh, J. L. (1990). Modulating effects of posttraining epinephrine on memory: Involvement of the amygdala in the noradrenergic system. *Brain Research, 368,* 125–133.

Marks, I. (1987). *Fears, phobias, and rituals: Panic, anxiety, and their disorders.* New York: Oxford University Press.

McAlonan, M., Wilkinson, L. S., Robbins, T. W., & Everitt, B. J. (1995). The effects of AMPA-induced lesions of the septo-hippocampal cholinergic projection on aversive conditioning to explicit and contextual cues and spatial learning in the water maze. *European Journal of Neuroscience, 7,* 281–292.

McFall, M., Murburg, M., & Ko, G. (1990). Autonomic response to stress in Vietnam combat veterans with post-traumatic stress disorder. *Biological Psychiatry, 27,* 1165–1175.

McFarlane, A. C., Atchison, M., & Yehuda, R. (1997). The acute stress response following motor vehicle accidents and its relation to PTSD. *Annals of the New York Academy of Sciences, 821,* 437–441.

McGaugh, J. L. (1989). Involvement of hormonal and neuromodulatory systems in the regulation of memory storage. *Annual Review of Neuroscience, 12,* 255–287.

Mountcastle, V. B. (1973). *Medical physiology* (13th ed.). St. Louis, MO: Mosby.

Munck, A., Guyre, P. M., & Holbrook, N. J. (1984). Physiological functions of glucocorticoids in stress and their relation to pharmacological actions. *Endocrinology Reviews, 5,* 25–44.

Murburg, M. M. (1994). *Catecholamine function in post-traumatic stress disorder: Emerging concepts, progress in psychiatry.* Washington, DC: American Psychiatric Press.

Ohman, A. (1992). Fear and anxiety as emotional phenomena: Clinical, henomenological, evolutionary perspectives, and information-processing mechanisms. In L. M. Haviland (Ed.), *Handbook of the emotions.* New York: Guilford Press.

O'Keefe, J. (1993). Hippocampus, theta, and spatial memory. *Current Opinions in Neurobiology, 3,* 917–924.

O'Keefe, J., & Nadel, L. (1978). *The hippocampus as a cognitive map.* Oxford, England: Clarendon Press.

Orr, S. P. (1990). Psychophysiologic studies of posttraumatic stress disorder. In E. L. Giller (Ed.), *Biological assessment and treatment of posttraumatic stress disorder* (pp. 135–160). Washington, DC: American Psychiatric Press.

Parkinson, J. K., Murray, E. A., & Mishkin, M. (1990). A selective mnemonic role for the hippocampus in monkeys: Memory for the location of objects. *Brain Research Bulletin, 24,* 293–296.

Perry, B. D. (1994). Neurobiological sequelae of childhood trauma: PTSD in children. In M. Murburg (Ed.), *Catecholamine function in post-traumatic stress disorder: Emerging concepts, progress in psychiatry.* Washington, DC: American Psychiatric Press.

Perry, B. D., Giller, E. L. Jr., & Southwick, S. M. (1987). Altered platelet alpha2-adrenergic binding sites in post-traumatic stress disorder. *American Journal of Psychiatry, 144,* 1511–1512.

Perry, B. D., Pollard, R. A., Blakley, T. L., Baker, W. L., & Vigilante, D. (1995). Childhood trauma, the neurobiology of adaptation and use-dependent development of the brain: How states become traits. *Infant Mental Health, 16,* 271–291.

Phillips, R. G., & LeDoux, J. E. (1992). Differential contribution of amygdala and hippocampus to cued and contextual fear conditioning. *Behavioral Neuroscience, 106,* 274–285.

Pitman, R. K. (1989). Posttraumatic stress disorder hormones, and memory [Editorial]. *Biological Psychiatry, 26,* 221–223.

Pitman, R. K., Orr, S. P., Forgue, D. F., Altman, B., de Jong, J. B., & Herz, L. R. (1990). Psychophysiologic responses to combat imagery of Vietnam veterans with posttraumatic stress disorder versus other anxiety disorders. *Journal of Abnormal Psychology, 99,* 49–54.

Post, R. M. (1992). Transduction of psychosocial stress into the neurobiology of recurrent affective disorder. *American Journal of Psychiatry, 49,* 999–1010.

Post, R. M., Weiss, S. R. B., & Smith, M. A. (1995). Sensitization and kindling: Implications for the evolving neural substrates of posttraumatic stress disorder. In M. J. Friedman, D. S. Charney, & A. Y. Deutch (Eds.), *Neurobiological and clinical consequences of stress: From normal adaptation to posttraumatic stress disorder* (pp. 203–224). Philadelphia: Lippincott–Raven.

Prins, A., Kaloupek, D. G., & Keane, T. M. (1995). Psychophysiological evidence for autonomic arousal and startle in traumatized adult populations. In M. J. Friedman, D. S. Charney, & A. Y. Deutch (Eds.), *Neurobiological and clinical consequences of stress: From normal adaptation to posttraumatic stress disorder* (pp. 291–314). Philadelphia: Lippincott–Raven.

Pynoos, R. S., Steinberg, A. M., & Wraith, R. (1995). A developmental model of childhood traumatic stress. In D. Cicchetti & D. J. Cohen (Eds.), *Manual of developmental psychopathology. Vol. 2. Risk, disorder, and adaptation* (pp. 72–95). New York: Wiley.

Rasmusson, A. M., & Charney, D. S. (1997). Animal models of relevance to PTSD. *Annals of the New York Academy of Sciences, 821,* 332–351.

Rauch, S. L., & Shin, L. M. (1997). Functional neuroimaging studies in posttraumatic stress disorder. *Annals of the New York Academy of Sciences, 821,* 83–98.

Reiser, M. (1991). *Memories in mind and brain: What dream imaging reveals.* New York: Basic Books.

Resnick, H. S., Yehuda, R., & Acierno, R. (1997). Acute postrape plasma cortisol, alcohol use, and PTSD symptom profile among recent rape victims. *Annals of the New York Academy of Sciences, 821,* 433–436.

Sapolsky, R. M. (1994). The physiological relevance of glucocorticoid endangerment of the hippocampus. *Annals of the New York Academy of Sciences, 743,* 294–304.

Selden, N. R. W., Everitt, D. J., Jarrard, L. E., & Robbins, T. W. (1991). Complementary roles for the amygdala and hippocampus in aversive conditioning to explicit and contextual cues. *Neuroscience, 42,* 335–350.

Smith, M. A., Davidson, J., & Ritchie, J. C. (1989). The corticotropin-releasing hormone test in patients with posttraumatic stress disorder. *Biological Psychiatry, 26,* 349–355.

Sorg, B. A., & Kalivas, P. W. (1995). Stress and neuronal sensitization. In M. J. Friedman, D. S. Charney, & A. Y. Deutch (Eds.), *Neurobiological and clinical consequences of stress: From normal adaptation to post-traumatic stress disorder* (pp. 83–102). Philadelphia: Lippincott–Raven.

Southwick, S. M., Bremner, D., Krystal, J. H., & Charney, D. S. (1994). Psychobiological research in post-traumatic stress disorder. *Psychiatric Clinics of North America, 17,* 251–264.

Southwick, S. M., Krystal, J. H., Bremner, J. D., Morgan, C. A., Nicolaou, A., Nagy, L. M., Johnson, D., Heninger, G. R., & Charney, D. S. (1997). Noradrenergic and serotonergic function in post traumatic stress disorder. *Archives of General Psychiatry, 54,* 749–758.

Southwick, S. M., Krystal, J. H., Johnson, D. R., & Charney, D. S. (1992). Neurobiology of posttraumatic stress disorder. In A. Tasman & M. B. Riba (Eds.), *Review of psychiatry* (Vol. 11). Washington, DC: American Psychiatric Press.

Southwick, S. M., Krystal, J. H., Morgan, C. A., Johnson, D., Nagy, L. M., Nicolaou, A., Heninger, G., & Charney, D. S. (1993). Abnormal noradrenergic function in post traumatic stress disorder. *Archives of General Psychiatry, 50,* 266–274.

Southwick, S. M., Yehuda, R., & Morgan, C. A. (1995). Clinical studies of neurotransmitter alterations in post-traumatic stress disorder. In M. J. Friedman, D. S. Charney, & A. Y. Deutch (Eds.), *Neurobiological and clinical consequences of stress: From normal adaptation to post-traumatic stress disorder* (pp. 335–349). Philadelphia: Lippincott–Raven.

Stein, M. B., Hanna, C., Koverola, C., Torchia, M., & McClarty, B. (1997). Structural brain changes in PTSD. Does trauma alter neuroanatomy? *Annals of the New York Academy of Sciences, 821,* 76–82.

True, W. R., Rice, J., Eisen, S. A., Heath, A. C., Goldberg, J., Lyons, M. J., & Nowak, J. (1993). A twin study of genetic and environmental contributions to liability for posttraumatic stress symptoms. *Archives of General Psychiatry, 50,* 257–263.

Yehuda, R. (1997). Sensitization of the hypothalamic–pituitary–adrenal axis in posttraumatic stress disorder. *Annals of the New York Academy of Sciences, 821,* 57–75.

Yehuda, R., Boisoneau, M., & Lowy, T. (1995). Dose-response changes in plasma cortisol and lymphocyte glucocorticoid receptors following dexamethasone administration in combat veterans with and without posttraumatic stress disorder. *Archives of General Psychiatry, 52,* 583–593.

Yehuda, R., Giller, E. L., Levengood, R. A., Southwick, S. M., & Siever, L. J. (1995). Hypothalamic–pituitary–adrenal functioning in posttraumatic stress disorder: Expanding the concept of the stress response spectrum. In M. J. Friedman, D. S. Charney, & A. Y. Deutch (Eds.), *Neurobiological and clinical consequences of stress: From normal adaptation to post-traumatic stress disorder* (pp. 351–365). Philadelphia: Lippincott–Raven.

Yehuda, R., Southwick, S. M., & Giller, E. L. (1992). Urinary catecholamine excretion and severity of PTSD symptoms in Vietnam combat veterans. *Journal of Nervous and Mental Disease, 180,* 321–325.

Yehuda, R., Southwick, S. M., & Krystal, J. H. (1993). Enhanced suppression of cortisol following dexamethasone administration in combat veterans with posttraumatic stress disorder and major depressive disorder. *American Journal of Psychiatry, 150,* 83–86.

Zigmond, M. J., Finlay, J. M., & Sved, A. F. (1995). Neurochemical studies of central noradrenergic responses to acute and chronic stress: Implications for normal and abnormal behavior. In M. J. Friedman, D. S. Charney, & A. Y. Deutch (Eds.), *Neurobiological and clinical consequences of stress: From normal adaptation to post-traumatic stress disorder* (pp. 45–60). Philadelphia: Lippincott–Raven.

6

Economic Models

AGNES RUPP and ELIOT SOREL

Health economists play a critical role in defining major public health problems and contributing to decisions regarding the allocation of public resources for research, treatment, and prevention. In recent years, research on estimating the costs of medical diseases and psychiatric conditions has included an emphasis on the social and economic consequences of traumatic stress. As mental health researchers explore the long-term consequences of traumatic stressors, including torture, the ability to look beyond the mental health effects of such experiences and examine the relationship between disorder, disability, and individual functioning will enable nations to address their most pressing public health concerns. In this chapter, we discuss several approaches to studying the economic consequences of disease and disorder and their relevance for understanding the broad social and economic consequences of torture and related violence and trauma.

Medical examination of survivors of torture and related violence and trauma often results in identifying physical or psychiatric illness, or both, in the survivor. Psychiatric outcomes can include posttraumatic stress disorder (PTSD), anxiety, depression, and substance abuse, among others. The economic consequences of such illnesses have traditionally been studied using a cost-of-illness methodology. The purpose of these studies is to enhance our understanding of the nature and extent of an illness and its economic consequences. Estimates of the economic impact associated with an illness are intended to assist policymakers in assigning priorities to specific interventions, including prevention, treatment, and rehabilitation of those affected by the illness.

AGNES RUPP • National Institute of Mental Health, Neuroscience Center Building, Bethesda, Maryland 20892.   ELIOT SOREL • Department of Psychiatry and Behavioral Sciences, George Washington University, 2021 K Street, NW, Washington, D.C. 20006.

The Mental Health Consequences of Torture, edited by Ellen Gerrity, Terence M. Keane, and Farris Tuma. Kluwer Academic/Plenum Publishers, New York, 2001.

From a cost-assessment standpoint, there are no differences in methodological approaches based on the cause of a medical or psychiatric illness. Whether the illness is the result of a natural (e.g., biological agent, earthquake) or human-caused (e.g., torture) disaster or event appears to be irrelevant. Therefore, applying the general economic concept of burden-of-illness to measure the economic consequences of torture and trauma can be a fruitful approach in this new field of policy-relevant scientific inquiry (Fairbank, Ebert, & Zarkin, 1999). In their pioneering literature review on the socioeconomic consequences of traumatic stress, Fairbank et al. apply specific components of the cost-of-illness approach to assess the economic consequences of trauma. In particular, the authors focus on the relationship between trauma and labor market outcomes, which are relevant to the economic productivity-loss issues addressed in the cost-of-illness literature. In reviewing the relatively small number of studies that focus on the relationship between trauma and labor market outcome, which includes studies of Holocaust survivors, childhood sexual and physical abuse survivors, combat veterans, and Southeast Asian refugees, Fairbank et al. provide preliminary evidence to support the association between traumatic stress and reduced labor market outcomes.

This chapter focuses on torture and related violence and trauma that are generally intentional, human-caused events (i.e., when one group of people intentionally damages the physical and psychological health and well-being of an individual or other groups of people) and studies of economic burden. Accordingly, the cost-effectiveness of treatment and preventive interventions is also relevant.

CONCEPTUAL FRAMEWORK

Economic Approaches to Valuing Human Life

Conceptually, to assess the magnitude of damage in the physical and mental health condition and functional economic capacity of an individual who has experienced an illness or trauma, values must be assigned to various aspects of human life, including health and functioning. Economists have generally employed three approaches to valuing human life: the human capital approach, the willingness-to-pay approach, and the utility loss approach. Estimating the economic value of human life is necessary to assess the economic burden of an illness or a disorder. Given that morbidity, disability, and premature mortality affect labor by causing persons to lose time from normal activities and effectiveness at work, in school, and in the household, illness creates an undeniable loss to individuals, families, communities, and the entire society. In the case of torture and trauma, this loss or damage is created intentionally by the torturer to control or punish the individual or group and reduce that person's or group's power.

The Human Capital Approach

The human capital approach places a value on an individual's contribution to national productivity and measures the indirect costs of illness in terms of the market valuation of lost wage earnings resulting from morbidity and mortality. The basic economic principles applied in this approach can be traced back to at least the 17th century (Patty, 1699). While the theory of human capital was developed by Becker (1964) and Mushkin (1962), who are also credited with bringing the human capital method to the health field, several others have contributed to its development and application as well (e.g., Hodgson & Meiers, 1982; Rice, 1996). In the mid-1980s, an advisory committee to the U.S. Public Health Service recommended the use of the human capital approach in cost-of-illness studies to ensure comparability among different estimates.

The Willingness-to-Pay Approach

This approach, proposed by Schelling (1968) and Mishan (1971), attempts to determine the subjective value that individuals would place on being free of the disease or, in this case, the consequences of torture and trauma. This approach, which is more aligned with conventional concepts of welfare economics, essentially values human life according to what individuals would be willing to pay for a change that reduces the probability or risk of the illness or death. Despite the difficulty of measuring the subjective preferences of individuals, which often generates criticism, several studies have been conducted based on this approach (e.g., Hu & Sandifer, 1981).

The Utility Loss Approach

A new disease burden measure, disability adjusted life years (DALYs), has recently been developed (Murray & Lopez, 1996) to measure the global burden of diseases. In Murray and Lopez's worldwide study, DALY was defined and used to provide a comparative index of the burden of 107 diseases and injuries. With this approach to utility loss, the unit of measurement is time rather than a monetary value. Although primarily a measure of burden, it also implicitly measures the value of life when the concepts of disability-free maximum life expectancy and the value of one additional disability-free year lived are introduced in constructing the DALY summary measure. The value of life is expressed in years and is derived from the capacity to generate utility. According to the weighting system of the DALY measure, the relative value of a year of life lived at different ages varies, increasing from birth until approximately the mid-30s, when it begins to decrease.

MAJOR ANALYTIC QUESTIONS

In general, cost-of-illness studies that measure the economic burden of disorder are concerned with two major questions: What are the measurable consequences of an illness, and what kind of economic values can be assigned to these consequences? The remainder of this section is organized around these two questions and is guided by a discussion of relevant research approaches.

What Are the Measurable Consequences of Torture and Related Violence and Trauma?

The following testimony of a torture survivor provides insight into how complex the economic impact of torture can be:

> My profession as a teacher brought me much fulfillment, but in my country, teaching literacy to children and adults was considered a subversive act. And so, they [soldiers] picked me up. I can't tell you everything they did to me. But I will tell you about the "hood." They tied it so tight to my neck, and the lime inside burned, it was like a blazing fire. I couldn't breathe, and I thought I would die. When they took the "hood" off, I still couldn't breathe, and the cell that they kept me in was so tiny I couldn't move. I couldn't breathe. There wasn't any air at all, at least that's how it seemed to me. Then they released me from this hell to the one I live in now.
>
> I was a loving and responsible husband and father and a dedicated teacher. With the money that I earned, I fed my children and bought them clothes. I devoted much of my time to teaching children and women how to read and write. Now that I'm here in this country, nothing is clear anymore. I can't do what I love most, and that is teaching. I'm no longer a good husband and father. With whatever money I can get, I buy liquor. I've even sold things out of our house, the television, canned food, my children's clothes, anything someone will buy, so I can get a drink. When I'm drunk, I can forget at least for a while. But then, later, I feel worse and I become abusive to my wife and children. I don't know why. I try to control this rage. But how can I, if I can't get control of my life? My wife, she's always complaining: "You need to get a job. We don't have money to pay this month's rent. The children need shoes." She doesn't say it, but I know what she means: It's my fault that I can't hold a steady job.
>
> I thought it might change this last time when I found a job in a shoe factory. But then I got fired again. Not because I wasn't doing my job but because there was something about the building that made me feel unsafe. How can I tell you? I felt so confined, and I would start to remember how they used the "hood." My face would start to burn again and I couldn't breathe. I would panic and run outside for air. Just like the soldiers, the supervisor took great pride in his authority and he would ridicule me in front of everyone. His arrogance seemed to imply that he knew everything about me. But he knew nothing of me or what I had been through. Then one day, I couldn't stand it anymore. I lost my temper and broke his nose. I am unemployed again, and we're back on welfare. My youngest son was injured by a land mine and needs an operation. The doctor told us that his condition may worsen if he doesn't have it soon. But without insurance he cannot have the surgery. Why does my son have to suffer? Once I was a teacher who could provide for his family; now I am nothing. (Used with permission.)

In general, studies of the economic impact of an illness focus on the health care costs related to prevention, treatment, rehabilitation, research, and the effect of an illness on productivity loss. Productivity loss that is due to illness and premature death can include educational attainment, labor force participation rate, and productivity and earnings. Ideally, the application of this methodology to cost-of-illness studies concerning torture and related violence and trauma would address the following questions:

1. What type of and how much health and mental health intervention would be required to address the consequences of trauma and torture in a given year and during the survivor's lifetime?
2. What effect does torture and related violence and trauma have on individual productivity in the home and the workplace?
3. How many people die as a result of torture and trauma, and what are the economic consequences of premature death?
4. What kind of loss (in assets, personal property, and accumulated wealth) is experienced by the survivors and victims, including the economic impact on the individual, family, and society?
5. What is the effect of torture and related violence and trauma on the educational attainment of youth?
6. What kind of economic burden is experienced by the family of survivors of torture and trauma; in other words, what is the economic contribution of the family to restore the well-being of the tortured or traumatized family member?
7. What other indicators of the economic impact of torture and related violence and trauma can be assessed (e.g., resources needed for repatriation, relocation, establishing and maintaining refugee camps, handling legal issues)?

Given the nature and variety of torture and trauma experienced by different individuals and groups, primary data collection is often needed to obtain detailed trauma-specific and culturally relevant information to answer the questions described above. This approach is exemplified by the survey work of the Harvard Program in Refugee Trauma on repatriation and disability issues among Khmer adults (Mollica et al., 1993). The primary aim of the Harvard survey was to identify groups at risk for psychosocial disability and economic collapse subsequent to their repatriation to Cambodia. This carefully designed research employed trained interviewers, a bilingual survey instrument based on recent scientific advances in crosscultural research, a sampling design sensitive to sampling requirements, culturally sensitive informed-consent procedures, and collaboration with several international agencies dealing with Cambodian refugees. Economic burden questions concerning family support, work opportunities, and school attendance were included in the questionnaire, which allowed the investigators to at least partially assess the economic consequences of trauma and torture in this refugee population.

Culturally relevant information concerning the consequences of torture and traumatic stress, including their effect on physical and mental health, disability, and functioning, can inform strategies for healing interventions and prevention. For example, several host countries of refugees, including survivors of trauma and torture, have developed guides to educate health professionals regarding the basic principles of working with survivors of torture and trauma and their families. In one such guide, Ferguson and Browne (1991) briefly summarize how torture and trauma may affect the individual, the community, and the family and provide information on how health and human services professionals can address these complex and challenging physical, psychological, social, economic, and family problems. As one indication of the problem, they report that in the late 1980s, about 10% to 30% of the 12,000 refugees annually resettled in Australia were survivors of torture. Focusing on migration policy in Europe in the 1990s, Purcell (1993) observed that many refugees and asylum-seekers were in transition for prolonged periods and emphasized the need for more and better data to develop policies that can successfully address the challenges associated with shifting migration. A 1996 World Health Organization publication, *Mental Health of Refugees*, provides information regarding the likely mental health impact of war, torture, natural disaster, and other traumatic experiences for those working with refugees and other displaced persons. This manual for front-line resettlement workers, planners, and other service providers offers practical advice on helping traumatized individuals and communities in the context of addressing a broad range of issues facing refugees and displaced persons.

Researchers have to make several conceptual and methodological decisions when collecting information about the economic consequences of an illness or a condition. These decisions include whether to focus on prevalence- or incidence-based information concerning exposure and outcomes of interest and whether to pursue causality in explaining the relationship of traumatic experiences, physical and mental health outcomes, and economic consequences.

Prevalence- and Incidence-Based Studies

Prevalence-based studies assess all existing (prevalent) cases of physical and mental health conditions resulting from torture and related violence and trauma in a given year or some other specified time period. The incidence-based approach focuses on new cases (incidence) during a given time period (Hodgson, 1983). The latter approach acquires knowledge about the onset and course of the disease, its duration, survival rates, and other consequences. In general, incidence-based studies require a relatively long study period and are more difficult and costly to conduct than are prevalence-based studies. A clear benefit of the incidence-based approach, however, is that by tracking new cases, the effectiveness of alternative interventions to prevent, treat, or manage a particular condition can be compared.

The following epidemiological data illustrate the importance of this type of information. A report on world mental health, referring to World Bank data of 1993, illustrates gender-specific DALYs, which are presented in Table 1 as a proportion of all years lived with disability for men and women (Desjarlais, Eisenberg Good, & Kleinman, 1995).

Violence and trauma with their potential sequelae of posttraumatic stress disorders, depression, anxiety, and substance abuse are a growing global concern. The manifestations of violence include violence directed against self, violence against others in a family context, random violence against strangers, and

Table 1. Gender-Specific Disability Adjusted Life Years as a Proportion of All Years Lived with Disability

Disability	Women (%)	Men (%)
Depression	25.6	10.4
Self-inflicted injuries	13.9	17.5
PTSD	6.6	3.2
Alcohol and drug dependence	6.1	25.7

Note. From *World Mental Health: Problems and Priorities in Low-Income Countries* (p. 181), by R. Desjarlais, L. Eisenberg, B. Good, and A. Kleinman, 1995, New York: Oxford University Press. Copyright 1995 by Oxford University Press. Reprinted with permission.

group- and state-sponsored terrorism and torture. In addition, PTSD and depression are often co-occurring conditions. According to a selected literature review of PTSD prevalence rates by the World Bank (1993), in all of the 11 studies reviewed, a varying, but significant, proportion of PTSD sufferers also had a diagnosis of major affective disorder. The lack of uniformity in methods used for coding one primary diagnosis over another highlights the need for research on the most meaningful ways of separating co-occurring disorders with the empirical tools of epidemiology, economics, and other disciplines.

Although detailed data on torture rates are not readily available, the epidemiology of broader violence and trauma may stimulate interest in developing economic burden studies and setting priorities for medical research, public health initiatives, and health services development. Similar undertakings could be initiated for refugee, migrant, and war-survivor populations. It seems reasonable that the continuum of public health initiatives and services developed based on the economic burden evidence would include primary, secondary, and tertiary prevention, as well as maintenance and rehabilitation components (Desjarlais et al., 1995). The development of these initiatives will benefit from feedback and collaboration between survivors and their families, care providers, and policymakers (Sorel, 1998). Decisions regarding resource allocation should be based not only on economic factors but also on clinical, ethical, and humane considerations.

Causality and Attribution

The focus of this section is on research to identify the economic consequences of torture and related violence and trauma. However, many of the consequences that follow torture and trauma may be further complicated by a variety of genetic, environmental, behavioral, or even unknown or random factors. The implications of the existence of preexisting conditions, other comorbidities, or both, are an important but often overlooked aspect of the cost estimation process. Whether the comorbidities are independent or interdependent phenomena also requires further inquiry, especially clinical inquiry, so as not to overestimate or underestimate the economic consequences of torture and trauma.

What Economic Values Can Be Assigned to Measurable Consequences?

Questions regarding the economic consequences of torture and related violence and trauma can be classified into three major categories: (a) costs related to physical and mental health care, (b) costs from productivity loss, and (c) other costs.

Economic theory and practice have developed several different approaches to assigning economic values to these three areas. Determining the actual health care expenditures for survivors of trauma and torture (or predicting the amount of health care expenditures that will be necessary) is essential not only to assess the burden of torture and trauma imposed on the health care system but also to inform policy, which will in turn guide efforts to restore the health and mental health of survivors. Conceptually, health care expenditures are assessed on the basis of the opportunity cost principle; the economic resources spent on treating an illness, whether caused by natural or human actions, could be spent on other activities. The more economic resources that are spent on the prevention and treatment of an illness, the larger are the opportunity costs and the more significant are the negative economic consequences of an illness (Heien & Pittman, 1989).

Both the collection of original targeted data and the mining of secondary data sources are useful approaches to assessing the actual value of the economic resources spent on health and mental health services. Asking survivors of torture and trauma how much they spent on health care and asking administrators of refugee camps, religious organizations, private independent foundations, and not-for-profit organizations about their expenditures on an individual or a per capita basis are examples of the use of primary collection strategies. This approach is likely to produce more focused estimates than attempting to extract information from secondary data sources that may have been designed for entirely different purposes (e.g., administrative data, payment records, and other sources that document health and mental health care expenditures or utilization).

Given the many ethical, legal, and political challenges of working with survivors of torture and trauma, the economist researcher is likely to benefit from the use of multiple sources in assessing the economic value of health services used or to be used to reduce the health and mental health damage of torture and trauma and to restore health. A combination of approaches, including special studies focusing on the value of resources and using expert judgment, is needed.

Techniques for Assessing the Costs Related to Health and Mental Health Care

Expenditures for health and related services are relatively straightforward to estimate, especially if the resources and services are exchanged in markets. These can be organized, legitimate markets or, in certain situations, black markets. Once the type and volume of utilization of services are known, this volume can be multiplied by the unit cost of the given service, which is determined by the market, especially the local market, because health care is primarily utilized in local markets.

Various treatment modalities have been proposed for working with survivors of torture and trauma. Interestingly, the reviewed literature regarding healing survivors of human rights violations places more emphasis on the role of nurses and social workers than other physical and mental health professionals (e.g., Laurence, 1992; Ferguson & Browne, 1991). This type of variation can have implications for the overall cost of services. For example, nurses and social workers have a primary role in providing mental health care for survivors of torture. The wage rates in these two professions are generally lower than those for psychologists or psychiatrists; thus, the cost of care per unit is likely to be less.

In the case of publicly provided services, market mechanisms do not apply. Because unit price and unit cost information is not available for a given service, the researcher has to obtain information about the budget of the given institution or program as well as about the number of people served. Once this information is known, the researcher can ascertain what part of the total budget was spent on survivors of torture and trauma or on mental health services for these survivors. Epidemiological data may help researchers in these cases. However, such data will provide only an average cost, and the researcher will not get information about the distribution of the population by the utilization and cost of mental health services. In other words, this technique will not allow the investigator to differentiate between those who make extensive use of the services and those who do not.

Anxiety and depression are two of the most prevalent mental disorders internationally and are frequently associated with torture and trauma. Treatment costs for these disorders have been estimated during the last decade. Stoudemire, Frank, Hedemark, Kamlet, and Blazer (1986), Rice and Miller (1993), Greenberg, Stiglen, Finkelstein, and Berndt (1993), and Kind and Sorensen (1993) have estimated the treatment costs of depression in the United States using different databases. The sole estimate for anxiety disorders (DuPont et al., 1996) is derived from the same database as Rice and Miller. Table 2 includes the most recent treatment cost estimates for several mental disorders in the United States.

The development of more data sources and estimation techniques has led to the refinement of the approaches used to study the economic burden of disease and disorder. However, it is unclear what proportion of these treatment costs can be attributed to mental health concerns associated with torture and related violence and trauma in the immigrant and nonimmigrant populations. It may be possible to statistically estimate what proportion of the user population experienced

Table 2. Treatment Costs of Mental Disorders in Billions of Dollars, United States, 1990

Mental disorder	Billions of dollars
All mental disorders	69.3
Schizophrenia	17.9
Depression	19.9
Anxiety disorders	11.0
Other	20.5

Note. From "Research Policy Implications of Cost-of-Illness Studies for Mental Disorders," by A. Rupp, E. M. Gause, and D. A. Regier, 1998, *British Journal of Psychiatry* (Suppl. 36), pp. 19–25. Copyright 1998 by *British Journal of Psychiatry*. Reprinted with permission.

torture or trauma by the creative use of different primary and secondary data sources. Once these statistics are available, a rough estimate can be developed regarding how much is spent on the treatment of anxiety and depression of patients who have been victims of torture and trauma. It may also lead to a rough cost per treated person estimate, which is an important component of the economic evaluation of health care programs.

As an example, one study (Miller, Cohen, & Rossman, 1993) estimated the medical and mental health treatment costs for rape victims. In 1989 the average medical treatment cost per rape victim in the United States was approximately $5,400, the majority of which involved psychological trauma costs.

Valuation Techniques for Assessing Costs Resulting From Lost Productivity

The Human Capital Approach

Using the human capital approach, a monetary value is assigned to production lost because of illness, impaired functioning in the labor market, and premature death (if torture results in death). These values are based on data regarding actual earnings found among survivors of torture and trauma and earnings of comparison populations (nontortured, nontraumatized) using age- and gender-adjusted national-level data. Fairbank et al. (1999) specifically identified studies that measure the labor market outcome of PTSD, using control or comparison groups and, in certain cases, sophisticated econometric modeling. In some studies, labor market outcomes were measured at a specific point in time (e.g., employment status, hours of work, wage level, occupational status), whereas in other studies, the focus was on labor market history variables (e.g., the number of different jobs in a period of time, periods of unemployment, longest period of time spent with the same employer).

To date researchers have examined associations between four types of traumatic exposure and labor market outcomes: trauma related to the Holocaust, sexual and physical abuse in childhood, combat exposure, and trauma experienced by Southeast Asian refugees. Fairbank et al. (1999) located two studies that compared labor market outcomes for Holocaust survivors with those of individuals who did not directly experience the Holocaust. In both studies, Holocaust survivors exhibited less occupational stability. On the basis of several studies, especially Russell (1986) and Hyman (1993), Fairbank et al. concluded that sexual abuse in childhood can adversely affect women's economic welfare. According to the Hyman study, women who were sexually abused as children earn 10% to 20% less than their nonabused counterparts.

Studies of the role of mental health in the trauma–labor market outcome relationship have most often involved individuals who have experienced combat and other forms of war stress. The most consistent finding in this domain is the relationship between current PTSD and reduced labor market participation among Vietnam veterans. The results of studies of Southeast Asian refugees are inconclusive; some studies report positive correlations between PTSD and negative labor market outcome, whereas others do not. In their summary, Fairbank et al. (1999) emphasized the importance of these studies in justifying the need for treating PTSD, which is a major issue in countries where psychiatric disorders are discriminated against in both privately and publicly financed programs. However, they also cautioned that at present definitive conclusions about the role of PTSD in the trauma–labor market outcome relationship would be premature. They emphasized the importance of improving research methodology concerning both the measurement of the severity of trauma and the development of more comprehensive conceptual models that specify other possible determinants of the trauma–labor market relationship beyond traditional socioeconomic variables. The methodology used to estimate indirect costs must be improved before it will be possible to estimate the full cost of traumatic stress to society.

Economic burden cost-assessment studies are critical to the development of cost–benefit, cost-effectiveness, and cost-utility studies in this area. The relationship between treatment cost and economic loss resulting from untreated depression has led to a cost–benefit analysis on the economic consequences of not treating depression (Rupp, 1995). This study used national-level epidemiological, clinical, and economic data and observed that every dollar spent on the treatment of mood disorders (untreated) yields 1 dollar in the net economic return on employment earnings. In this cost–benefit analysis, the effects of mental health treatment on the use and cost of medical services were also taken into consideration. There is some evidence that mental disorders, especially mood disorders, are associated with increased utilization of general medical care and that appropriate mental health care will reduce this utilization.

It has been argued that investing in and improving access to psychiatric care for a given population has a favorable tradeoff—the general medical care utilization of the same population will decrease. This tradeoff is known as the offset effect or offset hypothesis. The most widely known empirical estimates of the impact of the offset effect come from Mumford, Schlesinger, Glass, Patrick, and Cuerdon (1984), who found that treatment for mental disorders is usually accompanied by a 20% decrease in the use of general medical services. The empirical magnitude of the cost-offset effect in a well-designed study by Strain et al. (1991) is about 10%. A number of cost-offset studies relevant to substance abuse have been conducted over the past 20 years. Jones and Vischi (1979); Saxe, Dougherty, Esty, and Fine (1983); and Holder (1987) reviewed the literature and found evidence that alcohol abuse treatment can reduce the cost of general medical care. In their latest study, Holder and Blose (1992) found that the adjusted mean posttreatment costs of treated alcoholics were 24% lower than comparable costs for untreated alcoholics and that this difference was statistically significant. There have been far fewer drug abuse cost-offset studies. Lennox (1994) conducted a study of a 5-year treatment program and found that at the end of the 5th year the total health care costs of the treated drug abuse group were approximately only $50 higher than the mean costs of the nondependent group. During the pretreatment period, the difference in costs was $150 per month between the two groups.

Another cost-effectiveness study by Zhang, Rost, Fortney, and Smith (1996) on the treatment of depression demonstrates that the additional costs of treatment are more than balanced by reductions in the costs of lost productivity measured by wages. Without this and similar studies, it may be difficult to convince policymakers to allocate resources for the mental health treatment of survivors of torture and trauma beyond addressing the sometimes more dramatic and visible physical health consequences of torture.

The Willingness-to-Pay Approach

To date, the willingness-to-pay approach has not been used for any cost-of-mental-illness study (Rupp, 1995). This approach would measure what individuals would be willing to pay for a change that reduces the probability of torture and trauma and related physical and mental health consequences, including death and disability resulting from torture. Besides asking individuals how much they value the prevention of death and the avoidance of pain, suffering, and the mental and physical consequences of torture and trauma, the method could also determine how much the entire society is willing to pay. The two views may not necessarily be the same, that is, individual and societal values do not necessarily place emphasis on the same age group (in terms of avoidance of death). Different cultures may also have different values about the importance of the avoidance of torture and trauma at the societal and individual levels. Valuing life at different ages is an especially important component of the willingness-to-pay approach, as evidenced in empirical studies using a variety of measures to assess preferences (e.g., Busschbach, Jessing, & de Charro, 1993; Johannesson, 1992).

Another important issue is how much certain societies are willing to pay to care for the survivors of torture and trauma. For example, the United States was willing to pay for the physical and mental health care of Vietnamese refugees who arrived after the Vietnam War by making them eligible for Medicaid benefits through legislation. No previous immigrant or refugee groups have been eligible for this kind of public assistance in the United States. During the mid-1990s, the United States changed the eligibility rules for public assistance to immigrants, which is another indicator of what a society is willing to pay to help immigrants, refugees, asylum-seekers, and others who may be survivors of trauma and torture with health and mental health expenditures, disability benefits, housing costs, and other health and welfare services.

Studying the policies, rules, and regulations of countries that receive refugees regarding access to health and welfare services for torture and trauma survivors might be one approach for developing indicators of how much these recipient countries are willing to pay to help restore the physical and mental health of survivors of trauma and torture (Silove, Sinnerbrink, Field, Manicavasagar, & Steel, 1997). An equally important research question is how much these countries are willing to pay to prevent the politically motivated torture and trauma that frequently victimize disadvantaged individuals (or groups) with social, economic, demographic, biological, and psychological complexities (Akuwe, 1997). The same issue is emphasized by Basoglu (1993), who referred to an Amnesty International report on the global distribution of human rights violations whereby systematic torture and maltreatment were reported in 93 of the 204 countries examined. Reports of torture were more common from regions affected by political unrest, including mass demonstrations, riots, outbreaks of violence, coup attempts, civil war, armed tribal conflict, rebellions, and conflicts with various opposition groups demanding social and political reforms. According to Basoglu, these observations suggest that effective measures against torture and other human rights violations require a multilevel analysis of underlying social, political, cultural, and psychological factors. Such an analysis would entail a large-scale, long-term study and raises the question of how such an undertaking, as well as the implementation of its findings, would be funded. It is important to note that the World Bank (1993) has dealt with the health dimensions of dislocation by examining the places of dislocation, precipitators of distress, health consequences, and recommendations for policy, including a wide range of preventive and other actions. However, who should pay to carry out these policy recommendations is not discussed. Public financing of these activities is even more complex given the large economic disparities that exist not only between countries but also within the borders of certain countries. As the same World Bank report pointed out, global economic policies more often than not reinforce the economic status of the richest people in countries that struggle with great economic inequality.

The Utility Loss Approach

The comparative index of DALYs estimates the number of disability adjusted life years that are lost as a result of premature death measured by years of life lost (YLL) and years lived with disability (YLD) (see Table 3). One important application of the DALY is its use to measure the effect of violence and war in all of the involved countries for 1990. Volume I of *The Global Burden of Disease* series (Murray & Lopez, 1996) provides the only empirical data that may help to inform estimates of the economic burden of torture and related violence and trauma.

Table 3. Leading Causes of the Disability Adjusted Life Years (DALYs) at Ages 15–44 Years, 1990, World Statistics

Rank	Disease or injury	DALYs in thousands	Cumulative %
	All causes	419,144	
1	Unipolar major depression	42,972	10.3
2	Tuberculosis	19,673	14.9
3	Road traffic accidents	19,625	19.6
4	Alcohol use	4,848	23.2
5	Self-inflicted injuries	14,645	26.7
6	Bipolar disorder	13,189	29.8
7	War	13,134	32.9
8	Violence	12,955	36.0
9	Schizophrenia	12,542	39.0
10	Iron deficiency anemia	12,511	42.0

Note. From *The Global Burden of Disease* (Table 5.4), edited by C. J. L. Murray and A. L. Lopez, 1996, Cambridge, MA: Harvard University Press, pp. 433–469. Copyright 1996 by World Health Organization. Adapted with permission.

These data clearly indicate that violence and war generate a substantial economic burden on societies as measured by DALYs. The DALY methodology is complex and makes assumptions that are subject to debate and therefore refinement. For example, life expectancy is measured by the longest life expectancy in the world and assumes that every individual has an equal chance of living the longest possible life regardless of whether he or she is born in a more- or less-developed country. Another major methodological issue concerns the assessment of disability for the different disease and injury categories. These assessments are based on expert judgment for hypothetical cases. This methodology is currently being refined by a World Health Organization study on disability measurement. Despite such shortcomings, further application of this methodology may contribute to our understanding of the effect of trauma and torture on health. Table 4 provides more detailed data on the burden associated with war and violence.

Table 4. Deaths, Years of Life Lost (YLL), Years Lived With Disability (YLD), and Disability Adjusted Life Years (DALYs) by Cause in 1990

	Deaths	YLL	YLD	DALYs
	(in thousands)			
Established market economies				
Violence	30	778	214	993
War	—	1	1	2
Formerly socialist economies of Europe				
Violence	30	698	149	847
War	29	880	269	1,149
India				
Violence	56	1,328	182	1,510
War	3	95	23	119
China				
Violence	51	1,404	234	1,638
War	1	19	7	26
Other Asia and Pacific Islands				
Violence	51	1,356	179	1,534
War	15	452	141	598
Sub-Saharan Africa				
Violence	205	6,008	568	6,576
War	268	8,125	2,574	10,698
Latin America and the Caribbean				
Violence	102	2,825	347	3,172
War	17	522	166	698
Middle Eastern Crescent				
Violence	39	1,142	60	1,201
War	169	5,119	1,625	6,744
World				
Violence	563	15,540	1,932	17,472
War	502	15,213	4,807	20,019

Note. From *The Global Burden of Disease* (Annex Tables 6a through 6i), edited by C. J. L. Murray and A. L. Lopez, 1996, Cambridge, MA: Harvard University Press, p. 270. Copyright 1996 by World Health Organization. Reprinted with permission.

The DALY measure is expected to be used internationally for measuring the burden-of-illnesses and for normative health outcome measurement. Therefore, the use of DALYs in studying the consequences of torture and related violence and trauma has potential merit. Volume VIII in *The Global Burden of Disease* series, *The Global Burden of Injuries: Mortality and Disability from Suicide, Violence, War, and Unintentional Injuries* (Murray & Lopez, 1996), should be studied more closely to obtain information on specific injuries, including intentional injuries. This could include, for example, examining injuries that are coded two ways in the *International Statistical Classification of Diseases and Related Health Problems* (10th edition) (World Health Organization, 1992): according to the external cause of injury (E codes) and according to the nature of injury (N codes). Using DALYs, one can also estimate short- and long-term disabilities stemming from each source of injury. However, the available resources do not currently clarify the psychological components contributing to disability. An important methodological advance in the use of DALYs is to estimate the average duration of treated and untreated forms of each source of injury, which brings this approach relatively close to conducting cost-effectiveness analysis for different interventions. In short, further study of DALY methodology and consultation with the authors is necessary to fully exploit this approach in torture and trauma studies.

Other Costs

Several cost items associated with the consequences of torture and trauma may belong to the "other cost" category. For illustrative purposes, we focus on two areas: the cost to families and legal cost. As McGuire (1991) pointed out, the most significant innovation in the cost methodology of the large-scale cost-of-mental-illness study conducted by Rice (1996) is the inclusion of family costs. The focus of measurement here is on the value of time contributed by family members to care for their sick relative. The family contribution may include actual home care for the patient, leaving the labor force (thereby experiencing wage loss) to care for the relative, or, conversely, entering the labor force to pay for the health care costs of the relative; the value of time spent on transportation; and the like.

Often children are affected as well, particularly those in lower socioeconomic groups or those in situations where the entire family household collapses, which is referred to as property loss in cost-assessment studies. Additionally, years lost from school can have long-term consequences on the development of the economic capacity and well-being of children. In a study by Miller, Cohen, and Rossman (1993), the value of lost school days is calculated in monetary terms using administrative data from public schools. In 1993 each lost school day was valued at $23.96. This value is considered an economic loss because the student cannot use these available educational opportunities.

Contact of torture and trauma survivors with the legal system can be analyzed from two perspectives: (a) they meet lawyers to go through the refugee or asylum-seeking process or (b) as a consequence of torture and trauma, they come to the attention of the legal system of the receiving country. Some of these legal costs are financed by public resources; however, in other cases the survivor, the family, or both are responsible for paying these expenditures. Legally processing the cases of tens of thousands of refugees and asylum-seekers is not a negligible economic burden for the individual or the receiving country.

THE ROLE OF ECONOMIC BURDEN MEASURES

The purpose of conducting economic burden studies of various disorders is to assist policymakers in setting priorities for medical research and health care services. These studies measure the economic impact of an illness without paying specific attention to the effectiveness of the medical interventions or evaluating whether the population is undertreated or overtreated for a specific condition. Economic burden measures can play an important role in conducting cost–benefit, cost-effectiveness, and cost-utility analyses that evaluate the relative outcomes of various interventions. Keane (1998) urges researchers of PTSD treatment to employ measures that assess social and occupational functioning after treatment and without treatment interventions. As the DALY literature clearly indicates, without treatment intervention the lost productivity measured by DALYs or other methods can be higher than in cases where an illness is appropriately treated. Whether the additional cost of treatment is being offset in reduction of DALYs or other productivity-loss measures is an empirical question that can be analyzed with economic evaluation techniques (see the cost-offset studies discussed earlier). To mitigate the effect of torture and trauma, once it occurs, through treatment intervention is considered secondary prevention by public health policymakers. Policymakers and health professionals have a significant opportunity to learn from each other and effectively influence policy, the allocation of resources, and multisectoral collaboration (Sorel, 1997).

The role of primary prevention should not be overlooked, and it may be helpful to borrow successful approaches for studying and addressing natural disasters. For example, advances in architectural design used to build new structures can save human lives during earthquakes. Given the trend toward increasing incidents of violence, there is no reason not to invest in research on the prevention of torture, trauma, and violence. The cost-effectiveness of research to develop primary prevention methods for violence, torture, and trauma should be studied, including research on the tortured and the torturer. These studies can form the basis for local, national, and international policy concerning the prevention of torture and trauma.

CONCLUSIONS

In this chapter, we have borrowed from the general economic burden-of-illness literature and applied and adopted some of those concepts and methods specifically for torture and related violence and trauma. This represents a modest step toward integrating these fields of research at a time when torture and trauma are widespread in many parts of the world. The next step is to estimate the economic burden of torture and trauma in empirical studies. Many of the estimation issues are complex and exist in different conceptual frameworks that will benefit from the insights accumulated through empirical studies.

Regarding the literature discussed in this chapter, one can readily reach the following conclusions:

- Better methods and more detailed data are needed regarding the relative costs of physical and mental health services for treating survivors of torture, as well as approaches for estimating the indirect costs to individuals, families, and societies.
- Treatment for specific mental disorders has been accompanied by decreases in the use of general medical services; without treatment intervention, losses in productivity, measured by the DALY and other methods, can be higher than in cases when an illness is appropriately treated.
- Policymakers on a global basis are well advised by history to pay attention to the consequences of traumatic stress, including torture and human rights violations, not only for humanitarian reasons, but also for economic solvency and stability.

REFERENCES

Akuwe, C. (1997). Torture in the 21st century. *Torture, 7*(3), 82–87.

Basoglu, M. (1993). Prevention of torture and care of survivors: An integrated approach. *Journal of the American Medical Association, 270*(5), 606–611.

Becker, G. S. (1964). *Human capital: A theoretical and empirical analysis, with special reference to education.* New York: National Bureau of Economic Research, Columbia University Press.

Busschbach, J. J., Jessing, D. J., & de Charro, F. T. (1993). The utility of health at different stages of life: A quantitative approach. *Social Science and Medicine, 37*(2), 153–158.

Desjarlais, R., Eisenberg, L., Good, B., & Kleinman, A. (1995). *World mental health: Problems and priorities in low-income countries* (p. 181). New York: Oxford University Press.

DuPont, R. L., Rice, D. P., Miller, S. M., Shiraki, S., Rowland, C. R., & Harwood, R. J. (1996). The economic costs of anxiety disorders. *Anxiety, 2,* 167–172.

Fairbank, J. A., Ebert, L., & Zarkin, G. A. (1999). Socioeconomic consequences of traumatic stress. In P. A. Saigh & J. D. Bremmer (Eds.), *Posttraumatic stress disorder: A comprehensive text.* Boston: Allyn & Bacon.

Ferguson, B., & Browne, E. (1991). *Health care and immigrants: A guide for the helping professions.* Sydney, Australia: MacLennan and Petty.

Greenberg, P. E., Stiglen, L. E., Finkelstein, S. N., & Berndt, E. R. (1993). The economic burden of depression in 1990. *Journal of Clinical Psychiatry, 54*(11), 405–418.

Heien, D. M., & Pittman, D. J. (1989). The economic costs of alcohol abuse: An assessment of current methods and estimates. *Journal of Studies on Alcohol, 50,* 567–569.

Hodgson, T. A. (1983). The state of the art of cost-of-illness estimates. *Advances in Health Economics and Health Services Research, 4,* 129–164.

Hodgson, T. A., & Meirs, M. (1982). Cost-of-illness methodology: A guide to current practices and procedures. *Milbank Memorial Fund Quarterly, 60,* 429–462.

Holder, H. D. (1987). Alcoholism treatment and potential health care cost saving. *Medical Care, 25,* 52–70.

Holder, H. D., & Blose, J. O. (1992). The reduction of health care costs associated with alcoholism treatment: A 14-year longitudinal study. *Journal of Studies on Alcohol, 53,* 293–302.

Hu, T. W., & Sandifer, F. H. (1981). *Synthesis of cost of illness methodology.* Washington, DC: Public Services Library, Georgetown University.

Hyman, B. (1993). *The economic consequences of child sexual abuse in women.* Doctoral dissertation, Brandeis University, Waltham, MA. (UMI Dissertation Services, No. 9408865)

Johannesson, M. (1992). On the discounting of gained life-years in cost-effectiveness analysis. *International Journal of Technology Assessment in Health Care, 8*(2), 359–364.

Jones, D. R., & Vischi, J. R. (1979). Impact of alcohol drug abuse and mental health treatment of medical care utilization: A review of the research literature. *Medical Care, 17,* 1–82.

Keane, T. (1998). Psychological and behavioral treatment of posttraumatic stress disorder. In P. E. Nathan & J. M. Gorman (Eds.), *A guide to treatments that work.* New York: Oxford University Press.

Kind, P., & Sorensen, J. (1993). The costs of depression. *International Clinical Psychopharmacology, 7*(3–4), 191–195.

Laurence, R. (1992). Part II: The treatment of torture survivors: A review of the literature. *Issues in Mental Health Nursing, 13*(4), 311–320.

Lennox, R. D. (1994). *Health care costs reductions associated with drug abuse treatment financed under employment based health insurance.* Chapel Hill, NC: Pacific Institute for Research and Evaluation. Unpublished manuscript.

McGuire, T. G. (1991). Measuring the economic costs of schizophrenia. *Schizophrenia Bulletin, 17,* 375–388.

Miller, T. R., Cohen, M. A., & Rossman, S. B. (1993). Victim costs of violent crime and resulting injuries. *Health Affairs, 12*(4), 186–197.

Mishan, E. J. (1971). Evaluation of life and limb: A theoretical approach. *Journal of Political Economy, 79,* 687–705.

Mollica, R. F., Donelan, K., Tor, S., Lavelle, J., Elias, C., Frankel, M., & Blendon, R. J. (1993). The effect of trauma and confinement on functional health and mental health status of Cambodians living in Thailand–Cambodian border camps. *Journal of the American Medical Association, 270*(5), 581–586.

Mumford, E., Schlesinger, H. J., Glass, G. V., Patrick, C., & Cuerdon, T. (1984). A new look at evidence about reduced cost of medical utilization following mental health treatment. *American Journal of Psychiatry, 141*(10), 1145–1158.

Murray, C. J. L., & Lopez, A. L. (Eds.). (1996). *The global burden of disease.* Cambridge, MA: Harvard University Press.

Mushkin, S. J. (1962). Health as an investment. *Journal of Political Economy, 70*(5), 129–157.

Patty, W. (1699). *Political arithmetick, or a discourse concerning the extent and value of lands, people, buildings, etc.* London: Robert Cuel.

Purcell, J. N., Jr. (1993, November). Migration challenges of the 1990s. *The World Today,* 216–219.

Rice, D. P. (1996). Estimating the cost of illness. *Health Economics Series,* No. 6 (DHEW Pub. No. PHS 947-6). Rockville, MD: Department of Health, Education, and Welfare.

Rice, D. P., & Miller, S. M. (1993). The economic burden of affective disorders. In T. W. Hu & A. Rupp (Eds.), *Research in the economics of mental health* (pp. 37–53). Greenwich, CT: JAI Press.

Rupp, A. (1995). The economic consequences of not treating depression. *British Journal of Psychiatry, 166*(Suppl. 27), 29–33.

Rupp, A., Gause, E. M., & Regier, D. A. (1998). Research policy implications of cost-of-illness studies for mental disorders. *British Journal of Psychiatry, 173*(Suppl. 36), 19–25.

Russell, D. E. H. (1986). *The secret trauma: Incest in the lives of girls and women.* New York: Basic Books.

Saxe, L., Dougherty, D., Esty, K., Fine, M. (1983). *The effectiveness and costs of alcoholism treatment* (Report prepared under contract to the Office of Technology Assessment). Washington, DC: Congress of the United States.

Schelling, T. C. (1968). The life you save may be your own. In S. B. Chase (Ed.), *Problems in public expenditure analysis* (pp. 127–176). Washington, DC: Brookings Institution.

Silove, D., Sinnerbrink, I., Field A., Manicavasagar, V., & Steel, Z. (1997). Anxiety, depression and PTSD in asylum-seekers: Associations with pre-migration trauma and post-migration stressors. *British Journal of Psychiatry, 170*, 351–357.

Sorel, E. (1997). An invaluable asset for a robust economy and democracy. *Journal of the Pontifical Council for Pastoral Assistance to Health Care Workers, 12*(34), 86–87.

Sorel, E. (1998). Social psychiatry: A vision and a mission for the 21st century. *International Medical Journal, 4*, 237–249.

Stoudemire, A., Frank, R. G., Hedemark, N., Kamlet, M., & Blazer, D. (1986). The burden of depression. *General Hospital Psychiatry, 8*, 388–394.

Strain, J. J., Lyons, J. S., Hammer, J. S., Fahs, M., Lebovits, A., Paddison, P. L., Snyder, S., Strauss, E., Burton, R., & Nuber, G. (1991). Cost offset from a psychiatric consultation-liaison intervention with elderly hip fracture patients. *American Journal of Psychiatry, 148*(8), 1044–1049.

World Bank. (1993). *World development report: Investing in health.* New York: Oxford University Press.

World Health Organization. (1992). *International statistical classification of diseases and related health problems.* (10th edition). Geneva, Switzerland: Author.

World Health Organization. (1996). *Mental health of refugees.* Geneva, Switzerland: Author.

Zhang, M., Rost, K. M., Fortney, J. C., & Smith, G. R. (1996, September). *Economic returns on treatment for depression.* Paper presented at the Eighth Biennial Research Conference on the Economics of Mental Health, Bethesda, MD.

III

Torture and the Trauma of War

7

Refugees and Asylum-Seekers

J. DAVID KINZIE and JAMES M. JARANSON

The trauma stories of refugees are told in many different ways. Because of the complexity and difficulty of the experiences, the stories often are related as unstructured, and sometimes confusing, narratives. Some memories have been forgotten. Some are pronounced, intrusive, and painful. The story is rarely coherent or chronologically straightforward. Those providing care have a responsibility on hearing these stories to help organize them in a way that makes sense to the patient and that will help guide health care decisions. One story follows here.

The patient, Sue, is a 38-year-old Cambodian woman with four children. She entered the clinic and complained of a severe headache that had been present for 7 years. She said that she has had trouble with dizziness since the age of 13, but it has been much worse since she arrived in the United States in 1989. None of the medical evaluations have determined what was wrong. Sue has had very poor concentration, decreased sleep, and poor appetite resulting in a 16-pound weight loss. She had no interest in anything, and nothing gave her any pleasure. Sue states if she didn't have children, she feels that she should die. Since leaving Cambodia, she has had marked nightmares, involving scenes of Pol Pot beating her and threatening to cut her throat. She becomes terrified every night. She is irritable with herself and [her] children. Sue has marked intrusive thoughts about the problems she suffered in Cambodia and tries to avoid all thoughts and to keep them out of her mind. These efforts have been unsuccessful.

Sue says her earlier life had always been bad. She was born poor and always felt inferior. Even at the time of her wedding, bombs went off and ruined that occasion. She was expecting her second child when Pol Pot came to power in 1975. Her husband was then executed and her father died of starvation. Sue herself had to endure 4 years of hard labor, where she was frequently beaten and denied food and was sick much of the time.

J. DAVID KINZIE • Department of Psychiatry, Oregon Health Sciences University, Portland, Oregon 97201.   JAMES M. JARANSON • Department of Psychiatry, University of Minnesota, St. Paul, Minnesota 55108-1300.

The Mental Health Consequences of Torture, edited by Ellen Gerrity, Terence M. Keane, and Farris Tuma. Kluwer Academic/Plenum Publishers, New York, 2001.

In 1979, she learned her name was on the execution list, but the Vietnamese invaded before death occurred. She married again in 1980. When Sue and her family tried to escape to Thailand, a land mine exploded and blew off her husband's leg. The family suffered a devastating robbery in the Thai camp, and her life was threatened. Sue cried softly throughout the interview, appeared extremely sad, and was very overwhelmed by the interview. Her primary problems most recently were missing her mother, who died in Cambodia, and feeling unappreciated by her husband and her children. She did agree that the many severe life events she described may be affecting her now. (Used with permission.)

Information gathered through research, clinical and case reports, and service programs has documented the challenging psychological and social problems faced by refugees, immigrants, and asylum-seekers. The psychological challenges faced by these groups are further complicated by the demands of adjustment to a new country and dealing with the losses of homeland, culture, social ties, and former economic status (Ekblad, Ginsburg, Jansson, & Levi, 1994). Many of these individuals migrated because of the forces of war and ethnic strife and had difficult experiences in concentration camps, refugee camps, or both, including systematic torture and trauma. Asylum-seekers are those requesting refuge in a new country because of the political circumstances in their homeland and because their lives and the lives of others are threatened if they are forced to return. Documentation of the experiences of these groups has provided the growing evidence of the challenges they face, including high rates of psychological trauma, torture, and murder, sometimes resulting in serious psychological and psychiatric problems for survivors.

SCOPE OF THE PROBLEM

The number of refugees in forced migration circumstances has risen to a world crisis level, with a 1992 estimate reaching 16 million people. This figure does not include the 2 million refugees involved in the Yugoslavia crisis (Leopold & Harrell-Bond, 1994). An additional 15 to 25 million internally displaced persons did not cross political borders (and therefore are not classified as "refugees") and are also not included in this estimate. Thus, the world situation now includes about 40 to 50 million migrants. Among the recognized groups of forced migrants, the largest group (almost 10 million) is located in Middle Eastern and South Asian countries. The second largest group (about 5 million) is distributed throughout Africa.

The experiences of some refugee groups have been more extensively documented; thus, information on psychological problems and psychiatric disorders of these groups is more available. For example, the aftermath of the Vietnam War resulted in 700,000 refugees from Vietnam, Cambodia, and Laos who sought a secondary country for asylum (Mollica, 1994). Civil war in Nicaragua, El Salvador, and Guatemala displaced 2 million people (Farias, 1991). Many Kurds, Afghans, and Palestinians are living as refugees in their own lands (Dadfur, 1994; El-Sarraj, Tawahina, & Heine, 1994; Karadaghi, 1994). Genocide in the former Yugoslavia has displaced millions (Weine, 1997). Information about these refugee groups has been relatively more accessible.

STUDIES OF PSYCHOLOGICAL PROBLEMS
IN REFUGEE POPULATIONS

Formal research on refugees began after World War II with studies of the Jewish survivors of the brutal effects of the Nazi concentration camps. Some studies documented the serious and chronic effects of massive trauma, including fear, paranoia, depression, anxiety, and personality change (Benshein, 1960; Eitinger, 1960; Klein, 1974; Mattusek, 1975; Niederland, 1964; Ostwald & Bittner, 1968; Venzlaff, 1967). A "concentration camp syndrome," characterized by fatigue, irritability, restlessness, anxiety, and depression, was observed. A study in Norway found the post–World War II rate of schizophrenia among refugees to be five times higher than the rate among the nonrefugee Norwegian population (Eitinger, 1959). A high rate of schizophrenia was also found among European refugees in Australia but not among Jewish refugees, who instead had a high rate of "concentration camp syndrome" (Krupinski, Stoller, & Wallace, 1973).

The arrival of Indo-Chinese refugees in the United States after 1975 sparked additional research with refugees. With the introduction of the third edition of the *Diagnostic and Statistical Manual of Mental Disorders* diagnostic criteria (American Psychiatric Association, 1980), reliable psychiatric diagnoses became possible. Depression and then posttraumatic stress disorder (PTSD) among Southeast Asian refugees began to be documented more systematically (Boehnlein, Kinzie, Rath, & Fleck, 1985; Kinzie, Fredrickson, Rath, & Fleck, 1984; Kinzie, Tran, Breckenridge, & Bloom, 1980; Kroll et al., 1989; Westermeyer, 1988). Research studies with Vietnamese refugees, following the brutal Cambodian regime of Pol Pot from 1975 to 1979, revealed the effects of severe trauma and particularly high rates of PTSD. A diagnosis of PTSD was found among 50% of the clients at a Southeast Asian clinic. A differential effect was found in a similar clinic, in which PTSD was found to be 92% among Cambodians, 93% among Mien, and about 54% among Vietnamese (Kinzie et al., 1990). In community samples of Cambodians, rates of PTSD have ranged from 12% (Chung & Kagawa-Singer, 1993) to 50% (Kinzie, 1988) to 86% (Carlson & Rosser-Hogan, 1991).

In a longitudinal study of Cambodian adolescent refugees, rates of both depression and PTSD were also at about 50%. However, depressive symptoms diminished over time, whereas PTSD symptoms were more persistent and episodic (Kinzie, Sack, Angell, & Clarke, 1989; Kinzie, Sack, Angell, & Manson, 1986). Among Cambodian refugees, children with PTSD were less disabled than the adults, who had more symptoms (Sack et al., 1994). In one study of refugees along the Thai border, reports of traumatic mental health consequences were most extensive among the more highly educated people. Symptoms of clinical depression appeared in two thirds of the participants; PTSD was documented in one third of participants (Mollica, Poole, & Tor, 1998). Additionally, 15% to 20% of these refugees reported health impairments, limited activity, and moderate to severe bodily pain, with the remaining 80% reporting only fair or poor health (Mollica et al., 1993). Another study of Cambodian adolescents along the Thailand–Cambodia border revealed a high level of cumulative trauma and a positive dose–effects association of trauma exposure and symptoms (Mollica, Poole, Son, Murray, & Tor, 1997). The most common symptoms were somatic complaints, social withdrawal, attention problems, anxiety, and depression. No predictable relationship was found between trauma exposure and physical health or social functioning with this group.

Notably, some refugee studies have indicated that schizophrenia seems to be related to exposure to massive trauma. In a diagnostic study of the first 100 Cambodian refugee patients at a mental health clinic, 7 had schizophrenia and most also had PTSD (Kinzie & Boehnlein, 1993). The behavior and symptoms of all 7 of the patients diagnosed with schizophrenia were severe and extremely distressing to their families—all required hospitalization because of bizarre, agitated, threatening, and disruptive behavior. Three were threatening their own lives or those of others with knives. All had auditory hallucinations and delusions unrelated to the Pol Pot trauma. These patients were treated with antipsychotic medicine and, over the next several years, had reduction in delusions, hallucinations, and agitation, but they remained isolated, withdrawn, and socially impaired. One committed suicide 18 months after evaluation despite intensive treatment. Another large clinic with a higher proportion of Vietnamese refugees reported that about 20% of the patients were diagnosed with schizophrenia. Although not a widespread finding, the association between extreme trauma and severe symptoms such as these warrants further research.

Psychological problems and symptoms have been reported in other refugee studies. One study with refugees from El Salvador described men as having problems with nightmares, alcohol abuse, and loss of control, whereas the women reported angry feelings, somatic complaints, and crying (Farias, 1991). Of 30 children exposed to warfare in Central America, 10 had PTSD (Arroyo & Eth, 1985). Among Chilean and Salvadoran migrants, those who had experienced torture had higher rates of PTSD than those who had experienced neither torture nor trauma (Thompson & McGorry, 1995). Of the 87 Ethiopian Jews who journeyed to Israel, 27% had moderate to severe psychological symptoms (Arieli & Aycheh, 1992). Among 38 young Afghan refugees, 13 had PTSD, depression, or both (Mghir, Freed, Raskin, & Katon, 1995). Reports of Afghan refugees in Pakistan indicated a high prevalence of severe trauma and torture. The most common psychological symptoms were anxiety and depression, the latter of which was more often found among the torture survivors. Substance abuse had also increased in this group (Dadfur, 1994).

Studies of Bosnian refugees have shown that among the Bosnian survivors of "ethnic cleansing," 65% had PTSD and 35% had depression (Weine et al., 1995). Bosnian family life has been disrupted because of the massive trauma (Weine, Vojvoda, Hartman, & Hyman, 1997).

As a rule, asylum-seekers arrive in a country on a temporary visa and request refugee status. During a lengthy waiting period, while their refugee status claims are reviewed, basic services are not allowed, and they live under threat of forced repatriation (Silove, Sinnerbrink, Field, Manicavasagar, & Steel, 1997). In a study of 104 Burmese political dissidents who escaped to Thailand and survived without legal protection, the participants reported experiencing an average of 30 traumatic events (Allden et al., 1996). Of the 104 individuals, 38% had elevated depressive symptoms, and 23% met criteria for PTSD. Symptoms of avoidance and increased arousal were positively related to the cumulative trauma exposure, and ongoing symptoms were related to their unclear future and legal status. In a study of Tamil migrants in Australia, asylum-seekers had similar trauma and psychiatric symptoms as other refugees, but they had increased postmigration stress related to their insecure residency status (Silove, Steel, McGorry, & Mohan, 1997). These authors concluded that premigration trauma accounted for 20% of the variance in PTSD, whereas postmigration stress, including loss of culture and support, problems with health care and welfare, and adjustment difficulties, contributed 14% of the variance (Silove et al., 1997). Among Cambodian adolescents, war trauma was found to relate to PTSD symptoms, whereas postmigration stress related to depression (Sack, Clarke, & Seeley, 1996).

BIOLOGICAL, SOCIAL, AND CULTURAL EFFECTS OF TORTURE AND TRAUMA

Studies have shown that survivors of torture and trauma experience many of the same psychological symptoms, even when they are from different cultures and are exposed to different traumatic events. These symptoms include hyperarousal, reexperiencing of the event, avoidance behavior, amnesic episodes, difficulty concentrating, and poor memory. Difficulties with concentration and memory (both symptoms of PTSD) are very common and are subjectively very distressing to refugees. In some instances, these symptoms are related to head injury, a very common experience of survivors of torture (Goldfeld, Mollica, Pesavento, & Faraone, 1988).

Medication is helpful in some instances. For example, clonidine, a central nervous system antagonist of norepinephrine, appears to decrease nightmares and improve sleep (Kinzie, Sack, & Riley, 1994). Reactivation tests with Cambodian refugees showed increased cardiovascular response to traumatic videotapes, which was not found in similar studies with Vietnam veterans (Kinzie et al., 1998). Irritability, along with numbing and the lack of ability to handle frustration, may lead to serious marital distress, even domestic violence and divorce (Masaki & Wong, 1997).

Over time, treatment of Cambodian and Vietnamese inpatient and community samples has been successful in reducing both intrusive and hyperarousal symptoms. However, a large number of people have reactivation of these symptoms with moderate or severe stress, such as accidents, assault, surgery, family disruption, and even exposure to violence in the media. This tendency to reactivation, even 18 years after the original trauma, is a troubling and challenging aspect of the disorder and clearly indicates its chronicity even in those who are functioning well (Kinzie, 1988).

The long-term relationship of physical disease and PTSD among torture survivors is complicated and challenging for researchers. One recent report indicated that cardiovascular, cerebrovascular, and gastrointestinal diseases were more common in World War II and Korean War veterans with PTSD (Schnurr, Spiro, & Paris, 1997). However, another study compared rates of hypertension, diabetes, cerebrovascular accidents, or myocardial infarction among prisoners of war and the general population but did not find significant differences (Eberly & Engdahl, 1991). Many refugees reported marked somatic distress (Mollica et al., 1993), and 15% to 20% of refugees reported health impairments. To determine the long-term effects and disability of traumatized refugees, more detailed longitudinal studies are needed.

Among refugees, reported rates of substance abuse appear to be the primary symptom difference linked to cultural differences. For example, unlike the higher rates seen with American veterans, Asians tend to have lower rates of alcoholism. But among Central American refugee males, substance abuse is fairly common (Farias, 1991). A second cultural difference seems to be the personal need for detail recall and recollection of the torture experience and the willingness to re-member or report such information. In some reports, the Indo-Chinese tend to minimize their problems and are reluctant to talk about the events. When they have been compelled to tell their stories, they tend to have marked reexacerbation of nightmares and intrusive thoughts. This reexacerbation may relate to their Bud-dhist culture, with its sense of fate and a personal sense of shame about terrible deeds done by their countrymen. Alternatively, South American refugees seem to be more willing and perhaps even helped by the experience of recalling and de-scribing the trauma in detail (Morris & Silove, 1992).

RESEARCH RECOMMENDATIONS

These early studies have revealed areas for future research, including the following:

- Long-term study of the symptoms of patients, including the persistence of PTSD symptoms, concentration and learning problems, ability to work, and health problems, is needed. Many studies have shown that participants may experience increased vulnerability to stress with reactivation of the symptoms. This vulnerability needs to be documented further. Such vul-nerability has important implications for treatment philosophy and dis-ability evaluations.

- The effects of recalling the trauma itself in the absence of treatment or other consistently supportive environments need to be evaluated. It is possible that by breaking down avoidance and numbing, symptoms may actually increase. This effect of recall is particularly important when many individuals are be-ing required or urged to make public statements about the atrocities in-flicted on them in the past. Such statements may, in fact, exacerbate symptoms. Legal and social needs may be at variance with the personal needs of patients who may be fearful or made vulnerable by such demands for expression. The effects of these public or even private expressions of past experiences need to be better understood, with a goal of developing poli-cies for these requirements in different settings and procedures for appro-priately supporting patients who experience increased symptoms.

- The effects of pharmacotherapy need to be studied. Medication has been shown to be helpful for certain symptoms, particularly intrusive symptoms of sleep disturbance in PTSD. The effects of pharmacotherapy should be further explored with survivors of torture in various cultures.
- Evidence and nature of comorbidity among refugees needs to be documented. Much of the American experience with veterans has been heavily focused on related problems of substance abuse. This focus seems to be less true for many refugees and asylees, although for some, such as Afghans and Central Americans, this problem may be increasing and would require changes in the course of treatment efforts.
- The effectiveness of insight therapy needs to be studied. Many therapists have emphasized psychodynamic insight, understanding, and reintegration of the trauma as major components of treatment. Other therapists working with similar patients have found this approach less helpful. The differential effects of psychotherapy should be studied with particular emphasis on long-term follow-up studies, the value of group therapy, and the value of indigenous treatments. Many indigenous treatments have never been systematically evaluated.
- The psychological costs and benefits of "avoidance" for those coping with extreme trauma need to be evaluated. It is apparent that many traumatized patients cope through techniques involving active suppression, that is, avoidance behavior, refusal to talk about the event, avoidance of any reminders of the events, and other forms of numbing. Because these kinds of techniques are so frequently used, the utility of "avoidance" should be studied, and the benefits and problems for refugees of various cultures should be determined.

REFERENCES

Allden, K., Poole, C., Chantavanich, S., Ohmar, K., Aung, N., & Mollica, R. F. (1996). Burmese political dissidents in Thailand: Trauma and survival among young adults in exile. *American Journal of Public Health, 86*(11), 1561–1569.

American Psychiatric Association. (1980). *Diagnostic and statistical manual of mental disorders* (3rd ed.). Washington, DC: Author.

Arieli, A., & Aycheh, S. (1992). Psychopathology among Jewish Ethiopian immigrants to Israel. *Journal of Nervous and Mental Disease, 180,* 465–466.

Arroyo, W., & Eth, S. (1985). Children traumatized by Central American warfare. In S. Eth & R. S. Pynoos (Eds.), *Post-traumatic stress disorders in children.* Washington, DC: American Psychiatric Association Press.

Benshein, H. (1960). Die K.Z. Neurose den rassischen Verfolger: Ein Eintrag zur Psychopathologie der Neurosen [The concentration camp neurosis of the racially persecuted: A contribution on the psychopathology of neuroses]. *Der Nervenarzt, 31,* 462–469.

Boehnlein, J. K., Kinzie, J. D., Rath, B., & Fleck, J. (1985). One year follow-up study of posttraumatic stress disorder among survivors of Cambodian concentration camps. *American Journal of Psychiatry, 142,* 956–959.

Carlson, E. B., & Rosser-Hogan, R. (1991). Trauma experiences, post-traumatic stress, dissociation, and depression in Cambodian refugees. *American Journal of Psychiatry, 148,* 1548–1551.

Chung, R. C., & Kagawa-Singer, M. (1993). Predictors of psychological distress among Southeast Asian refugees. *Social Science and Medicine, 36*(5), 631–639.

Dadfur, A. (1994). The Afghans: Bearing the scars of a forgotten war. In A. J. Marsella, T. H. Bornemann, S. Ekblad, & J. Orley (Eds.), *Amidst peril and pain: The mental health and well-being of the world's refugees* (pp. 125–140). Washington, DC: American Psychological Association.

Eberly, R. E., & Engdahl, B. E. (1991). Prevalence of somatic and psychiatric disorders among former prisoners of war. *Hospital and Community Psychiatry, 42,* 807–813.

Eitinger, L. (1959). The incidence of mental disorders among refugees in Norway. *Journal of Mental Science, 105,* 326–338.

Eitinger, L. (1960). The symptomatology of mental disease among refugees in Norway. *Journal of Mental Science, 106,* 947–966.

Ekblad, S., Ginsburg, B. E., Jansson, B., & Levi, L. (1994). Psychosocial and psychiatric aspects of refugee adaptation and care in Sweden. In A. J. Marsella, T. H. Bornemann, S. Ekblad, & J. Orley (Eds.), *Amidst peril and pain: The mental health and well-being of the world's refugees.* Washington, DC: American Psychological Association.

El-Sarraj, E. R., Tawahina, A. A., & Heine, F. A. (1994). The Palestinians: An uprooted people. In A. J. Marsella, T. H. Bornemann, S. Ekblad, & J. Orley (Eds.), *Amidst peril and pain: The mental health and well-being of the world's refugees* (pp. 141–152). Washington, DC: American Psychological Association.

Farias, P. J. (1991). Emotional distress and its socio-political correlates in Salvadoran refugees: Analysis of a clinical sample. *Culture, Medicine, and Psychiatry, 15,* 167–192.

Goldfeld, A. E., Mollica, R. F., Pesavento, B. H., & Faraone, S. V. (1988). The physical and psychological sequelae of torture: Symptomatology and diagnosis. *Journal of the American Medical Association, 259,* 2725–2729.

Karadaghi, P. (1994). The Kurds: Refugees on their own land. In A. J. Marsella, T. H. Bornemann, S. Ekblad, & J. Orley (Eds.), *Amidst peril and pain: The mental health and well-being of the world's refugees* (pp. 115–124). Washington, DC: American Psychological Association.

Kinzie, J. D. (1988). The psychiatric effects of massive trauma on Cambodian refugees. In J. P. Wilson, Z. Harel, & B. Kahana (Eds.), *Human adaptation of extreme stress: From the Holocaust to Vietnam* (pp. 305–317). New York: Plenum Press.

Kinzie, J. D., & Boehnlein, J. K. (1993). Psychotherapy of the victims of massive violence: Countertransference and ethical issues. *American Journal of Psychotherapy, 47,* 90–102.

Kinzie, J. D., Boehnlein, J. K., Leung, P. K., Moore, L. J., Riley, C., & Smith, D. (1990). The prevalence of posttraumatic stress disorder and its clinical significance among Southeast Asian refugees. *American Journal of Psychiatry, 147,* 913–917.

Kinzie, J. D., Denney, D., Riley, C., Boehnlein, J., McFarland, B., & Leung, P. (1998). A cross-cultural study of reactivation of posttraumatic stress disorder symptoms. *Journal of Nervous and Mental Disease, 186,* 670–676.

Kinzie, J. D., Fredrickson, R. H., Rath, B., & Fleck, J. (1984). Post-traumatic stress disorder among survivors of Cambodian concentration camps. *American Journal of Psychiatry, 141,* 645–650.

Kinzie, J. D., Sack, W. H., Angell, R. H., & Clarke, G. (1989). A three-year follow-up of Cambodian young people traumatized as children. *Journal of the American Academy of Child and Adolescent Psychiatry, 28,* 501–504.

Kinzie, J. D., Sack, W. H., Angell, R. H., & Manson, S. (1986). The psychiatric effects of massive trauma on Cambodian children: I. The children. *Journal of the American Academy of Child Psychiatry, 25*(3), 370–376.

Kinzie, J. D., Sack, R. L., & Riley, C. M. (1994). The polysomnographic effects of clonidine on sleep disorders in posttraumatic stress disorder: A pilot study with Cambodian patients. *Journal of Nervous and Mental Disease, 182,* 585–587.

Kinzie, J. D., Tran, K. A., Breckenridge, A., & Bloom, J. D. (1980). An Indo-Chinese refugee psychiatric clinic: Culturally accepted treatment approaches. *American Journal of Psychiatry, 137*, 1429–1432.

Klein, H. (1974). Delayed effects and after-effects of severe traumatization. *Israel Annals of Psychiatry, 12*, 293–303.

Kroll, J., Habenicht, M., Mackenzie, T., Yang, M., Chan, S., Vang, T., Nguyen, T., Ly, M., Phommasouvanh, B., Nguyen, H., Vang, Y., Souvannasoth, L., & Cabugao, R. (1989). Depression and posttraumatic stress disorder in Southeast Asian refugees. *American Journal of Psychiatry, 146*(12), 1592–1597.

Krupinski, J., Stoller, A., & Wallace, L. (1973). Psychiatric disorders in East European refugees now in Australia. *Social Science and Medicine, 7*, 331–349.

Leopold, M., & Harrell-Bond, B. (1994). An overview of the world refugee crisis. In A. J. Marsella, T. H. Bornemann, S. Ekblad, & J. Orley (Eds.), *Amidst peril and pain: The mental health and well-being of the world's refugees* (pp. 17–32). Washington, DC: American Psychological Association.

Masaki, B., & Wong, L. (1997). Domestic violence in Asian community. In E. Lee (Ed.), *Working with Asian Americans: A guide for clinicians* (pp. 439–451). New York: Guilford Press.

Mattusek, P. (1975). *Internment in concentration camps and their consequences*. New York: Springer-Verlag.

Mghir, R., Freed, W., Raskin, L., & Katon, W. (1995). Depression and post-traumatic stress disorder among a community sample of adolescent and young Afghan refugees. *Journal of Nervous and Mental Disease, 183*, 24–30.

Mollica, R. (1994). Southeast Asian refugees migration, history and mental health issues. In A. J. Marsella, T. H. Bornemann, S. Ekblad, & J. Orley (Eds.), *Amidst peril and pain: The mental health and well-being of the world's refugees* (pp. 83–100). Washington, DC: American Psychological Association.

Mollica, R. F., Donelan, K., Tor, S., Lavelle, J., Elias, C., Frankel, M., & Blendon, R. J. (1993). The effect of trauma and confinement on functional health and mental health status of Cambodians living in Thailand–Cambodian border camps. *Journal of the American Medical Association, 270*, 581–586.

Mollica, R. F., Poole, C., Son, L., Murray, C., & Tor, S. (1997). Effects of war trauma on Cambodian refugee adolescents' functional health and mental health status. *Journal of American Child and Adolescent Psychiatry, 36*, 1098–1106.

Mollica, R. F., Poole, C., & Tor, S. (1998). Symptoms, functioning, and health problems in massively traumatized populations: The legacy of Cambodian tragedy. In B. P. Dohrenwend (Ed.), *Adversity, stress, and psychopathology* (pp. 34–51). New York: Oxford University Press.

Morris, P., & Silove, D. (1992). Cultural influences in psychotherapy with refugee survivors of torture and trauma. *Hospital and Community Psychiatry, 43*, 820–824.

Niederland, W. G. (1964). Psychiatric disorders among persecution victims. *Journal of Nervous and Mental Disease, 139*, 458–474.

Ostwald, P., & Bittner, E. (1968). Life adjustment after severe persecution. *American Journal of Psychiatry, 124*(110), 1393–1400.

Sack, W. H., Clarke, G. N., & Seeley, J. (1996). Multiple forms of stress in Cambodian adolescent refugees. *Child Development, 67*(1), 107–116.

Sack, W. H., McSharry, S., Clarke, G. N., Kinney, R., Seeley, J., & Lewinsohn, P. (1994). The Khmer adolescent project: I. Epidemiologic findings in two generations of Cambodian refugees. *Journal of Nervous and Mental Disease, 182*, 387–395.

Schnurr, P. P., Spiro, A., & Paris, A. H. (1997, November). *PTSD and cardiovascular, cerebrovascular, and gastrointestinal disorders in the normative aging study*. Paper presented at the annual meeting of the International Society for Traumatic Stress, Montreal, Quebec, Canada.

Silove, D., Sinnerbrink, I., Field, A., Manicavasagar, V., & Steel, Z. (1997). Anxiety, depression and posttraumatic stress disorder in asylum-seekers: Associations with pre-migration trauma and post-migration stressors. *British Journal of Psychiatry, 170*, 351–357.

Silove, D., Steel, Z., McGorry, P., & Mohan, P. (1997). Trauma exposure, postmigration stressors, and symptoms of anxiety, depression and posttraumatic stress in Tamil asylum-seekers: Comparisons with refugees and immigrants. *Acta Psychiatrica Scandinavica, 97*(3), 175–181.

Thompson, M., & McGorry, P. (1995). Psychological sequelae of torture and trauma in Chilean and Salvadorean migrants: A pilot study. *Australia and New Zealand Journal of Psychiatry, 29*, 84–95.

Venzlaff, V. (1967). *Die psychoreaktiven Störungen nach entschädigungspflichtigen ereignissen: Die sogenannten Unfallneurosen* [Psychoreactive disturbances following compensable events: The so-called accident neuroses]. Berlin: Springer-Verlag.

Weine, S. (1997, May). *Bosnian survivors: Memories and witnessing: After Dayton.* Paper presented at the annual meeting of the American Psychiatric Association, San Diego, CA.

Weine, S., Becker, D. F., McGlashan, T. H., Laub, D., Lazrove, S., Vojvoda, D., & Hyman, L. (1995). Psychiatric consequences of "ethnic cleansing": Clinical assessments and trauma testimonies of newly resettled Bosnian refugees. *American Journal of Psychiatry, 152*(4), 536–542.

Weine, S., Vojvoda, D., Hartman, S., & Hyman, L. (1997). A family survives genocide. *Psychiatry, 60*, 24–39.

Westermeyer, J. (1988). *DSM-III* psychiatric disorders among Hmong refugees in the United States: A point prevalence study. *American Journal of Psychiatry, 145*(2), 197–202.

8

Veterans of Armed Conflicts

JOHN A. FAIRBANK, MATTHEW J. FRIEDMAN, and STEVEN SOUTHWICK

In this chapter basic and clinical research findings are presented on the effect of armed conflicts on the veterans of such conflicts. For this discussion, "veterans" are defined as people who were participants—whether as active combatants or in support roles—in wars or related activities. The overall focus is on the mental health and functional outcomes of exposure to war stress emanating from studies of war veterans. The relatively abundant body of research examining the epidemiological (i.e., prevalence, comorbidities, and risk factors) and clinical characteristics of posttraumatic stress disorder (PTSD) is highlighted.

SCOPE OF PARTICIPATION IN ARMED CONFLICTS

Because of the number and distribution of veterans of armed conflicts throughout the world, it is important to study their experiences and psychosocial adjustment. There have been, and continue to be, so many wars and warlike events that vast numbers of people have participated and will continue to participate in armed conflicts. In the history of armed conflicts involving just European countries since 1918, there have been more than 60 instances of war between countries, civil wars, episodes of terrorism, and military interventions (Orner, 1992). Zwi (1991) counted 127 wars and more than 20 million war-related deaths in the world since World

JOHN A. FAIRBANK • Department of Psychiatry, Duke University Medical Center, Durham, North Carolina 27710.   MATTHEW J. FRIEDMAN • Dartmouth University, and the National Center for Post-Traumatic Stress Disorder, White River Junction, Vermont 05009.   STEVEN SOUTHWICK • Department of Psychiatry, Yale University School of Medicine, West Haven, Connecticut 06516.

The Mental Health Consequences of Torture, edited by Ellen Gerrity, Terence M. Keane, and Farris Tuma. Kluwer Academic/Plenum Publishers, New York, 2001.

War II. More recently, the scale of participation in the armed conflict in South Africa is substantial, as documented in written testimony submitted to the South African Truth and Reconciliation Commission by representatives of the African National Congress and its armed forces and by members of the former apartheid government and its military and other security structures.

IMPACT

Case Study

One case example, abstracted from the public-domain of the National Vietnam Veterans Readjustment Study (NVVRS) (Kulka et al., 1988), typifies the effect of war-related PTSD on the social functioning of some veterans. This case is one example of the human experience of participants in armed conflicts and illustrates how these experiences may affect all of society.

> J.S., a Hispanic male veteran in his late 30s, has been married for almost 20 years, has three children, and works as a semiskilled laborer. He lives in a large metropolitan area in the northeastern region of the United States. He is the eldest of four children and grew up in a poor but stable and supportive family environment. He was drafted into the U.S. Army in 1966 and served one tour of duty in Vietnam, which ended in 1968. His primary duty was reconnaissance in an infantry unit. He experienced high and sustained war-zone stress exposure; he walked at the point of the squad, was frequently under fire, witnessed the death and injury of close buddies, witnessed the mutilation of the bodies of American troops, and was wounded in combat. He received several decorations, including the Purple Heart.

> J.S. reports that his experience in Vietnam matured him, but that he had difficulty coping and began to drink heavily for the first time during his tour. On his return to civilian life, his problems with alcohol intensified; he was treated medically for alcohol-related pancreatic disease several years after his return. Alcohol abuse remains a serious problem to the present time.

> With respect to the psychological impact of the war, he reported, "I developed a nasty temper, became very nervous, and have bad dreams that take me back into the war, like it's happening all over—then I can't get back to sleep." When reminded of the war, he becomes upset and vividly imagines the sights and smells of the battlefield, including the discovery of bodies that had been left for several days in the forest heat. He describes himself as frightened by his urges, easily startled, frequently on guard for no reason, emotionally withdrawn, and using alcohol to help forget about his wartime memories. His wife concurs, reporting that he has frequent nightmares, becomes enraged over minor irritations, avoids reminders of the war, and is reluctant to be emotionally close. He says he is fortunate that his wife continues to be supportive, despite his volatility and withdrawal (Kulka et al., 1988, pp. iv–16 to v–17). (Used with permission.)

Posttraumatic Stress Disorder

It was largely through the study of the postwar experiences of soldiers exposed to combat that the syndrome known today as PTSD (American Psychiatric

Association, 1987) was identified. Although accounts of postwar problems of combat veterans have long been known (Da Costa, 1871), the medical and scientific communities' efforts to describe and understand these problems did not achieve a critical mass until World War I (e.g., Hyams, Wignall, & Roswell, 1996; Kolb, 1943; Rivers, 1920). The prevalence of war-related mental health problems such as PTSD has been shown to vary as a function of the nature of the exposure (i.e., the experiences that people had while in war) and the characteristics of the participants (Kulka et al., 1990; Litz, Orsillo, Friedman, Ehlich, & Batres, 1997; Solomon, Weisenberg, Schwarzwald, & Mikulincer, 1987; Spiro, Schnurr, & Aldwin, 1994). These findings underscore the notion that each individual's experience of a given war is different and that the nature of a war's specific "risk profile" (i.e., how many people are exposed to which kinds of events) is an important determinant of each war's psychological and emotional sequelae (Schlenger, Fairbank, Jordan, & Caddell, 1999).

Therefore, prevalence rates of PTSD and other health problems are presented by conflict and by participants' characteristics and roles within a given conflict. Estimates of the prevalence of PTSD among U.S. Vietnam veterans are based on findings from several major community epidemiological studies. These include findings from the NVVRS (Kulka et al., 1990; Schlenger et al., 1992) that indicated that 15.2% of men and 8.5% of women who served with U.S. military forces in Vietnam had current PTSD, that is, met the criteria of the third revised edition of the *Diagnostic and Statistical Manual of Mental Disorders* (DSM-III-R; American Psychiatric Association, 1987) during the 6 months prior to the interview. These rates were significantly higher than the PTSD prevalence rates reported for two comparison groups: (a) male and female veterans who did not serve in Southeast Asia and (b) civilians who did not serve in the military. Lifetime prevalence rates (i.e., the estimated proportion who had met the DSM-III-R criteria for PTSD at any time in their lives, whether they met the criteria currently) among Vietnam veterans were 30.9% for men and 26.9% for women (Weiss et al., 1992).

NVVRS findings also indicated significant differences in the prevalence of PTSD among African-American, Hispanic, and White male Vietnam veterans. Rates of current PTSD were 20.6% for African-American men, 27.9% for Hispanic men, and 13.7% for White men. A recent study of two American Indian samples also found significantly higher rates of lifetime and current PTSD among American Indians than among White Vietnam veterans (Friedman et al., 1997). Overall, findings from these studies indicate that ethnicity and race are risk factors for exposure to war stress and development of PTSD.

The Centers for Disease Control and Prevention Vietnam Experience Study (1988) estimated a lifetime PTSD prevalence of 14.7% and a current (past month) prevalence of 2.2%. In the Department of Veterans Affairs (VA) Twin Study (Goldberg, True, Eisen, & Henderson, 1990), the current prevalence of PTSD among a sample of twins who served in Vietnam was 16.8% compared with 5.0% among those who served elsewhere. Findings from the St. Louis site of the National Institute of Mental Health Epidemiologic Catchment Area program suggested a lifetime PTSD prevalence of 6.3% for Vietnam veterans (Helzer, Robins,

& McEvoy, 1987), adjusted to 11.8% when sampling and response rates were accounted for (Keane & Wolfe, 1990). In a study of Vietnam veteran members of a national veterans' organization (American Legion), current PTSD prevalences ranging from 1.8% to 15% were reported, depending on how exposure to combat was operationalized. Although the estimates of current PTSD prevalence in these and other major studies ranged from 1.8% to more than 25%, the estimates from the majority of studies lie very nearly within the 95% confidence interval of the NVVRS estimates (13.0% to 17.4%). These findings suggest that postwar PTSD among American Vietnam veterans is a significant and chronic public health problem (Schlenger et al., 1999).

O'Toole et al. (1994) estimated the prevalence of PTSD in a national sample of Australian veterans of the Vietnam war. Findings indicated a lifetime prevalence ranging from 11.7% to 20.9%, depending on how exposure to trauma and PTSD were assessed. The current (1-month) estimate of PTSD prevalence among Australian Vietnam veterans was 11.6%. In a study of Israeli veterans of the Lebanon war, Solomon et al. (1987) reported a PTSD prevalence rate of 16% 1 year after the war among soldiers who had not experienced an acute stress reaction during the war and a PTSD prevalence of 59% for soldiers who had experienced acute combat stress.

Follow-ups at 2 years (Solomon & Mikulincer, 1988) and 3 years (Solomon, 1989) postwar showed that soldiers who had experienced an acute stress reaction during military service continued to have significantly higher rates of PTSD than the comparison group. In both groups, rates of PTSD prevalence declined somewhat over time. Studies of American veterans of the Persian Gulf War and recent peacekeeping missions in Somalia and Bosnia have also shown elevated rates of PTSD among veterans exposed to hazardous conditions in these conflicts (Litz et al., 1997; Perconte, Wilson, Pontius, Dietrick, & Spiro, 1993; Southwick & Morgan, 1995; Southwick et al., 1993; Stretch et al., 1996; Sutker, Uddo, Brailey, & Allain, 1993; Wolfe, Brown, & Kelley, 1993). A longitudinal study of PTSD prevalence among Persian Gulf War veterans reported increasing rates of PTSD over 1-month, 6-month, and 24-month assessments following return to the United States from the Persian Gulf (Southwick & Morgan, 1995; Southwick et al., 1993).

Comorbidity of PTSD with Other Disorders

Psychiatric comorbidity has been examined among clinical and community samples of veterans with PTSD. Keane and Wolfe (1990) studied patients in the Boston VA Medical Center's PTSD program and found high rates of comorbid substance abuse, major depression, dysthymic disorder, and antisocial personality disorder. Kulka et al. (1990) found that virtually all Vietnam veterans with PTSD had met criteria for one or more other psychiatric disorders at some time during their lives, and half were characterized by a current comorbid disorder. In men, the most prevalent comorbid disorders were alcohol abuse or dependence (75% lifetime, 20% current), generalized anxiety disorder (44% lifetime, 20% current), and major depression (20% lifetime, 16% current). Among women veterans, the most frequent disorders co-occurring with PTSD were major depression (42% lifetime, 23% current), generalized anxiety disorder (38% lifetime, 20% current), and dysthymic disorder (33% lifetime). Thus, war-related PTSD assessed in veterans 15 or more years after their participation in an armed conflict is associated with high levels of comorbid psychiatric disorder. More recently, PTSD has been found to play an important role in veterans' functioning independent of a variety of comorbid psychiatric and physical disorders to which impaired functioning might be attributable (Schlenger et al., 1999).

Other Psychological Outcomes

For men, participation in armed conflicts is associated with increased risk for developing antisocial personality disorder, even when a history of childhood behavior problems, PTSD diagnosis, and military factors are controlled in the analysis (Barrett et al., 1996; Resnick, Foy, Donahoe, & Miller, 1989). Compared with male Vietnam veterans exposed to low levels of war stress, men exposed to high levels were more likely to meet diagnostic criteria for major depression, dysthymia, obsessive-compulsive disorder, generalized anxiety disorder, and alcohol abuse and dependence (Jordan et al., 1991). For women who served in the American military in Vietnam, fewer disorders are associated with exposure to war stress. However, women exposed to high levels of war stress reported higher rates of major depression and dysthymia than female veterans who experienced less war trauma in Vietnam (Jordan et al., 1991).

Neurobiological Findings

A substantial body of research has found evidence of abnormalities in brain structure and function in war veterans with PTSD (Friedman, Charney, & Deutch, 1995). These findings are reviewed and synthesized in chapter 5 in this volume.

Physical Health

There is a growing body of research describing the long-term effects of trauma exposure and PTSD on veterans' physical health and utilization of medical services (e.g., Beckham et al., 1997; Centers for Disease Control and Prevention Vietnam Experience Study, 1988; Friedman et al., 1997; Friedman & Schnurr, 1995; Kulka et al., 1990; Long, Chamberlain, & Vincent, 1992; Shalev, Bleich, & Ursano, 1990; Solomon & Mikulincer, 1988). Shalev et al. (1990) found that Israeli veterans with PTSD reported more somatic symptoms than did matched controls but that groups did not differ on laboratory test findings. This study and others have also shown a greater frequency of adverse health practices (e.g., smoking, alcohol use) among veterans with PTSD. Analysis of American NVVRS (Kulka et al., 1990) and Mutsunaga Vietnam Veterans Project (Friedman et al., 1997) cohorts indicates that for White, Black, Hispanic, American Indian, Native Hawaiian, and Japanese-American theater veterans, exposure to war-zone stress and PTSD symptomatology predict a lower perceived health status and a greater utilization of both physical and mental health services as indicated by the volume of inpatient admissions and outpatient visits.

Economic Impact

Several studies have examined associations between exposure to war stress, PTSD, and labor market outcomes among military veterans (Kulka et al., 1990; McCarren et al., 1995; Vincent, Long, & Chamberlain, 1994; Zatzick, Marmar, et al. 1997; Zatzick, Weiss, et al., 1997). Findings from these studies indicate that traumatic war experiences not only compromise mental and physical health, but also have deleterious consequences on labor market functioning. In two large samples of Vietnam veterans in the United States and a third sample in New Zealand, veterans receiving a diagnosis of PTSD were more likely to be unemployed than were those without the disorder (Kulka et al., 1990; McCarren et al., 1995; Vincent et al., 1994; Zatzick, Marmar, et al., 1997; Zatzick, Weiss, et al., 1997). Additionally, PTSD has been found to be associated with greater occupational instability among Vietnam veterans (Kulka et al., 1990). However, the relationship between PTSD and income and earnings in veterans is equivocal given that studies have reported mixed findings. Analysis of NVVRS data by Zatzick, Marmar, et al. (1997) and Zatzick, Weiss, et al. (1997) strongly suggests that the relationship between war trauma and labor market outcomes is in part mediated by PTSD.

Social Consequences

A number of studies have examined the social consequences of participation in armed conflicts (Barrett et al., 1996; Carroll, Rueger, Foy, & Donahoe, 1985; Jordan et al., 1992; Roberts et al., 1982; Yager, Laufer, & Gallops, 1984). Particularly noteworthy is the finding that participation in armed conflict is associated with postwar involvement in the criminal justice system, including arrests for violent crimes (Yager et al., 1984). In a study that compared families of male Vietnam veterans with PTSD with families of male veterans without PTSD, families of veterans with PTSD showed much higher levels of severe and diffuse problems with marital and family adjustment, parenting skills, and violent behavior (Jordan et al., 1992).

Risk and Protective Factors

Risk for PTSD among military veterans separates into premilitary, military, and postmilitary factors (Keane et al., 1985; Kulka et al., 1990; Yehuda, 1999). Cumulative evidence across decades of research with war veterans emphasizes the importance of the stressor in predicting health outcomes, with an approximate dose–response relationship: higher levels of exposure to war stressors are associated with poorer health outcomes. Among war-related factors, variables such as serving in an enlisted rank, being drafted or conscripted into the military (versus volunteering), and receiving wounds in action have been shown to increase risk for PTSD (Helzer et al., 1987; Kulka et al., 1990).

Specific dimensions of war stressor exposure that have been found to directly affect PTSD are a malevolent environment, perceived threat, or participating in or witnessing atrocities or abusive violence (D. W. King, King, Gudanowski, & Vreven, 1995). Participation in traditional combat activities (e.g., firing a weapon, receiving incoming rounds) appears to have an effect on PTSD, although recent research suggests that combat affects PTSD indirectly through perceived threat (D. W. King, King, Foy, & Gudanowski, 1996). Identified risk factors that predate military service include a positive family history of psychiatric disorder and instability (e.g., Fontana & Rosenheck, 1994; Kulka et al., 1990); emotional or psychological disorder as a youth, such as conduct disorder (Kulka et al., 1990); previous trauma history, including sexual or physical abuse during childhood (Engel et al., 1993; Fontana, Schwartz, & Rosenheck, 1997); and developmental maturity at the time of entry into armed conflict (Kulka et al., 1990). Orr and Pittman (1999) have recently provided evidence that poorer intellectual ability or a compromised neurodevelopmental history constitutes a neurocognitive risk factor for PTSD. Genetic studies involving veterans with PTSD show that even after controlling for factors that influence exposure to trauma, there may be a genetic influence on vulnerability for PTSD (True & Lyons, 1999).

A host of other factors have been shown to affect PTSD in military veterans. These factors include social cognitive variables, such as self-efficacy, attributional style, and coping (Mikulincer & Solomon, 1988; Solomon, Benbenishty, & Mikulincer, 1991; Solomon, Mikulincer, & Benbenishty, 1989); hardiness (Sutker, Davis, Uddo, & Ditta, 1995); functional and structural social support variables; and stressful life events that occur after participation in armed conflict, including repeated exposures to violent events (L. A. King, King, Fairbank, Keane, & Adams, 1998; Wolfe, Brown, & Bucsela, 1992); and postwar homecoming experiences (Fontana & Rosenheck, 1995).

RECOMMENDATIONS FOR FUTURE RESEARCH

- Research is needed to develop and evaluate approaches for effectively reintegrating large numbers of veterans into societies that have limited economic resources available for providing veterans with medical, educational, and housing benefits.
- Symptoms, signs, and ill-defined conditions of veterans of armed conflicts, such as joint pain, fatigue, headaches, memory loss, rash or dermatitis, and so forth, continue to be poorly understood and require systematic epidemiologic and clinical study.
- Research is needed on methods for improving the use of information on risk factors for war-related health problems to prevent such consequences among men and women who serve in military forces.

- There is currently a lack of empirical information on the types of problems associated with reintegrating demobilized armed forces from formerly opposing parties into a society.
- The longitudinal course of traumatic stress reactions among veterans of armed conflicts is still poorly understood. Research is needed that prospectively follows the course of traumatic stress reactions from acute stress disorder to end-stage chronic PTSD, as well as the course of other behavioral and health problems.

REFERENCES

American Psychiatric Association. (1987). *Diagnostic and statistical manual of mental disorders* (3rd ed., rev.). Washington, DC: Author.

Barrett, D. H., Resnick, H. S., Foy, D. W., Dansky, B. S., Flanders, W. D., & Stroup, N. E. (1996). Combat exposure and adult psychosocial adjustment among U.S. army veterans serving in Vietnam, 1965–1971. *Journal of Abnormal Psychology, 105*(4), 575–581.

Beckham, J. C., Kirby, A. C., Feldman, M. E., Hertzberg, M. A., Moore, S. D., Crawford, A. L., Davidson, J. R. T., & Fairbank, J. A. (1997). Prevalence and correlates of heavy smoking in Vietnam veterans with chronic posttraumatic stress disorder. *Addictive Behaviors, 22*, 637–647.

Carroll, E. M., Rueger, D. B., Foy, D. W., & Donahoe, C. P. (1985). Vietnam combat veterans with posttraumatic stress disorder: Analysis of marital and cohabiting adjustment. *Journal of Abnormal Psychology, 94*, 329–337.

Centers for Disease Control and Prevention Vietnam Experience Study. (1988). Health status of Vietnam veterans: I. Psychosocial characteristics. *Journal of the American Medical Association, 259*(18), 2701–2707.

Da Costa, J. M. (1871). On irritable heart: A clinical study of a form of functional cardiac disorder and its consequences. *American Journal of the Medical Sciences, 61*(121), 17–52.

Engel, C. C., Engel, A. L., Campbell, S. J., McFall, M. E., Russo, J., & Katon, W. (1993). Posttraumatic stress disorder symptoms and precombat sexual and physical abuse in Desert Storm veterans. *Journal of Nervous and Mental Disease, 181*, 683–688.

Fontana, A., & Rosenheck, R. (1994). Posttraumatic stress disorder among Vietnam theater veterans: A causal model of etiology in a community sample. *Journal of Nervous and Mental Disease, 182*, 677–684.

Fontana, A., & Rosenheck, R. (1995). Attempted suicide among Vietnam veterans: A model of etiology in a community sample. *American Journal of Psychiatry, 152*, 102–109.

Fontana, A., Schwartz, L. S., & Rosenheck, R. (1997). Posttraumatic stress disorder among female Vietnam veterans: A causal model of etiology. *American Journal of Public Health, 87*, 169–175.

Friedman, M. J., Ashcraft, M. L., Beals, J. L., Keane, T. M., Manson, S. M., & Marsella, A. J. (1997). *Final report: Matsunaga Vietnam Veterans Project* (Vol. 1). White River Junction, VT: National Center for Post-Traumatic Stress Disorder and National Center for American Indian and Alaska Native Mental Health Research.

Friedman, M. J., Charney, D. S., & Deutch, A. Y. (Eds.). (1995). *Neurobiological and clinical consequences of stress: From normal adaptation to post-traumatic stress disorder.* Philadelphia: Lippincott–Raven.

Friedman, M. J., & Schnurr, P. P. (1995). The relationship between trauma, post-traumatic stress disorder, and physical health. In M. J. Friedman, D. S. Charney, & A. Y. Deutch (Eds.), *Neurobiological and clinical consequences of stress: From normal adaptation to post-traumatic stress disorder* (pp. 507–524). Philadelphia: Lippincott–Raven.

Goldberg, J., True, W. R., Eisen, S. A., & Henderson, W. G. (1990). A twin study of the effects of the Vietnam War on posttraumatic stress disorder. *Journal of the American Medical Association, 263*, 1227–1232.

Helzer, J. E., Robins, L. N., & McEvoy, L. (1987). Post-traumatic stress disorder in the general population: Findings of the Epidemiologic Catchment Area Survey. *New England Journal of Medicine, 317*, 1630–1634.

Hyams, K. C., Wignall, F. S., & Roswell, R. (1996). War syndromes and their evaluation: From the U. S. Civil War to the Persian Gulf War. *Annals of Internal Medicine, 125*(5), 398–405.

Jordan, B. K., Marmar, C. R., Fairbank, J. A., Schlenger, W. E., Kulka, R. A., Hough, R. L., & Weiss, D. S. (1992). Problems in families of male Vietnam veterans with posttraumatic stress disorder. *Journal of Consulting and Clinical Psychology, 60*(6), 916–926.

Jordan, B. K., Schlenger, W. E., Hough, R., Kulka, R., Weiss, D., Fairbank, J. A., & Marmar, C. R. (1991). Lifetime and current prevalence of specific psychiatric disorders among Vietnam veterans and controls. *Archives of General Psychiatry, 48*, 207–215.

Keane, T. M., Fairbank, J. A., Caddell, J. M., Juesta, M., Zimering, R. T., & Bender, M. E. (1985). A behavioral approach to assessing and treating post-traumatic stress disorder in Vietnam veterans. In C. R. Figley (Ed.), *Trauma and its wake. Vol. I: The study and treatment of post-traumatic stress disorder* (pp. 257–294). New York: Brunner/Mazel.

Keane, T. M., & Wolfe, J. (1990). Comorbidity in post-traumatic stress disorder: An analysis of community and clinical studies. *Journal of Applied Social Psychology, 20*(21), 1776–1788.

King, D. W., King, L. A., Foy, D. W., & Gudanowski, D. M. (1996). Prewar factors in combat-related posttraumatic stress disorder: Structural equation modeling in a national sample of female and male Vietnam veterans. *Journal of Consulting and Clinical Psychology, 64*, 520–531.

King, D. W., King, L. A., Gudanowski, L. A., & Vreven, D. L. (1995). Alternative representations of war zone stressors: Relationships to post-traumatic stress disorder in male and female Vietnam veterans. *Journal of Abnormal Psychology, 104*, 184–196.

King, L. A., King, D. W., Fairbank, J. A., Keane, T. M., & Adams, G. A. (1998). Resilience/recovery factors in posttraumatic stress disorder among female and male Vietnam veterans: Hardiness, postwar social support, and additional stressful life events. *Journal of Personality and Social Psychology, 74*(2), 420–434.

Kolb, L. (1943). Postwar psychiatric perspectives. In F. J. Sladen (Ed.), *Psychiatry and the war: A survey of the significance of psychiatry and its relation to disturbances in human behavior to help provide for the present war effort and for postwar needs* (pp. 299–310). Springfield, IL: Thomas.

Kulka, R. A., Fairbank, W. E., Hough, R. I., Jordan, B. K., Marmar, C. R., & Weiss, D. S. (1990). *Trauma and the Vietnam War generation: Report of findings from the National Vietnam Veterans Readjustment Study*. New York: Brunner/Mazel.

Kulka, R. A., Schlenger, W. E., Fairbank, J. A., Hough, R. L., Jordan, B. K., Marmar, C. R., & Weiss, D. S. (1988). *Contractual report of findings from the National Vietnam Veterans Readjustment Study*. Research Triangle Park, NC: Research Triangle Institute.

Litz, B. T., Orsillo, S. M., Friedman, M., Ehlich, P., & Batres, A. (1997). Posttraumatic stress disorder associated with peacekeeping duty in Somalia for U.S. military personnel. *American Journal of Psychiatry, 154*(2), 178–184.

Long, N., Chamberlain, K., & Vincent, C. (1992). The health and mental health of New Zealand Vietnam War veterans with posttraumatic stress disorder. *New Zealand Medical Journal, 105*(944), 417–419.

McCarren, M., Janes, G. R., Goldberg, J., Eisen, S., True, W. R., & Henderson, W. G. (1995). A twin study of the association of post-traumatic stress disorder and combat exposure with long-term socioeconomic status in Vietnam veterans. *Journal of Traumatic Stress, 8*, 111–124.

Mikulincer, M., & Solomon, Z. (1988). Attributional style and combat-related posttraumatic stress disorder. *Journal of Abnormal Psychology, 97*, 303–313.

Orner, R. J. (1992). Post-traumatic stress disorders and European war veterans. *British Journal of Clinical Psychology, 31*, 387–403.

Orr, S. P., & Pitman, R. K. (1999). Neurocognitive risk factors for posttraumatic stress disorder. In A. Yehuda (Ed.), *Risk factors for posttraumatic stress disorder* (pp. 125–141). Washington, DC: American Psychiatric Association Press.

O'Toole, B. I., Marshall, R. P., Grayson, D. A., Schureck, R. I., Dobson, M., French, M., Pulvertaft, B., Meldrum, L., Bolton, J., & Vennard, J. (1994). *The Australian Vietnam Veterans health study: III. Psychology health of Australian Vietnam Veterans and the relationship to combat*. Unpublished manuscript.

Perconte, S. T., Wilson, A. T., Pontius, E. B., Dietrick, A. L., & Spiro, K. J. (1993). Psychological and war stress symptoms among deployed and nondeployed reservists following the Persian Gulf War. *Military Medicine, 158,* 516–521.

Resnick, H. S., Foy, D. W., Donahoe, C. P., & Miller, E. N. (1989). Antisocial behavior and posttraumatic stress disorder in Vietnam veterans. *Journal of Clinical Psychology, 45,* 860–866.

Rivers, W. H. R. (1920). Repression and suppression. In H. C. Miller (Ed.), *Functional nerve disease: An epitome of war experience for the practitioner* (pp. 88–98). London: Frowde, Hodder, & Stroughton.

Roberts, W. R., Penk, W. E., Gearing, M. L., Robinowitz, R., Dolan, M. P., & Patterson, E. T. (1982). Interpersonal problems of Vietnam combat veterans with symptoms of posttraumatic stress disorder. *Journal of Abnormal Psychology, 91*(6), 444–450.

Schlenger, W. E., Fairbank, J. A., Jordan, B. K., & Caddell, J. M. (1999). Combat-related posttraumatic stress disorder: Prevalence, risk factors, and comorbidity. In P. A. Saigh & J. D. Bremner (Eds.), *Posttraumatic stress disorder: A comprehensive text* (pp. 69–91). Boston: Allyn & Bacon.

Schlenger, W. E., Kulka, R. A., Fairbank, J. A., Hough, R. I., Jordan, B. K., Marmar, C. R., & Weiss, D. S. (1992). The prevalence of post-traumatic stress disorder in the Vietnam generation: A multimethod, multisource assessment of psychiatric disorder. *Journal of Traumatic Stress, 5,* 333–363.

Shalev, A., Bleich, A., & Ursano, R. J. (1990). Posttraumatic stress disorder: Somatic comorbidity and effort tolerance. *Psychosomatics, 31,* 197–203.

Solomon, Z. (1989). Psychological sequelae of war: A 3-year prospective study of Israeli combat stress reaction casualties. *Journal of Nervous and Mental Disease, 177,* 342–346.

Solomon, Z., Benbenishty, R., & Mikulincer, M. (1991). The contribution of wartime, pre-war, and post-war factors to self-efficacy: A longitudinal study of combat stress reaction. *Journal of Traumatic Stress, 4,* 345–361.

Solomon, Z., & Mikulincer, M. (1988). Psychological sequelae of war: A 2-year follow-up study of Israeli combat stress reaction casualties. *Journal of Nervous and Mental Disease, 176,* 264–269.

Solomon, Z., Mikulincer, M., & Benbenishty, R. (1989). Locus of control and combat-related posttraumatic stress disorder: The intervening role of battle intensity, threat appraisal, and coping. *British Journal of Clinical Psychology, 28,* 131–144.

Solomon, Z., Weisenberg, M., Schwarzwald, J., & Mikulincer, M. (1987). Posttraumatic stress disorder frontline soldiers with combat stress reaction: 1982 Israeli experience. *American Journal of Psychiatry, 144,* 448–454.

Southwick, S. M., & Morgan, C. A. (1995). Trauma-related symptoms in veterans of Operation Desert Storm: A 2-year follow-up. *American Journal of Psychiatry, 152,* 1150–1155.

Southwick, S. M., Morgan, A., Nagy, L. M., Brenner, D., Nicolaou, A. I., Johnson, D. R., Rosenheck, R., & Charney, D. S. (1993). Trauma-related symptoms in veterans of Operation Desert Storm: A preliminary report. *American Journal of Psychiatry, 150,* 1524–1528.

Spiro, A., Schnurr, P. P., & Aldwin, C. M. (1994). Combat-related posttraumatic stress disorder symptoms in older men. *Psychology and Aging, 9*(1), 17–26.

Stretch, R. H., Marlowe, D. H., Wright, K. M., Bliese, P. D., Knudson, K. H., & Hoover, C. H. (1996). Post-traumatic stress disorder symptoms among Gulf War veterans. *Military Medicine, 161,* 407–410.

Sutker, P. B., Davis, J. M., Uddo, M., & Ditta, S. R. (1995). War zone stress, personal resources, and posttraumatic stress disorder in Persian Gulf War returnees. *Journal of Abnormal Psychology, 104,* 444–452.

Sutker, P. B., Uddo, M., Brailey, K., & Allain, A. N. (1993). War-zone trauma and stress-related symptoms in Operation Desert Shield/Storm (ODS) returnees. *Journal of Social Issues, 49*, 33–49.

True, W., & Lyons, M. (1999). Genetic risk factors for post-traumatic stress disorder: A twin study. In R. Yehuda (Ed.), *Risk factors for posttraumatic stress disorder* (pp. 61–78). Washington, DC: American Psychiatric Association Press.

Vincent, C., Long, N., & Chamberlain, K. (1994). Relation of military service variables to posttraumatic stress disorder in New Zealand war veterans. *Military Medicine, 159*, 322–326.

Weiss, D. S., Marmar, C. R., Schlenger, W. E., Fairbank, J. A., Jordan, B. K., Hough, R. L., & Kulka, R. A. (1992). The prevalence of lifetime and partial post-traumatic stress disorder in Vietnam theater veterans. *Journal of Traumatic Stress, 5*, 365–376.

Wolfe, J., Brown, P. J., & Bucsela, M. L. (1992). Symptom responses of female Vietnam veterans to Operation Desert Storm. *American Journal of Psychiatry, 149*, 676–679.

Wolfe, J., Brown, P. J., & Kelley, J. M. (1993). Reassessing war stress: Exposure and the Persian Gulf War. *Journal of Social Issues, 49*, 15–31.

Yager, T., Laufer, R., & Gallops, M. (1984). Some problems associated with war experience in men of the Vietnam generation. *Archives of General Psychiatry, 41*, 327–333.

Yehuda, R. (Ed.). (1999). *Risk factors for posttraumatic stress disorder.* Washington, DC: American Psychiatric Association.

Zatzick, D. F., Marmar, C. R., Weiss, D. S., Browner, W., Metzler, T. J., Golding, J. M., Stewart, A., Schlenger, W. E., & Wells, K. B. (1997). Posttraumatic stress disorder and functioning and quality of life outcomes in a nationally representative sample of male Vietnam veterans. *American Journal of Psychiatry, 154*(12), 1690–1695.

Zatzick, D. F., Weiss, D. S., Marmar, C. R., Metzler, T. J., Wells, K., Golding, J. M., Stewart, A., Schlenger, W. E., & Browner, W. S. (1997). Posttraumatic stress disorder and functioning and quality of life outcomes in female Vietnam veterans. *Military Medicine, 7*, 262–268.

Zwi, A. B. (1991). Militarism, militarization, health, and the third world. *Medicine and War, 7*, 262–268.

9

Former Prisoners of War
Highlights of Empirical Research

BRIAN ENGDAHL and JOHN A. FAIRBANK

Former prisoners of war (POWs) endured grave physical and emotional conditions during their internment. Often they experienced a variety of traumatic events, including torture. For these reasons, research on former POWs is directly related to the problems of survivors of torture. The conditions POWs survived—enforced captivity, fear and terror, pain and suffering, and shame and humiliation—all parallel reports from survivors of torture. Clearly, torture survivors share many life experiences with former POWs, and the research conducted on POWs in many different countries may be very relevant to understanding the specific mental health consequences of torture. The research on POWs has previously been comprehensively reviewed (Engdahl & Eberly, 1990). What follows is an update highlighting POW research of particular relevance to the experiences of torture survivors.

WORLDWIDE POW RESEARCH

Wars, political unrest, and civil upheavals in the 20th century led hundreds of thousands of individuals to experience enforced captivity and attendant maltreatment. Stenger (1996) estimated that there are 58,800 American former POWs and 7,000 Canadian former POWs. Worldwide, the number of former POWs is many times these figures. Many POWs were intentionally subjected to beatings and torture at the hands of their captors; still others suffered untreated medical

BRIAN ENGDAHL • Veterans Administration Medical Center, Minneapolis, Minnesota 55417.   JOHN A. FAIRBANK • Department of Psychiatry, Duke University Medical Center, Durham, North Carolina 27710.
The Mental Health Consequences of Torture, edited by Ellen Gerrity, Terence M. Keane, and Farris Tuma. Kluwer Academic/Plenum Publishers, New York, 2001.

conditions, food and shelter deprivation, armed attack, and forced relocations. Civilian prisoners taken during international conflicts include an estimated 75,000 European Jewish Nazi concentration camp survivors (Epstein, 1979) and about 1 million non-Jews (Ruge, as cited in Thygesen, Hermann, & Willanger, 1970). For compelling social and economic reasons, these survivors of internment constitute subgroups of the general population requiring study to determine their status and needs. As a result, studies come from many parts of the industrialized world. These studies will be described in the next several paragraphs.

Denmark

Many Danish survivors of Nazi prison camps were extensively interrogated and tortured; the physical torture comprised primarily blows or kicks to the head (Thygesen et al., 1970). Moreover, these prisoners were detained for up to 4 years under conditions of overcrowding, inadequate shelter and hygiene, and poor diets combined with excessive work requirements. Threats of execution or reprisals against their families were common. These former POWs were found to be still experiencing many severe symptoms even 15 to 20 years postinternment. These symptoms included frequent nightmares of particularly heinous events, memory impairment, libido loss, irritability, emotional instability, and mental dullness and apathy.

Australia

In a random study of selected Australian World War II POW and non-POW combatant samples, the POWs were found to be experiencing significantly more depressive symptoms and affective disorders even 40 years after repatriation as compared with the non-POW group (Tennant, Goulston, and Dent, 1986). The investigators suggested that over the long follow-up period, symptoms of anxiety diminished, but depression increased as a reaction to chronic posttraumatic impairment.

Israel

A 20-year follow-up of Israeli combat veterans ($N = 296$) and POWs ($N = 164$) was conducted by Solomon, Neria, Ohry, Waysman, and Ginzburg (1994). Posttraumatic stress disorder (PTSD) and psychophysiological complaints (primarily anxiety symptoms) were especially frequent among POWs (Ohry et al., 1994). Importantly, Ohry et al. (1994) found that PTSD was particularly persistent among POWs: fewer than half of those who had developed PTSD at any time had recovered some 20 years after the POW experience. These findings support the notion that the psychological effects of internment are adverse and enduring.

Bosnia-Herzegovina

In one of the few treatment outcome studies on concentration camp survivors, Drozdek (1997) assigned 120 refugees now living in the Netherlands to 6 months of (a) group psychotherapy, (b) nonsystematic pharmacological therapy, or (c) a combination of the two therapies in the treatment of PTSD. Treatment was initiated within 3 months of release from the prison camps. Psychotherapy incorporated psychodynamic and abreactive (trauma discussion) components. All treatments (i.e., group therapy and drugs, group therapy alone, or drugs alone) yielded positive short-term effects, with some long-term positive effects observable at 3 years postintervention. Elderly participants benefited less from the interventions than did younger participants. More treatment research is needed to identify those interventions that are most effective for particular survivor groups.

Canada

Among POWs held by the Japanese during World War II, Canadian investigators documented long-standing impairments in the central nervous system and psychological functioning (Klonoff, McDougall, Clark, Kramer, & Horgan, 1976; Richardson, 1965). For example, 84% of the Canadian POWs reported a history of neurologic damage sustained during internment; neurologic damage was still evident in 51% after they returned to Canada (Crawford & Reid, 1947).

Other Countries

Depression, PTSD, and a wide range of anxiety symptoms were observed among POWs in reports from Great Britain (Newman, 1944), France (Crocq, Macher, Barros-Beck, Rosenberg, & Duval, 1993), Russia (Galitski, 1991), and Germany (Paul, 1986). Persistent PTSD was a frequent outcome among Dutch resistance fighters in Holland who were studied decades after the war ended; many of these fighters were imprisoned as a result of their actions during the Nazi occupation of the Netherlands (Op den Velde et al., 1996).

United States

Research from the United States on POWs has greatly expanded in the past 20 years as a result of public interest and supportive public policy toward those interred during war. Uniformly, these studies demonstrate that former POWs manifest high rates of persistent and debilitating psychiatric disorder. In 1950, the U.S. Department of Veterans Affairs began a series of POW studies examining a large national sample of POWs and non-POW combat veteran controls. Hospitalizations for psychoneurosis were found to be four to five times greater among World War II POWs of Japan and Germany compared with controls; in addition, excess mortality was found among POWs of Japan, primarily due to accidents and tuberculosis (Cohen & Cooper, 1954).

In a later study that included POWs held by North Korea, POWs of Japan suffered significantly more psychiatric hospitalizations for anxiety reactions, alcoholism, "nervousness and debility," psychoneurotic reactions, and schizophrenic disorders (Beebe, 1975). Findings from this study suggest that POWs held by

Japan sustained more significant negative physical and mental health effects than POWs held by Germany or North Korea, as evidenced by weight loss, neurologic diagnoses, body wounds, skin abnormalities, and other conditions. Terrorizing executions, beatings and torture, constant semistarvation, and untreated disease characterized the experience of POWs of Japan.

This same cohort of POWs and controls was followed by Page, Engdahl, and Eberly (1991). They found that depressive symptoms were still greatly elevated among the POWs 20 to 40 years after release from captivity. These symptoms were directly related to captivity maltreatment and inversely related to education and age at time of capture and the amount of social support received on return from military service. Depression appeared to be a consequence of the severe anxiety initially observed in the cohort.

In a community sample of POWs (N= 426), Eberly and Engdahl (1991) learned that anxiety disorders (particularly PTSD) and affective disorders were more frequent among POWs than in the general population. Disorders less likely to be a function of trauma exposure (e.g., schizophrenia and bipolar disorders) were not. In another community sample of POWs (N = 262) from World War II and the Korean War, more than half met lifetime criteria for PTSD, and 30% met criteria for current PTSD, even 40 to 50 years after the traumatic events (Engdahl, Dikel, Eberly, & Blank, 1997). The most severely traumatized group (POWs held by Japan) had lifetime rates of PTSD of 84% and current rates of 58%. Those who were tortured or who witnessed the torture of others were at particular risk for PTSD, even 40 to 50 years later. Very few of these survivors had ever sought mental health treatment.

A recent survey of U.S. civilians held as POWs by the Japanese (N=129) included the largest number of female POWs yet reported (N= 58) (Potts, 1994). The female survivors had a 37% lifetime and a 15% current rate of PTSD, confirming high rates of this disabling condition secondary to internment irrespective of the gender of the survivor.

COURSE AND COMPLICATIONS

In a community sample of 262 POWs, nearly two thirds of lifetime PTSD cases were complicated by at least one other Axis I psychiatric disorder; almost half of current PTSD cases also met criteria for another psychiatric condition (Engdahl, Dikel, Eberly, & Blank, 1998). PTSD almost always emerged soon after trauma exposure. Lifetime PTSD increased the risk for lifetime panic disorder, major depression, alcohol abuse or dependence, and social phobia. Current PTSD increased the risk for current panic disorder, dysthymia, social phobia, major depression, and generalized anxiety disorder. The types of comorbid diagnoses and their patterns of onset for PTSD secondary to POW experiences were comparable to the diagnoses and patterns observed for PTSD in general (Kessler, Sonnega, Bromet, Hughes, & Nelson, 1995). Specifically, PTSD nearly always arose soon after trauma exposure; alcohol abuse arose at the same time as PTSD; panic disorder arose equally often at the time of PTSD onset and after PTSD onset; and depression most often arose following PTSD. From these studies of the course of the disorder, it appears that the majority of POWs experience significant problems with anxiety on release from captivity. For some, these symptoms tended to decrease over time; for others (especially those who developed PTSD), there was a persistent symptom course for decades; and for still other individuals, the occurrence of subsequent stressful life events often led to a secondary depression or to the exacerbation of an existing depression.

BIOLOGICAL CORRELATES OF CAPTIVITY SURVIVORS' IMPAIRMENTS

PTSD has known biological correlates (see chapter 5), and, accordingly, disruptions in various physiological and neuropsychological systems are expected. The emphasis on neuropsychological sequelae among concentration camp survivors in the Danish (Thygesen et al., 1970) and Norwegian studies (Eitinger, 1985) coincides with the recent research among refugees (Mollica & Caspi-Yavin, 1992) and POWs. In a sample of American POWs of Japan, PTSD correlated with measures of brain cell loss and sleep abnormalities—specifically, increased awakenings and a lack of Stage 4 (deep) sleep (Peters, van Kammen, van Kammen, & Neylan, 1990). Further, Sutker, Winstead, Galina, and Allain (1991) contrasted POWs and combat veterans of the Korean War and reported that the POWs evidenced not only increased rates of psychopathology when compared to the combat controls, but also increased cognitive deficits that were primarily a function of captivity weight loss. With the high incidence of head injuries, malnutrition, and inadequately treated disease during captivity among former POWs, it is crucial to partial out the effects of each to obtain a full understanding of the long-term biological effects of captivity in this population.

THE CAPTOR–CAPTIVE RELATIONSHIP AND COPING

Reports detailing the torture, coping, and recovery problems faced by U.S. POWs held by North Vietnam (Hunter, 1992; Nice, Garland, Hilton, Baggett, & Mitchell, 1996; Ursano, Wheatley, Sledge, Rahe, & Carlson, 1986) may be relevant to the concerns of countries affected by war and social turmoil. Problems faced by families of POWs and families of soldiers missing in action are also relevant (Hunter, 1993). The results of this work are reviewed here.

Farber, Harlow, and West (1957) analyzed the tactics of captors to compromise the functioning of POWs and identified three components: (a) debility, induced through starvation, fatigue, infliction of pain, and failure to adequately treat diseases and injuries; (b) dread, the anticipatory anxiety induced through unrelenting uncertainty and threat of death, pain, and nonrelease; and (c) dependency, developed because captors totally control resources for alleviating the first two states. The power relationships developed by captors have several components, including isolation, deprivation, abuse, and interrogation (Hinkle & Wolff, 1956). Isolation and the denial of access to communication are induced through solitary confinement and psychological removal from previous sources of identification. Understanding the specific components of POWs' captivity and how they coped with efforts to isolate and demean them are important to initiating any clinical interventions. Appreciating the methods employed to cope with the strategies of the captors will assist the clinician in identifying strengths on which to build additional coping skills in the postcaptivity period.

Deprivation of food and medical care, physical and sexual abuse, and seemingly endless periods of interrogation are characteristics of captivity that are frequent enough to explore with all POWs who have been released (Suedfeld, 1990). To more fully understand the experience of any individual's captivity, therapists are encouraged to assess the context of the captivity and both the successful and unsuccessful coping efforts of the survivor. These assessments will communicate to the survivor a genuine effort to understand the experience and an appreciation of the issues involved in recovery.

RECENT ATTENTION TO U.S. POWS

The capacities of a society to confront and understand its traumatic past and to recognize and assist its survivors are attributes of progressive, caring nations. POW research in the countries noted earlier may be interpreted as a society's recognition that what happened to these survivors is significant, worthy of recognition by the greater society, and important to address in systematic and thoughtful ways. In the United States, the major boost for POW research and services came from the 1981 Former Prisoners of War Benefits Act (Public Law 97–31). This act offered health examinations and certain benefits to all POWs. Using repatriation records and veterans service organizations, all locatable POWs were registered, provided medical examinations, and offered follow-up physical and mental health care to address their needs. Use of a standard examination format and a medical history questionnaire helped to provide uniform data for the more than 23,000 POWs examined in the first years of the program (Veterans Administration, 1987). As a result, there has been a nationwide increase in services and benefits for POWs and their families. Even though they had experienced significant health problems since repatriation, most POWs did not seek treatment until the implementation of the mandated protocol exams.

Many former POWs who could benefit from psychiatric and psychological treatment have not accessed available assistance. Some researchers have hypothesized that this is due directly to the captivity experiences. For example, these past experiences often created a mindset of passivity and resignation, while some POWs developed survivor guilt and questioned whether they deserved benefits of any kind (Farber et al., 1957). Further, some POWs felt abandoned by their government when they were taken captive ("we were expendable") and rejected governmental efforts at aid. Still others perceived that they were treated with indifference and rejection by society because of their status as "soldiers who surrendered to the enemy." For individuals who were held captive, and in particular those who developed PTSD, outreach activities are needed to identify and assist those at greatest risk for disability and in need of assistance.

Elias (1986), in noting the advances made by the Department of Veterans Affairs toward POWs, stated that interventions were developed that "beckon victims to help liberate themselves." The mandated exam process and the community-based efforts to encourage POWs to seek these exams resulted in widespread participation. Many former POWs and their families who now are being served never would have sought medical and psychological treatment without community encouragement, which often came from fellow veterans who knew of their situation and unresolved needs. Together with increases in treatment and benefits, research was authorized that helped determine links between captivity maltreatment and later medical and psychiatric disorders, including PTSD, other anxiety disorders, depression, and ischemic heart disease. Accordingly, benefits and treatment have been granted for these conditions.

The following account illustrates the experiences of one POW who suffered nearly 50 years with untreated PTSD until offered services as a result of the initiatives described above:

A 74-year-old white male reported a normal childhood, leaving school after 10th grade to work and play semiprofessional baseball. His National Guard unit was activated in 1941 and sent to the Philippines. Japan attacked on December 8, 1941. Following fierce combat with heavy casualties, mainland Allied forces were surrendered April 9, 1942. Together with more than 10,000 ill and underfed Americans, he was forced onto the Bataan Death March. As a POW, he witnessed senseless executions and endured beatings, death threats, malnutrition, and multiple untreated medical diseases. While laboring, his weight dropped from 155 to 80 pounds until he was too ill to work. In December 1944, he and 1,600 other POWs were forced into the hold of one of the last ships to leave the Philippines. Only half were to survive transport to Japan. The unmarked ship was sunk by American planes after leaving port; he swam to shore. He was recaptured and put on another ship that was hit by American planes near Formosa; he again swam to shore. The journey to Japan on these "hell ships" included 49 days of confinement in the overcrowded, intensely hot holds of three different ships with little food, water, or sanitation. Many POWs became delirious, attacked fellow POWs, and were killed.

In Japan he labored in a coal mine for 12 hours per day, 10 days at a time followed by 1 day off. Rations were about 1,000 calories per day. Anyone too ill to work was placed on half rations. Camp officials made it clear that they were under orders to execute all POWs if America invaded Japan. Instead, the officials abandoned the camp following the nuclear bombings of Hiroshima and Nagasaki and the Japanese surrender.

Throughout his captivity and postwar life he has maintained an inner posture of resistance. He returned home, married, recuperated from tuberculosis, and began work for the Postal Service, where he remained a clerk for 36 years, failing to be promoted "because of my personality." He and his wife raised three children.

His only Axis 1 disorder was PTSD, lifetime and current. He recalled complaining of nervousness to several nonpsychiatric physicians after World War II but was not referred for mental health services. He reported being told he would "have to live with it." His records indicate that he refused tranquilizers. He suffers a trauma-related phobia of closed spaces and experiences most of the PTSD symptoms, chiefly daily intrusive recollections, frequent nightmares, hypervigilance, and survivor guilt. His only friends are a few other POWs of Japan.

After participation in the POW protocol examination and a POW research study, he joined a POW support group that meets twice monthly. Although he at times appears anxious and speaks rapidly, he describes decreased distress and has become more comfortable in discussing personal concerns as a result of participating in the group. (Used with permission.)

In summary, POW research demonstrates the links between captivity maltreatment and persistent psychiatric disorders. The POW literature also reveals the continuing needs of many POWs and their families for support and treatment. Community support for treatment is an important element in assisting these survivors to access and optimally use any services that are available.

REFERENCES

Beebe, G. W. (1975). Follow-up studies of World War II and Korean War prisoners, II: Morbidity, disability, and maladjustments. *American Journal of Epidemiology, 101*, 400–422.

Cohen, B. M., & Cooper, M. Z. (1954). *A follow-up study of World War II prisoners of war.* Washington, DC: U.S. Department of Veterans Affairs.

Crawford, J. N., & Reid, J. A. G. (1947). Nutritional disease affecting Canadian troops held prisoners of war by the Japanese. *Canadian Journal of Research, 25*, 53–85.

Crocq, M. A., Macher, J. P., Barros-Beck, J., Rosenberg, S. J., & Duval, F. (1993). Posttraumatic stress disorder in World War II prisoners of war from Alsace-Lorraine who survived captivity in the USSR. In J. P. Wilson & B. Raphael (Eds.), *International handbook of traumatic stress syndromes* (pp. 253–261). New York: Plenum Press.

Drozdek, B. (1997). Follow-up study of concentration camp survivors from Bosnia-Herzegovina: Three years later. *Journal of Nervous and Mental Disease, 185*, 690–694.

Eberly, R. E., & Engdahl, B. E. (1991). Prevalence of somatic and psychiatric disorders among former prisoners of war. *Hospital and Community Psychiatry, 42*, 807–813.

Eitinger, L. (1985). The concentration camp syndrome: An organic brain syndrome? *Integrative Psychiatry, 3*, 115–126.

Elias, R. (1986). *The politics of victimization: Victims, victimology, and human rights.* New York: Oxford University Press.

Engdahl, B. E., Dikel, T., Eberly, R. E., & Blank, Jr., A. (1997). Posttraumatic stress disorder in a community sample of former prisoners of war: A normative response to severe trauma. *American Journal of Psychiatry, 154*, 1576–1581.

Engdahl, B. E., Dikel, T., Eberly, R. E., & Blank, Jr., A. (1998). The comorbidity and course of psychiatric disorders in a community sample of former prisoners of war. *American Journal of Psychiatry, 155*(12), 1740–1745.

Engdahl, B. E., & Eberly, R. E. (1990). The effects of torture and other captivity maltreatment: Implications for psychology. In P. Suedfeld (Ed.), *Psychology and torture* (pp. 31–48). Washington, DC: Hemisphere Press.

Epstein, H. (1979). *Children of the Holocaust.* New York: Putnam.

Farber, I., Harlow, H., & West, L. (1957). Brainwashing, conditioning, and DDD (debility, dependency, and dread). *Sociometry, 20*, 271–285.

Former Prisoners of War Benefits Act of 1981 (Title 38, U.S.C.), Pub. L. No. 97–31, 95 Stat. 935 (August 14, 1981).

Galitski, V. P. (1991). Social-psychological aspects of POWs. *Sotsiologicheskie Issledovaniya [Sociological Studies], 10,* 48–63.

Hinkle, L., & Wolff, H. (1956). Communist interrogation and indoctrination of "enemies of the state." *Archives of Psychiatry and Neurology, 76,* 115–174.

Hunter, E. J. (1992). The Vietnam prisoner of war. In J. P. Wilson & B. Raphael (Eds.), *International handbook of traumatic stress syndromes* (pp. 297–303). New York: Plenum Press.

Hunter, E. J. (1993). Long-term effects on children of a parent missing in wartime. In F. W. Kaslow (Ed.), *The military family: In peace and war.* New York: Springer.

Kessler, R. C., Sonnega, A., Bromet, E., Hughes, M., & Nelson, C. B. (1995). Posttraumatic stress disorder in the National Comorbidity Survey. *Archives of General Psychiatry, 52,* 1048–1060.

Klonoff, H., McDougall, G., Clark, G., Kramer, P., & Horgan, J. (1976). The neuropsychological, psychiatric, and physical effects of prolonged and severe stress: 30 years later. *Journal of Nervous and Mental Disease, 163,* 246–252.

Mollica, R. F., & Caspi-Yavin, Y. (1992). Overview: The assessment and diagnosis of torture events and symptoms. In M. Basoglu (Ed.), *Torture and its consequences: Current treatment approaches* (pp. 253–276). New York: Cambridge University Press.

Newman, F. H. (1944). The prisoner of war mentality: Its effect after repatriation. *British Medical Journal, 1,* 8–10.

Nice, D. S., Garland, C. F., Hilton, S. M., Baggett, J. C., & Mitchell, R. E. (1996). Long-term health outcomes and medical effects of torture among U.S. Navy prisoners of war in Vietnam. *Journal of the American Medical Association, 276,* 375–381.

Ohry, A., Solomon, Z., Neria, Y., Waysman, M., Bar-On, Z., & Levy, A. (1994). The aftermath of captivity: An 18-year follow-up of Israeli ex-POWs. *Behavioral Medicine, 20,* 27–33.

Op den Velde, W., Hovens, J. E., Aarts, P. G., Frey-Wouters, E., Falger, P. R., van Duijn, H., & de Groen, J. H. (1996). Prevalence and course of posttraumatic stress disorder in Dutch resistance veterans of the civilian resistance during World War II: An overview. *Psychological Reports, 78,* 519–529.

Page, W. F., Engdahl, B. E., & Eberly, R. E. (1991). Prevalence and correlates of depressive symptoms among former prisoners of war. *Journal of Nervous and Mental Disease, 179,* 670–677.

Paul, H. A. (1986). *Einflüsse extremer Belastungen auf die psychischen und psychosozialen Verhältnisse ehemaliger Kriegsgefangener* [The influence of extreme stress on the psychological and psychosocial life circumstances of former prisoners of war]. Stuttgart, Germany: Gentner.

Peters, J., van Kammen, D. P., van Kammen, W. P., & Neylan, T. (1990). Sleep disturbance and computerized axial tomographic scan findings in former prisoners of war. *Comprehensive Psychiatry, 31,* 535–539.

Potts, M. K. (1994). Long-term effects of trauma: Posttraumatic stress among civilian internees of the Japanese during World War II. *Journal of Clinical Psychology, 50,* 681–698.

Richardson, H. J. (1965). *Report of a study of disabilities and problems of Hong Kong veterans 1964–1965.* Ottawa: Canadian Pensions Commission.

Solomon, Z., Neria, Y., Ohry, A., Waysman, M., & Ginzburg, K. (1994). PTSD among Israeli former prisoners of war and soldiers with combat stress reaction: A longitudinal study. *American Journal of Psychiatry, 151,* 554–559.

Stenger, C. A. (1996). *American prisoners of war in WWI, WWII, Korea, Vietnam, Persian Gulf, and Somalia.* Washington, DC: Department of Veterans Affairs Advisory Committee on Former Prisoners of War.

Suedfeld, P. (Ed.). (1990). *Psychology and torture.* Washington, DC: Hemisphere Press.

Sutker, P. B., Winstead, M. D., Galina, Z. H., & Allain, A. N. (1991). Cognitive deficits and psychopathology among former prisoners of war. *American Journal of Psychiatry, 148,* 67–72.

Tennant, C. C., Goulston, K. J., & Dent, O. F. (1986). The psychological effect of being a prisoner of war: Forty years after release. *American Journal of Psychiatry, 143,* 618–621.

Thygesen, P., Hermann, K., & Willanger, R. (1970). Concentration camp survivors in Denmark: Persecution, disease, disability, compensation. *Danish Medical Bulletin, 17,* 65–108.

Ursano, R. J., Wheatley, R. D., Sledge, W., Rahe, A., & Carlson, E. (1986). Coping and recovery styles in the Vietnam era prisoner of war. *Journal of Nervous and Mental Disease, 174,* 707–714.

Veterans Administration. (1987, May). Services provided to former POWs. *The VA Today,* 6.

10

Holocaust Trauma and Sequelae

BOAZ KAHANA and EVA KAHANA

The Nazi Holocaust is recognized as representing the ultimate culture of terror (Lewin, 1993). It has been argued that the effects of torture and maltreatment entered the scientific consciousness in its aftermath (Engdahl & Eberly, 1990). The enormity of the suffering of survivors of Nazi concentration camps and other atrocities has led to pioneering research on the long-term effects of massive psychic trauma. The history and contributions of the literature on survivors of the Nazi Holocaust also poignantly illustrate the complexities, ethical dilemmas, and scientific challenges inherent in understanding and documenting the role of perpetrators, bystanders, rescuers, and healers at various points in the experience and aftermath of trauma (Hilberg, 1992). The ethical and moral implications of focusing on alternative perspectives must also be acknowledged. A focus on documenting adverse impacts may serve to revictimize survivors, whereas a focus on their adaptability, strength, and resiliency may be construed as trivializing the horrors that they have endured (Davidson & Charny, 1992).

Garwood (1996) suggested that the four major elements of trauma suffered by Holocaust survivors are powerlessness, fear of annihilation, object loss, and torture. In addition to the original trauma suffered during the Holocaust, long-term survivors are also confronted with chronic stresses residual to the trauma. These stresses include intrusive memories of trauma, social and psychological isolation, and stigma (Kahana et al., 1997). In addition, survivors, like others, also confront normative chronic life stresses along with the possibility of nonnormative, post-Holocaust trauma, such as the Gulf War Scud missile attacks on Israel (Solomon &

BOAZ KAHANA • Department of Psychology, Cleveland State University, Cleveland, Ohio 44115.   **EVA KAHANA** • Department of Sociology, Case Western Reserve University, Cleveland, Ohio 44106.

The Mental Health Consequences of Torture, edited by Ellen Gerrity, Terence M. Keane, and Farris Tuma. Kluwer Academic/Plenum Publishers, New York, 2001.

Prager, 1992). Understanding the effect of the original trauma involves an appreciation of such cumulative life stresses.

In this chapter we consider evidence regarding the long-term impact of experiencing the Nazi Holocaust. We review factors that were found to ameliorate the negative physical, psychological, and social consequences of extreme maltreatment and torture during the Holocaust. We also note the problems that survivors face in coping with normative stresses of the life course, chronic stresses residual to the trauma, and new episodes of traumatization. Finally, we briefly address broader social issues relevant to other manifestations of maltreatment or torture, as illuminated by the experiences and adaptations of Holocaust survivors.

IMPACT OF TRAUMA

The traumatic events experienced by survivors of the Holocaust left an indelible mark on every aspect of their subsequent existence. The early and even longer-term impact of these events on the well-being, personality, and peace of mind of survivors has been extensively documented by the clinical psychiatric literature and more recently by more quantitative social science research. Whereas the conclusions of clinicians have emphasized deep emotional disturbances among survivors, empirical studies have provided evidence of resilience and resourcefulness along with psychological distress (Whiteman, 1993).

Our research studies (B. Kahana, Harel, & Kahana, 1989) were among the first empirical investigations to focus on the long-term sequelae of experiencing the Holocaust. We conducted individual interviews with more than 300 Holocaust survivors, divided evenly between those living in the United States and those living in Israel. A comparison group of 300 non-Holocaust survivors who immigrated to the United States or to Israel just before World War II was included in the study. Differences were considered between survivors and the comparison group in terms of physical health, psychiatric symptomatology, and social functioning. The following discussion will draw on a review of diverse published studies as well as our own data in addressing the impact of the trauma and adaptation of survivors.

In addition to nomothetic approaches documenting the impact of trauma on groups of survivors, it is also important to acknowledge the valuable qualitative information available from ideographic approaches based on eyewitness accounts (e.g., Eisenberg, 1982; Tory, 1990; Wijze, 1997) and oral histories (e.g., Fisher, 1991; Langer, 1991).

Psychological Impact

Based on survivor accounts and psychiatric evaluations of those seeking help or compensation after the Holocaust, an extensive psychodynamic literature documented severe psychic damage, referred to as the "KZ syndrome," among Holocaust survivors (Chodoff, 1963; Krystal, 1968; Niederland, 1981). Numerous case studies revealed chronic states of depression and anxiety, anhedonia (inability to enjoy life), survivor guilt, unresolved grief, and hypermnesia (inability to suppress memories of persecution). These studies were subsequently critiqued on the basis of bias resulting from their focus on clinical populations, their lack of reliance on standard and replicable assessment techniques, the absence of control groups, and their failure to focus on coping and strengths of survivors (Harel, Kahana, & Kahana, 1988).

Eitinger and associates conducted the first large-scale studies of Holocaust survivors, which provided data on psychological sequelae of the trauma during the decades immediately following the Holocaust. On the basis of data collected in the 1960s (Eitinger, 1980; Eitinger & Strom, 1973), Holocaust survivors who were treated in Oslo psychiatric facilities exhibited significant somatic and psychological scars.

Community surveys of nonclinical populations of Holocaust survivors were initiated in the United States, Canada, and Israel during the 1980s, almost 40 years after the trauma. In an early study—based on 135 survivors and a comparison group of 133 immigrants to Canada—Eaton, Sigal, and Weinfeld (1982) observed significant elevations in psychological symptom distress among survivors, using the Langner index of mental health. Four or more symptoms were reported by 43% of survivors, compared with 28% of the comparison group.

One of the largest community-based studies of Holocaust survivors in Israel was reported by Carmil and Carel (1986) involving a group of 1,150 Holocaust survivors and a comparison group of 2,159 respondents. On the basis of selective questions from the Cornell Medical Index, small but statistically significant differences in psychological distress were found. Thirty-three percent of survivors reported three or more areas of distress versus 25% of the comparison group.

Our own study (Harel et al., 1988; B. Kahana et al., 1989, 1997; B. Kahana, Harel, & Kahana, 1988) remains the only investigation that simultaneously focused on the psychological distress among Holocaust survivors as well as a comparison group both in the United States and in Israel. In terms of psychological distress, survivors' Symptom Checklist-90 primary symptom dimension profiles were elevated relative to both comparison participants and standardized norms. In terms of morale, respondents' responses to Lawton's 17-item Morale Scale indicated striking differences between the survivor and comparison groups on 7 of the 17 items. Our overall findings portray significantly greater symptomatology among survivors than among those in the comparison group. However, there is considerable overlap between these two groups, and many survivors exhibit fewer symptoms or appear no different from those in the comparison group. Whereas such overlap in distributions is not surprising, it raises an important note of caution against stereotyping the Holocaust survivor as being psychologically impaired.

Few reports in the literature on the Holocaust use formal criteria for posttraumatic stress disorder (PTSD). In Kuch and Cox's (1992) study of 124 Holocaust survivors, 46.8% met the third edition *Diagnostic and Statistical Manual of Mental Disorders* (DSM-III; American Psychiatric Association, 1980) PTSD criteria. In a recent small-scale study of Holocaust survivors in Poland, PTSD criteria based on DSM-III-Revised (American Psychiatric Association, 1987) were found in all 21 survivors assessed (Orwid, Domagalska, & Pietruzewski, 1995).

Taken together, diverse studies considering the psychological impact of the Holocaust among long-term survivors reveal a consistent picture of a small, but statistically significant, elevation in indicators of psychological distress. Nevertheless, there is a noteworthy overlap in distributions between survivors and normal nontraumatized comparison groups.

Cognitive Impact

Early evidence of cognitive problems among Holocaust survivors was found by Eitinger (1980) in a sample of Norwegian patients who demonstrated poor memory and inability to concentrate. Encephalopathy was diagnosed in 81% of these survivors. The work of Shanan and Shahar (1983) still stands as a singular effort to consider differences in cognitive functioning between Holocaust survivors and those who did not endure the trauma of the Holocaust. In comparing matched groups of concentration camp inmates with persons who spent the Holocaust in hiding and those who lived in Israel during the Holocaust, these investigators found no significant differences in Wechsler Adult Intelligence Scale subscales (verbal or performance). Nevertheless, concentration camp survivors ranked lowest, those in hiding scored somewhat higher, and the nontraumatized group that lived in Israel ranked the highest. In a follow-up study of this cohort 8 years later, Shanan (1988–1989) observed age-appropriate cognitive functioning and active coping styles in the 25 remaining survivors compared with the remaining members of the control group. In a study of 44 concentration camp survivors and 31 matched control subjects, Lomranz, Shmotkin, Zechovoy, and Rosenberg (1985) found Holocaust survivors to be more past-oriented and less future-oriented than the comparison group.

Neuropsychological Impact

Although considerable work has been done on neurotransmitter functions among Vietnam veterans suffering from PTSD, relatively little research has focused on Holocaust survivors in this regard. In one recent study (Yehuda, Giller, Kahana, & Southwick, 1994), significant elevations in dopamine metabolites were found among Holocaust survivors, which was similar to findings among Vietnam veterans. The role of neurotransmitters in Holocaust survivors suffering from PTSD is currently being studied, as is the hypothalamic–pituitary–adrenocortical axis (Yehuda, Boisneau, Lowy, & Giller, 1996). Additionally, systematic studies are needed on the effectiveness of psychopharmacological medications for Holocaust survivors (e.g., antidepressants, benzodiazepines, and antipsychotic medications).

Physical Health Impact

Eitinger and Strom (1973) initially investigated the physical health sequelae of the Holocaust. In research based on Norwegians who were detained in German concentration camps, survivors showed higher mortality rates, more frequent hospitalizations, and higher incidence of sick periods. In a study based on Holocaust survivors applying for reparations in Germany, Matussek (1975) found evidence of somatic disorders that were related to the severity of trauma endured. Physical symptoms persist even in the long-term aftermath of the Holocaust among individuals who continue to survive into late life. Among 124 survivors studied by Kuch and Cox (1992) 50 years after the Holocaust, 89.5% reported severe headaches, 50.8% had persistent dizziness, and 33.1% reported gastrointestinal distress. Holocaust survivors in our study (B. Kahana et al., 1989) reported significantly more physical symptoms than respondents in the comparison group. Thus, significantly greater proportions of survivors reported symptoms that may have a psychogenic component, such as headaches and abdominal cramps. Conversely, few significant differences emerged between the survivors and those in the comparison groups for diagnosed illnesses such as arthritis, cancer, and Parkinson's disease. Furthermore, 89% of survivors reported that the Holocaust had adversely affected their physical health, although only 31% said that the negative effects were extreme.

Our data about the nature of physical symptoms among Holocaust survivors are consistent with reports by Goldfeld, Mollica, Pesavento, and Faraone (1988) about prevalent symptoms derived from a meta-analysis of research involving victims of torture. These studies noted headaches, hearing impairments, gastrointestinal distress, and joint pain as the most prevalent symptoms.

Social Adaptation

Two recent studies have addressed the social adaptation of Holocaust survivors from a sociological perspective. Helmreich (1992) and Hass (1995) each conducted in-depth qualitative interviews with nonclinical volunteers who survived the Holocaust. Their research has documented the social achievements and resilience of American Holocaust survivors who built productive lives and developed cohesive families in spite of the extreme trauma they had endured. This research contrasts with psychiatric studies that have focused on intergenerational transmission of trauma (Kestenberg, 1972; Russell, 1974).

Our own research, based on more quantitative data, also supports the findings of Helmreich and Hass. Thus, we find that Holocaust survivors who generally have much more limited educational attainment than the comparison group (average of high school versus average of college education), nevertheless, do not differ in terms of income, occupational status, or work history. Many survivors also maintain stable marriages and close family ties.

INDIVIDUAL DIFFERENCES

Research has shown that the consequences of maltreatment are likely to be conditioned both by predisposing chronic tensions and resources of individual victims and by the duration and severity of maltreatment (Engdahl & Eberly, 1990). It is noteworthy that in the literature on Holocaust survivors, the focus has generally been on the overall impact of the trauma, with little research interest directed toward individual or situational differences in experience or impact of trauma.

Degree of Trauma

There has been only limited research differentiating the impact of surviving extreme trauma on the basis of specific types of trauma endured. It has often been noted that when maltreatment is overwhelming and horrendous, there is little value in attempting to categorize the magnitude of maltreatment. Nevertheless, a few studies have focused on differences in psychological distress among those who survived the Holocaust in death camps versus those hiding in other settings (Robinson, Rapaport-Bar-Sever, & Rapaport, 1994). Research has found some evidence that psychological distress is correlated with intensity of trauma. Accordingly, death camp survivors exhibited more depression and anhedonia than did survivors who were not incarcerated in such settings (Robinson et al., 1994). In a study of sleep disturbances among Holocaust survivors, Rosen, Reynolds, Yaeger, Houck, and Hurwitz (1991) found that Holocaust survivors who were incarcerated longer reported significantly more sleep disturbances and awakenings resulting from bad dreams than did those who experienced less extensive trauma.

A study of the files of Holocaust survivors who applied for compensation from Germany found that survivors who had been in the Auschwitz concentration camp had significantly more symptoms and were three times more likely to meet PTSD diagnostic criteria than a comparison group who did not spend time in a concentration camp (Kuch & Cox, 1992). In a Canadian community survey (Eaton et al., 1982), a small but notable difference was observed in responses to the Langner mental health scale, with concentration camp survivors showing a higher incidence of psychological distress than those who survived in other contexts. On balance, the data showed only small effects based on distinguishing different magnitudes of Holocaust-related suffering. Furthermore, several studies did not discern significant differences between groups who spent the Holocaust in different settings (Shanan & Shahar, 1983; Yehuda, Elkin, et al., 1996).

Personal Background

Age and gender have been the major personal background variables considered as sources of diversity in adapting to the Holocaust.

Age

An Australian research study with 200 Holocaust survivors provides some evidence that those individuals who experienced persecution during their childhood exhibit greater psychological problems in selected areas such as "contact abnormalities" (Bower, 1994). Shanan and Shahar's (1983) research also suggests that Holocaust survivors who were children during the Holocaust exhibited greater difficulties in its aftermath. In one recent study, Yehuda, Elkin, et al.

(1996) reported a significant negative relationship between age at the time of trauma and PTSD symptoms, with the exception of intrusive thoughts, which showed a positive relationship with age.

Gender

Studies of Holocaust survivors also found that the long-term effect of the Holocaust differed by gender. In a large-scale survey of Holocaust survivors and a comparison group in Israel, Carmil and Carel (1986) reported that women Holocaust survivors were significantly more likely to report psychological distress than were men, with 85% of women endorsing some emotional distress items versus 65% of men.

COPING WITH LIFE STRESSES SUBSEQUENT TO THE TRAUMA OF THE HOLOCAUST

Latent PTSD may be activated by new life crises or by particularly stressful events (Christenson, Walker, Ross, & Maltbie, 1981). A number of empirical studies conducted in the long-term aftermath of the Holocaust have explored the issue of the potential vulnerability of victims of this trauma in response to later stresses. There is evidence that Holocaust survivors exhibit more severe reactions when facing life-threatening stressors, such as major illness or war (Rosenbloom, 1985).

Peretz, Baider, Ever-Hadani, and DeNour (1994) compared symptoms of psychological distress among cancer patients who were survivors of the Holocaust with comparison groups of cancer patients who did not endure the Holocaust and Holocaust survivors who were healthy. The findings revealed much greater incidence of distress among Holocaust survivors coping with the stress of cancer than among the nontraumatized respondents.

Research conducted in the aftermath of the Gulf War found evidence that survivors of the Holocaust were vulnerable to retraumatization. Studies focusing on wartime stress showed that Holocaust survivors whose homes were damaged by Scud missile attacks during the Persian Gulf War exhibited dramatically more distress than did Holocaust survivors whose homes did not sustain such damage or persons who did not endure the Holocaust but whose homes did sustain such damage. Furthermore, research comparing 61 Holocaust survivors with a matched group of 131 elderly persons who did not suffer the trauma of the Holocaust reveals that Holocaust survivors perceived higher levels of danger and exhibited greater anxiety than the comparison group after the Gulf War (Solomon & Prager, 1992). In an important study focusing on children of survivors, Solomon (1989) found greater evidence of PTSD among soldiers who participated in the 1982 Lebanon War and whose parents were Holocaust survivors than in a comparison group of soldiers whose parents were not in the Holocaust.

These data are also consistent with earlier reports by Eaton et al. (1982), who had observed a correlation between psychological distress among Holocaust survivors on the Langner mental health scale and their perception of increased anti-Semitism in Montreal, Canada. These data suggest a reawakening of the psychiatric consequences of earlier trauma in the face of the potential reemergence of ethnic persecution.

PROTECTIVE FACTORS FACILITATING HEALING

Psychotherapy

Extensive literature exists on psychotherapy with Holocaust survivors (Danieli, 1981). However, much of this work is in the psychoanalytic tradition, and data on the efficacy of these therapies are limited. Also, research has shown that only a small proportion of survivors have received psychotherapy. In a study of 124 Holocaust survivors seeking compensation, a majority of whom showed symptoms of PTSD (DSM-III criteria), only 17.7% had received any form of psychotherapy (Kuch & Cox, 1992). On the basis of our data on more than 300 U.S. and Israeli Holocaust survivors (B. Kahana et al., 1997), less than 10% of the survivors had received psychotherapy or counseling. We recently collected data on Holocaust survivors who have remained in Hungary since the end of World War II, where less than 2% had received any formal treatment. This low percentage suggests that political and social influences also play important roles in the access of survivors of trauma to formal services and in the acceptability of mental health services to the survivors. There is also some evidence that survivors do not readily benefit from traditional psychodynamic therapies (Krystal, 1991). However, there is insufficient systematic research evidence to evaluate these claims.

The problems of therapists in successfully treating Holocaust survivors may have complex etiologies, including the challenging nature of the posttraumatic stress problems addressed. Other barriers include insufficient prior treatment guidelines and countertransference (Danieli, 1981). Some suggest that therapists themselves, in spite of their generally positive attitudes (Ofri, Solomon, & Dasberg, 1995), reflect the social stigma and misunderstanding of Holocaust survivors and other traumatized groups (Solomon, 1995).

Social Relations

Social resources and integration represent the most important documented protective factors that were influential before, during, and after exposure to trauma. Strong family attachments before the trauma have been cited as protective factors in explaining the remarkable resilience of many survivors (Lee, 1988). There is strong evidence that even during the war, many victims formed helping dyads and friendships in the midst of terrible living conditions. Through such protective ties and social relationships, they could preserve a human identity or "human image" (Davidson & Charny, 1992). Postwar self-help groups also facilitated posttraumatic adaptation and normalization of life among survivors. Such social supports served as a substitute extended family and may have reduced the need for formal psychotherapy. Data from our research have also documented that survivors living in Israel, where they formed strong social ties to the community, show less evidence of psychological distress than their U.S. counterparts (B. Kahana et al., 1997).

In considering the therapeutic value of social integration for survivors of the Holocaust, Solomon (1995) has provided an incisive analysis. She points to paradoxes involved in the integration of Holocaust survivors in Israeli society. On the one hand, the ability to contribute to the building of a community and to participate in social initiatives may have been therapeutic for survivors of past socially induced trauma. On the other hand, the very efforts to draw survivors into these new initiatives could also lead to denying or delegitimizing their prior suffering. This could have been one mechanism that contributed to a conspiracy of silence. Such problems can be even more complex for survivors who must continue to live in the very societies where their trauma had been perpetrated (Friedlander, 1993) and where there is an upsurge in nationalization during the post-Communist era (Kovacs, 1997). Thus, our recent research on Hungarian Holocaust survivors demonstrates that this group has continued to grapple with dramatic social changes in a milieu that still includes individuals who were perpetrators of trauma or bystanders who are sympathetic to Nazis (E. Kahana & Kahana, n.d.). These challenges would also be clearly applicable to survivors of social victimization in South Africa.

Collective and Societal Healing Efforts

Collective or social mechanisms for healing have played an important role in the posttraumatic adjustment of Holocaust survivors. Meaningful communication with society can serve as a valuable therapeutic release. In this way Holocaust survivors can find meaning in survivorship through retelling their experiences and preserving the collective memory of their suffering. They can also celebrate survival by educating the next generation and by establishing museums or other war memorials. It is noteworthy that these efforts at healing have become fully realized only 40 or 50 years after the occurrence of the trauma. Survivors had to overcome the widely noted conspiracy of silence (Bergman & Jucovy, 1982; Solomon, 1995), as well as their own reluctance or inability to reminisce about the painful past.

Contrasted with the very limited reliance on formal mental health services, survivors have increasingly turned to informal healing experiences often shared with fellow survivors. These include bearing witness to the cataclysmic event of the Holocaust (Wiesenthal, 1986), participating in commemorative ceremonies (Hass, 1995), undertaking healing journeys to the sites of their former homes and of their persecution, and participating in efforts to bring former Nazis to justice (Blum, 1977). These are mostly bottom-up rather than top-down mechanisms for healing, as noted in other work on survivors of torture and atrocities in this volume. The social context for many of the healing activities noted by survivors is in the spheres of close affiliation with family, religious groups, and survivor groups. Patriotic affiliation with their adoptive countries and affiliation with ideologies that refute racism, such as socialism or the civil rights movement in the United States, have also been found to be meaningful (Dinnerstein, 1982). The broader social nexus within which the trauma is now considered includes a focus on rescuers (Fogelman, 1994; Tec, 1986; Wiesenthal, 1989). Similarly, growing attention has been directed at the resistance movement during the Holocaust (Ainsztein, 1975; Suhl, 1975). Such attention to forces of "good," even at a time when "evil" permeates social reality, can help enhance self-efficacy and diminish feelings of helplessness among survivors. In contrast to grass-roots initiatives, top-down services, including social or mental health services, have been used by survivors. Reparation, another top-down approach, could potentially promote reconciliation. However, implementation of reparations has had a checkered history, often serving to stigmatize and revictimize survivors. While some survivors benefited from such efforts, most survivors accepted them with much unease and conflict (Kestenberg, 1982).

CONTEXTUALIZING THE HOLOCAUST EXPERIENCE

With the elapse of time since the Holocaust, collective memories of trauma have more freely found expression. There has been a great upsurge of interest in better understanding the immense complexity of this cataclysmic event.

New insights have been gained from survivor testimonies and oral histories by individuals who were previously not ready to reflect on their experiences or whose experiences society was not ready to hear. The theoretical underpinnings of work on survivorship have also been increasingly diverse, bringing into play reflections of artists, poets, and humanists, along with social science perspectives (Amishai-Maisels, 1993; Avisar, 1988; Braham, 1980; Eliach, 1982). Finally, moving beyond the homogenizing effects of trauma, social scientists and clinicians alike are beginning to pay attention to the diversity in human experiences in responding to and interpreting the trauma. Thus, more attention has been given to the Holocaust experiences of women (DeSilva, 1993; Eibeshitz & Eilenberg-Eibeshitz, 1993) and children (Eisenberg, 1982; Fisher, 1991).

Researchers are also beginning to take a more process-oriented view, as in the book *Journey Back From Hell* (Gill, 1988), recognizing that we must look beyond outcomes of trauma such as PTSD and focus on the healing journey required of survivors as they move on with their lives. This temporal emphasis has also allowed us to take a closer look at the stages of the post-Holocaust journey. Thus, the initial period of resettlement and the social isolation of survivors as they tried to build new lives have been highlighted (Baumel, 1990; Dinnerstein, 1982).

In addition to temporal considerations of process, there is also conceptual development regarding mechanisms involved in dealing with stress and, in particular, in the central role of meaning and memory (Langer, 1991) in trauma. Finally, the literature is beginning to address the previously neglected broader social issues raised by torture and "man's inhumanity to man" as we focus on perpetrators (Lifton, 1986) and on social values that endorse violence (Pawelczynska, 1979). Issues regarding perpetrators have given rise to a debate about the degree to which perpetrators were misled or simply followed orders (Friedlander, 1993;

Gilbert, 1985) or, alternatively, served as Hitler's willing executioners (Goldhagen, 1996).

Deeper philosophical questions have also been raised to explore the occurrence of such gross inhumanity and the common roots of evil in all genocide (Staub, 1989; Wallimann & Dobkowski, 1987). Parallels have been drawn between Nazi atrocities and other examples of genocidal mentality (Fasching, 1993; Lifton & Markusen, 1990). There has also been recognition of society's frequent failure to censure perpetrators and its tolerance of their rising to leadership positions (Hazzard, 1990). The implications of the Holocaust for understanding Christian–Jewish relationships and, more generally, minority–majority relationships have been explored using both historical and sociological perspectives. Some of these works also grapple with issues of reconciliation (Bauer et al., 1989; Chalk & Jonassohn, 1990).

CONCLUSION

A review of the scientific literature on survivors of the Holocaust provides consistent evidence of lasting psychological scars left by the overwhelming maltreatment and torture that characterize the experience of survivors. Since formal studies of PTSD among Holocaust survivors are of recent origin (using DSM-III and other criteria), it is necessary to rely on other indicators of mental health problems and psychological distress in evaluating studies of the impact of the Holocaust. Community surveys and assessments based on clinical populations yield evidence of sleep disturbances, depression, anxiety, and intrusive memories even 50 years after the original trauma. The duration and intensity of traumatic experiences, as well as more recent life crises, are correlated with negative outcomes. New stresses, particularly of a life-threatening nature, tend to rekindle PTSD and psychological distress even among generally well-functioning survivors. In spite of strong and enduring evidence of survivors living with chronic stress as a residue of traumatic Holocaust experiences, there is also remarkable evidence of their social achievements, adaptability, and resilience. Major evidence of healing is associated with social supports and social integration rather than formal psychotherapy.

New developments in Holocaust scholarship have helped to contextualize survivorship. They also help us in recognizing the diversity and uniqueness of the survivor experience of each subgroup exposed to torture and inhumanity, while at the same time being able to assimilate that uniqueness into a collective understanding. In this process, universality no longer threatens uniqueness, and the message of Holocaust survivors can enlighten our understanding of other exemplars of torture and related violence and trauma.

REFERENCES

Ainsztein, R. (1975). *Jewish resistance in Nazi-occupied Eastern Europe.* New York: Barnes & Noble.

American Psychiatric Association. (1980). *Diagnostic and statistical manual of mental disorders* (3rd ed.). Washington, DC: Author.

American Psychiatric Association. (1987). *Diagnostic and statistical manual of mental disorders* (3rd ed., rev.). Washington, DC: Author.

Amishai-Maisels, Z. (1993). *Depiction and interpretation: The influence of the Holocaust on the visual arts.* New York: Pergamon Press.

Avisar, I. (1988). *Screening the Holocaust: Cinema's images of the unimaginable.* Bloomington, IN: Indiana University Press.

Bauer, Y., Eckardt, A., Little, F., Franklin, H., Maxwell, E., Maxwell, R., & Patterson, D. (Eds.). (1989). *Remembering for the future: Working papers and addenda.* New York: Elsevier Science.

Baumel, J. T. (1990). *Unfulfilled promise: Rescue and resettlement of Jewish refugee children in the United States, 1934–1945.* Juneau, AK: Denali Press.

Bergman, M., & Jucovy, M. (1982). *Generations of the Holocaust.* New York: Basic Books.

Blum, H. (1977). *Wanted! The search for Nazis in America.* New York: Quadrangle/New York Times.

Bower, H. (1994). The concentration camp syndrome. *Australian and New Zealand Journal of Psychiatry, 28*(3), 391–397.

Braham, R. L. (1980). *The politics of genocide: The Holocaust in Hungary.* New York: Columbia University Press.

Carmil, D., & Carel, R. (1986). Emotional distress and satisfaction in life among Holocaust survivors: A community study of survivors and controls. *Psychological Medicine, 16,* 141–149.

Chalk, F. R., & Jonassohn, K. (1990). *The history and sociology of genocide.* New Haven, CT: Yale University Press.

Chodoff, P. (1963). Late effects of the concentration camp syndrome. *Archives of General Psychiatry, 8,* 323–333.

Christenson, R., Walker, J., Ross, D., & Maltbie, A. (1981). Reactivation of traumatic conflicts. *American Journal of Psychiatry, 138,* 984–985.

Danieli, Y. (1981). The aging survivor of the Holocaust: On achievement of integration in aging survivors of the Nazi Holocaust. *Journal of Geriatric Psychiatry, 14,* 191–210.

Davidson, S., & Charny, I. (1992). *Holding on to humanity: The message of Holocaust survivors—The Shamai Davidson papers.* New York: New York University Press.

DeSilva, P. (1993). Post-traumatic stress disorder: Cross-cultural aspects. *International Review of Psychiatry, 5*(2–3), 217–229.

Dinnerstein, L. (1982). *America and the survivors of the Holocaust.* New York: Columbia University Press.

Eaton, W., Sigal, J., & Weinfeld, M. (1982). Impairment of Holocaust survivors after 33 years: Data from an unbiased community sample. *American Journal of Psychiatry, 139,* 773–777.

Eibeshitz, J., & Eilenberg-Eibeshitz, A. (1993). *Women in the Holocaust: A collection of testimonies.* Brooklyn, NY: Remember.

Eisenberg, A. (1982). *The lost generation: Children in the Holocaust.* New York: Pilgrim Press.

Eitinger, L. (1980). The concentration camp syndrome and its late sequela. In J. Dimsdale (Ed.), *Survivors, victims and perpetrators.* New York: Hemisphere Press.

Eitinger, L., & Strom, A. (1973). *Mortality and morbidity after excessive stress: A follow-up investigation of Norwegian concentration camp survivors.* New York: Humanities Press.

Eliach, Y. (1982). *Hasidic tales of the Holocaust.* New York: Vintage Books.

Engdahl, B. E., & Eberly, R. E. (1990). The effects of torture and other captivity maltreatment: Implications for psychology. In P. Suedfeld (Ed.), *Psychology and torture* (pp. 31–48). Washington, DC: Hemisphere Press.

Fasching, D. (1993). *The ethical challenge of Auschwitz and Hiroshima: Apocalypse or utopia?* Albany, NY: State University of New York Press.

Fisher, J. G. (1991). *The persistence of youth: Oral testimonies of the Holocaust.* New York: Greenwood Press.

Fogelman, E. (1994). *Conscience and courage: Rescuers of Jews during the Holocaust.* New York: Anchor Books.

Friedlander, S. (1993). *Memory, history, and the extermination of the Jews of Europe.* Bloomington, IN: Indiana University Press.

Garwood, A. (1996). The Holocaust and the power of powerlessness: Survivor guilt—An unhealed wound. *British Journal of Psychotherapy, 13*(2), 243–258.

Gilbert, M. (1985). *The Holocaust: A history of the Jews of Europe during the Second World War.* New York: Holt.

Gill, A. (1988). *The journey back from hell: Conversations with concentration camp survivors: An oral history.* New York: Avon Books.

Goldfeld, A., Mollica, R., Pesavento, B., & Faraone, S. (1988). The physical and psychological sequelae of torture: Symptomatology and diagnosis. *Journal of the American Medical Association, 259,* 2725–2729.

Goldhagen, D. J. (1996). *Hitler's willing executioners: Ordinary Germans and the Holocaust.* New York: Knopf.

Harel, Z., Kahana, B., & Kahana, E. (1988). Psychological well-being among Holocaust survivors and immigrants in Israel. *Journal of Traumatic Stress Studies, 1*(4), 413–428.

Hass, A. (1995). *The aftermath: Living with the Holocaust.* New York: Cambridge University Press.

Hazzard, S. (1990). *Countenance of truth: The United Nations and the Waldheim case.* New York: Viking Books.

Helmreich, W. (1992). *Against all odds.* New York: Simon & Schuster.

Hilberg, R. (1992). *Perpetrators, victims, bystanders: The Jewish catastrophe 1933–1945.* New York: Harper Collins.

Kahana, B., Harel, Z., & Kahana, E. (1988). Predictors of psychological well-being among survivors of the Holocaust. In J. Wilson, Z. Harel, & B. Kahana (Eds.), *Human adaptation to extreme stress: From the Holocaust to Vietnam* (pp. 171–192). New York: Plenum Press.

Kahana, B., Harel, Z., & Kahana, E. (1989). Clinical and gerontological issues facing survivors of the Nazi Holocaust. In P. Marcus & A. Rosenberg (Eds.), *Healing their wounds: Psychotherapy with Holocaust survivors and their families* (pp. 197–211). New York: Praeger.

Kahana, B., Kahana, E., Harel, Z., Kelly, K., Monahan, P., & Holland, L. (1997). A framework for understanding the chronic stress of Holocaust survivors. In B. Gottlieb (Ed.), *Coping with chronic stress* (pp. 315–342). New York: Plenum Press.

Kahana, E., & Kahana, B. (n.d.). *Coping with social change in the aftermath of the Holocaust: A study of Hungarian Holocaust survivors.* Unpublished manuscript.

Kestenberg, J. (1972). Psychoanalytic contributions to the problem of survivors from Nazi persecution. *Israeli Annals of Psychiatry and Related Disciplines, 10,* 311–325.

Kestenberg, M. (1982). Discriminatory aspects of the German indemnification policy: A continuation of persecution. In M. S. Bergmann & M. E. Jucovy (Eds.), *Generations of the Holocaust* (pp. 62–79). New York: Columbia University Press.

Kovacs, A. (1997). *A Különbség Köztünk Van: Az Antiszemitizmus És a Fiatal Elit.* Budapest: Cserépfalvi.

Krystal, H. (1968). *Massive psychic trauma.* New York: International Universities Press.

Krystal, H. (1991). Integration and self-healing in post-traumatic states: A ten year retrospective. *American Imago, 48*(1), 93–118.

Kuch, K., & Cox, B. (1992). Symptoms of PTSD in 124 survivors of the Holocaust. *American Journal of Psychiatry, 149,* 337–340.

Langer, L. (1991). *Holocaust testimonies: The ruins of memory.* New Haven, CT: Yale University Press.

Lee, B. (1988). Holocaust survivors and internal strengths. *Journal of Humanistic Psychology, 28*(1), 67–96.

Lewin, C. (1993). Negotiated selves in the Holocaust. *Ethos, 21*(3), 295–318.

Lifton, R. J. (1986). *The Nazi doctors: Medical killing and the psychology of genocide*. New York: Basic Books.

Lifton, R. J., & Markusen, E. (1990). *The genocidal mentality: Nazi Holocaust and nuclear threat*. New York: Basic Books.

Lomranz, J., Shmotkin, D., Zechovoy, A., & Rosenberg, E. (1985). Time orientation in Nazi concentration camp survivors: Forty years after. *American Journal of Orthopsychiatry, 55*(2), 230–236.

Matussek, P. (1975). *Internment in concentration camps and its consequences*. New York: Springer-Verlag.

Niederland, W. (1981). The survivor syndrome: Further observations and dimensions. *American Psychoanalytic Association Journal, 29,* 413–425.

Ofri, I., Solomon, Z., & Dasberg, H. (1995). Attitudes of therapists toward Holocaust survivors. *Journal of Traumatic Stress, 8*(2), 229–242.

Orwid, M., Domagalska, K., & Pietruzewski, K. (1995). The psychosocial effects of the Holocaust on Jewish survivors living in Poland. *Psychiatria-Polska, 29*(3), 29–48.

Pawelczynska, A. (1979). *Values and violence in Auschwitz: A sociological analysis*. Berkeley, CA: University of California Press.

Peretz, T., Baider, L., Ever-Hadani, P., & DeNour, A. (1994). Psychological distress in female cancer patients with Holocaust experience. *General Hospital Psychiatry, 16*(6), 413–418.

Robinson, S., Rapaport-Bar-Sever, M., & Rapaport, J. (1994). The present state of people who survived the Holocaust as children. *Acta Psychiatrica Scandinavica, 89*(4), 242–245.

Rosen, J., Reynolds, C., Yaeger, A., Houck, P., & Hurwitz, L. (1991). Sleep disturbances in survivors of the Nazi Holocaust. *American Journal of Psychiatry, 148,* 62–66.

Rosenbloom, M. (1985). The Holocaust survivor in late life. In G. S. Getzel & M. J. Mellor (Eds.), *Gerontological social work practice in the community*. Wheeling, IL: Hawthorne Press.

Russell, A. (1974). Late psychosocial consequences in concentration camp survivors' families. *American Journal of Orthopsychiatry, 44,* 611–619.

Shanan, J. (1988–1989). Surviving the survivors: Late personality development of Jewish Holocaust survivors. *International Journal of Mental Health, 17*(4), 42–71.

Shanan, J., & Shahar, O. (1983). Cognitive and personality functioning of Jewish Holocaust survivors during the midlife transition (46–65) in Israel. *Archiv für Psychologie, 135,* 275–294.

Solomon, Z. (1989). A three year prospective study of posttraumatic stress disorder in Israeli combat veterans. *Journal of Traumatic Stress, 2,* 59–73.

Solomon, Z. (1995). From denial to recognition: Attitudes towards Holocaust survivors from WWII to the present. *Journal of Traumatic Stress, 8*(2), 2–15.

Solomon, Z., & Prager, E. (1992). Elderly Israeli Holocaust survivors during the Persian Gulf War: A study of psychological distress. *American Journal of Psychiatry, 149,* 1707–1710.

Staub, E. (1989). *The roots of evil: The origins of genocide and other group violence*. New York: Cambridge University Press.

Suhl, Y. (1975). *They fought back: The story of the Jewish resistance in Nazi Europe*. New York: Schocken.

Tec, N. (1986). *When light pierced the darkness: Christian rescue of Jews in Nazi-occupied Poland*. New York: Oxford University Press.

Tory, A. (1990). *Surviving the Holocaust: The Kovno Ghetto diary*. Cambridge: Harvard University Press.

Wallimann, I., & Dobkowski, M. N. (Eds.). (1987). *Genocide and the modern age: Etiology and case studies of mass death*. New York: Greenwood Press.

Whiteman, D. (1993). Holocaust survivors and escapees: Their strengths. *Psychotherapy, 30*(3), 443–451.

Wiesenthal, S. (1986). *Every day remembrance day: A chronicle of Jewish martyrdom*. New York: Holt.

Wiesenthal, S. (1989). *Justice, not vengeance.* Mahwah, NJ: Paulist Press.

Wijze, L. de. (1997). *Only my life: A survivor's story.* New York: St. Martin's Press.

Yehuda, R., Boisneau, D., Lowy, M., & Giller, E. (1996). Dose–response changes in plasma cortisol and lymphocyte glucocorticoid receptors following dexamethasone administration in combat veterans with and without posttraumatic stress disorder. *Archives of General Psychiatry, 52,* 583–593.

Yehuda, R., Elkin, A., Binder-Brynes, K., Kahana, B., Southwick, S., Schmeidler, J., & Giller, E. L. (1996). Dissociation in aging Holocaust survivors. *American Journal of Psychiatry, 153,* 3935–3940.

Yehuda, R., Giller, E., Kahana, B., & Southwick, S. (1994). Depressive features in Holocaust survivors with and without post-traumatic stress disorder. *Journal of Traumatic Stress, 7,* 699–704.

11

Survivors of War Trauma, Mass Violence, and Civilian Terror

DERRICK SILOVE and J. DAVID KINZIE

A 55-year-old Bosnian refugee, newly arrived in Australia, attended a trauma treatment service complaining of frightening flashbacks, difficulties concentrating, extreme anxiety, nightmares, and insomnia. During the war, he had been drafted into the local militia and soon found himself on the front line. He spoke with guilt about the deaths of those he felt forced to shoot ("I was forced to kill my countrymen in a war that I never supported"). After a few days, a mortar shell landed in his trench, killing several of his friends and inflicting horrific injuries on others. The front was overrun, and he fled to his home, hiding with his family in the cellar.

The family was discovered, and he was apprehended and taken to a concentration camp. His wife and daughters were sexually assaulted and evicted, being forced to march for several days to a remote area of the country. In the camp, he was deprived of food and water and was forced to labor 18 hours a day. Around him, friends were beaten, interrogated, tortured, and killed in summary executions. He believed that he was spared partly because of his age and partly because he knew one of the guards. The sense of injustice and humiliation was intense, but he knew that any protest would result in instant death. In the treatment sessions he received at the trauma center, he repeatedly returned to the issue of anger, stating that he could live with many of his symptoms, but not with the memories of the humiliation and injustices he had suffered. (Used with permission.)

DERRICK SILOVE • School of Psychiatry, Southwestern School, University of New South Wales, Sydney, Australia.   J. DAVID KINZIE • Department of Psychiatry, Oregon Health Sciences University, Portland, Oregon 97201.

The Mental Health Consequences of Torture, edited by Ellen Gerrity, Terence M. Keane, and Farris Tuma. Kluwer Academic/Plenum Publishers, New York, 2001.

INTRODUCTION

In recent decades, more than 100 regions around the world have been disrupted by war or social conflict. Groups of civilians continue to be exposed to sporadic acts of terror such as mass shootings, bombings, and hijackings. Although less is known about the psychosocial effects of such mass trauma on entire communities, evidence does exist that individuals directly exposed to trauma are at increased risk for substantial psychological disturbances.

Several recent studies have focused on the consequences of terrorist attacks (Abenhaim, Dab, & Salmic, 1992), mass shootings (Creamer, Burgess, Buckingham, & Pattison, 1993), aircraft hijackings (Cremniter et al., 1997), and bombings of civilian targets (Tucker, Dickson, Pfefferbaum, McDonald, & Allen, 1997). Research has also been undertaken on the social and health-related effects of political violence and war in countries such as Northern Ireland, Lebanon, and Sri Lanka. Most of the research on populations from developing countries has focused on refugees or displaced persons, particularly from Southeast Asia (see Kinzie, 1993, for an overview). In the last 5 years, the diversity and number of ethnic groups participating in such research has been growing, particularly the war-affected populations from the former Yugoslavia, Afghanistan, Sri Lanka, Burma, and Central America.

In many of these studies, it is difficult to categorize the various groups under study, as such groups are often not mutually exclusive. Perpetrators of violence, survivors of torture or sexual abuse, refugees, and other war-affected populations often overlap. In contemporary internecine conflicts, such as those that have taken place in Bosnia and Africa, civilians commonly serve as irregulars in local militia. Therefore, individuals may at times be combatants as well as victims of torture, trauma, persecution, and displacement. This fact is important to recognize in research design as well as in treatment development, as these multiple and often conflicting roles can be an important factor in recovery.

Because the effects of torture are evaluated extensively in other chapters of this book, studies that make explicit reference to torture in their titles have been deliberately excluded from this chapter, as have reports relating to the effect of trauma on children and adolescents, to Holocaust survivors, and to treatment issues. The major areas considered in the present overview are as follows: (a) methodological issues raised by recent research, especially in relation to sampling; (b) measurement of trauma and the relationship of traumatic experiences to psychiatric outcomes, particularly posttraumatic stress disorder (PTSD); (c) rates of trauma-related psychiatric disorders and possible reasons for their variability across studies; and (d) the respective roles of pretraumatic, peritraumatic, and posttraumatic factors as possible moderators of traumatic effects.

METHODOLOGY

Sampling

Approaches to sampling have varied considerably across research studies, with the nature of the trauma and the characteristics of the study population being important in determining the rigor and feasibility of the research design. For example, studies involving sudden acts of civilian terror have varied in their ability to achieve high participation rates. Creamer et al. (1993) studied 391 of 838 potential trauma victims occupying a building attacked by a gunman in Melbourne, Australia. Others (e.g., North, Smith, & Spitznagel, 1997) were able to include an even higher percentage of survivors. Many studies—for example, the Tucker et al. (1997) study of the Oklahoma City bombing—have focused on self-selected subjects presenting for assistance at a clinic. Studies undertaken in fully accessible populations, such as those residing in refugee camps (e.g., Mollica et al., 1993), have allowed researchers to use random sampling techniques, thereby producing more generalizable estimates of the prevalence of mental disorders. By contrast, refugee populations in resettlement countries are dispersed across the population, making it difficult to apply rigorous epidemiological sampling methods, although a few notable studies have succeeded in achieving such standards (e.g., Abe, Zane, & Chun, 1994; Beiser, Cargo, & Woodbury, 1994; Beiser, Johnson, & Turner, 1993).

Certain high-risk groups constitute "hidden" populations that necessitate different approaches to sampling. For example, Allden et al. (1996) used the "snowball sampling" technique to recruit Burmese dissidents living under precarious conditions in Thailand. Asylum-seekers living in western countries can be particularly difficult to recruit because of their undefined status and their understandable caution about disclosing personal information. Thus, "convenience sampling" and related techniques have often been used. For example, in a study of the psychosocial well-being of asylum-seekers in Australia, Silove, Sinnerbrink, Field, Manicavasagar, and Steel (1997) interviewed asylum-seekers attending a welfare center supported by a religious group. In a subsequent study (Silove, Steel, McGorry, & Mohan, 1998), a list of names from a community ethnic organization was used to disseminate questionnaires to asylum-seekers, thereby allowing subjects to respond anonymously. Other, more conventional, approaches have been used to study refugees utilizing specialty mental health clinics or hospital services (Delimar, Sivik, Korenjak, & Delimar, 1995; Ekblad & Roth, 1997; Kozaric-Kovacic, Folnegovic-Smalc, Skrinjaric, Szajnberg, & Marusic, 1995; Silove, McIntosh, & Becker, 1993). The method of sampling is an important factor in determining what we know about prevalence rates of disorders such as PTSD in survivors of war and mass violence.

Measurement

Approaches to measuring risk factors, psychiatric status, and levels of psychosocial functioning vary substantially across studies. Some studies have based their findings on very general indices of the level of stress manifested by survivor groups (Cremniter et al., 1997). Other investigations, such as those conducted in Ireland, have attempted to use broad indices such as hospital admission rates and patterns of psychotropic drug usage to evaluate the social effect of widespread political violence (Cairns & Wilson, 1993). In the refugee literature, differences in the methods used to diagnose PTSD may account for some of the variability in prevalence rates reported across such studies. Sources of potential measurement disparities may include (a) differences across such instruments and nosological systems in the criteria for diagnosing PTSD, (b) the extent to which instruments have been accurately recalibrated when translating measures into other languages, and (c) variations in recall relating to the time lapse between trauma exposure and psychiatric assessment.

Notwithstanding these limitations, research methods have converged in recent years, particularly in relation to the diagnostic criteria used for measuring key psychiatric outcomes such as PTSD, anxiety, and depression. For example, in the last 5 years, structured instruments such as the Structured Clinical Interview for the *Diagnostic and Statistical Manual of Mental Disorders* (DSM) have been used to provide diagnoses according to the recent versions of the *Diagnostic and Statistical Manual of Medical Disorders* (DSM-III, DSM-III-R, or DSM-IV) (American Psychiatric Association, 1980, 1987, 1994). Self-report measures have been translated into several languages and are being used across populations from diverse cultural backgrounds. The Harvard Trauma Questionnaire (HTQ) (Mollica & Caspi-Yavin, 1991) for measuring PTSD was originally calibrated to provide a threshold for assigning a DSM-III-R diagnosis in Indo-Chinese populations. More recently, the measure has been shown to correspond closely to the diagnostic domains of the DSM-IV category of PTSD (Smith-Fawzi et al., 1997). Similarly, the Hopkins Symptom Checklist-25 (Mollica, Wyshak, de Marneffe, Khuon, & Lavelle, 1987), a measure of anxiety and depression, has been applied widely across diverse refugee groups. Other measures for depression (Kinzie et al., 1982), as well as anxiety and somatization (Beiser & Fleming, 1986), have been developed for use among Indo-Chinese populations.

Crosscultural Validity of Western Diagnoses

The following is a comment by a refugee who recently escaped from a war situation when interviewed about PTSD symptoms:

> All the villagers have nightmares and trouble sleeping. Everyone is fearful of wandering too far from the village and no one talks about the bad things that have happened. It is better not to think about the past ... there is too much trouble right now. We are always nervous, on guard, and suspicious. We have to be ... the military attack any time and usually at night. These things you ask about are natural in all of us. (Used with permission.)

An important debate is under way about the validity of applying western-derived notions such as "trauma" and "PTSD" across cultures. Opinions remain polarized across the emic–etic divide, with some researchers (e.g., Bracken, Giller, & Summerfield, 1995) pointing out that the "symptoms" of PTSD may have different meanings across diverse cultures—the so-called categorical fallacy. Others, such as Beiser et al. (1994), have found that symptom constellations such as depression and panic show a high degree of construct stability across cultures. Some studies have attempted to incorporate both emic and etic constructs in developing diagnostic assessments (Beiser & Fleming, 1986; Kinzie et al., 1982; Mollica et al., 1993). The "emic" perspective refers to the "insider's" or "native's" interpretation of particular customs or beliefs. The "etic" perspective refers to the external viewpoint, for example, the views of an outside researcher. Nevertheless, since the emic–etic debate rests on fundamental differences in the conceptualization and evaluation of psychopathology across cultures, it seems unlikely that consensus can be reached easily on the key issues in contention.

TRENDS IN TRAUMA ASSESSMENT

The accuracy of individual recall of trauma events and associated PTSD symptoms is a matter of growing scientific discussion in both civilian and war settings. Identifying survivors and confirming their exposure to trauma is potentially more accurate in a civilian context, for example, after acts of terror such as shootings and bombings, particularly since corroborative eyewitness reports can confirm details regarding sequence of events (Creamer et al., 1993; North et al., 1997; Tucker et al., 1997). Such information can facilitate accurate assessment and grouping of survivors according to key variables such as the extent and duration of exposure to threat and their experiences in the immediate posttraumatic period (Cremniter et al., 1997). Alternatively, most studies of refugees rely on recall of multiple trauma events that occurred over extended periods of time, often several years before the survivor is interviewed. With only a few exceptions, longitudinal designs have not been feasible in the study of refugee groups, although such studies of survivors of other civilian and natural disasters have been conducted (Creamer et al., 1993; McFarlane, 1988; North et al., 1997).

Also, in studies of refugee groups, trauma exposure assessment almost always relies on the reports of individual participants. In general, for logistical reasons, the individual's reports of trauma are not validated, for example, by interviewing a family member or another witness. The passage of time may affect the details of memories in a number of ways, and much research is still needed in this area. One recent study (Southwick, Morgan, Nicolau, & Charney, 1997) undertaken on Gulf War veterans suggests that persistent PTSD symptoms may lead to the elaboration of memories of past trauma over time, resulting in variations in the recall of salient events by affected survivors. Such findings are consistent with emerging knowledge about the dynamic nature of the neurophysiological processes involved in the storage of memory over time (Zola, 1997). PTSD sufferers may also underreport early posttraumatic symptoms when interviewed some time after the event (North et al., 1997), possibly because of the memory changes known to be associated with the disorder (Yehuda et al., 1995). Such findings should alert researchers to the inherent difficulties that may emerge in relying entirely on the histories of individual trauma survivors, particularly when they are interviewed many years after exposure to war, mass violence, or other related trauma.

A number of studies (Chung & Kagawa-Singer, 1993; Hauff & Vaglum, 1993; Hinton et al., 1993; Mollica et al., 1993) have derived indices of total trauma exposure by adding across various categories of trauma experienced by participants. In all instances, such trauma "scores" do not reflect the total number of trauma events per se, but rather the number of categories of trauma experienced, such as being exposed to direct threat or injury; witnessing killings, violence, or abuses; having food or water withheld; being imprisoned; experiencing brainwashing; being separated from family members; and being tortured. It is also noteworthy that some of the "trauma" items included in the HTQ, such as lack of access to shelter or medical care, may not fulfill the DSM-IV definition for a trauma.

Unlike studies that focus explicitly on torture (e.g., Basoglu, Paker, Osmen, Tasdemir, & Sahin, 1994; Thompson & McGorry, 1995) or in which torture was a central issue (El-Sarraj, Punamaki, Salmi, & Summerfield, 1996; Ramsay, Gorst-Unsworth, & Turner, 1993), those that deal primarily with war-affected populations tend to give less attention to torture as a specific form of trauma. Some studies (Allden et al., 1996; Hauff & Vaglum, 1993; Mollica et al., 1993; Silove et al., 1997; Smith-Fawzi et al., 1997) include measures such as the HTQ that will identify those who have been tortured. Other studies (e.g., Chung & Kagawa-Singer, 1993; Hauff & Vaglum, 1993; McKelvey, Webb, & Mao, 1993) do not assess torture as a separate category of trauma. Why have investigators undertaken large epidemiological studies on war-affected populations, but have not included torture as a separate variable in their data analyses? One obvious reason may be that war-affected populations are often exposed to multiple traumas, either simultaneously or in rapid succession, thus making it difficult or impossible to disentangle the consequences of any single trauma. The emphasis on a wide range of traumas may also reflect the reality of the multiple experiences of war-affected populations.

TRAUMA AS A RISK FACTOR

Mass Shootings, Bombings, and Terrorist Attacks

Although the overall rate of PTSD in survivors of human-made, technological, and natural disasters is on the order of 30% (Green, 1996), there is much variability across studies. For example, rates of PTSD in populations exposed to shootings, bombings, or terrorist attacks in civilian settings have varied from 10% (Abenhaim et al., 1992) to 74% (Creamer, Burgess, Buckingham, & Pattison, 1989). Variability in PTSD rates across these types of studies may be attributable in part to the diagnostic system used, with DSM-III-R tending to yield fewer cases than DSM-

III (Creamer et al., 1989; Schwartz & Kowalski, 1991), as well as the method and particular instrument of assessment.

In some studies the extent of the physical injuries following mass attacks may increase the risk of PTSD. In a study of civilian survivors of terrorist attacks in France from 1982 to 1987, of 254 survivors, PTSD was present in 10.5% of the uninjured, in 8.3% of the moderately injured, and in 30.7% of the severely injured (Abenhaim et al., 1992). Some survivors appear to be free of any posttraumatic symptoms. For example, following the crash of a Pan Am jet into the Scottish town of Lockerbie in 1988, the mental health consequences of 66 adults were examined. PTSD was present to a modest or severe degree in 44% of those assessed, but 18 subjects showed no evidence of any psychiatric disturbance (Brooks & McKinley, 1992).

Evidence is emerging that the immediate psychic reaction to trauma may prove to be a good predictor of long-term adaptation. In April 1995, terrorists bombed a U.S. federal building in Oklahoma City, Oklahoma, killing 168 people and injuring more than 800 people. A recent report described 86 adults who sought help 6 months after the bombing (Tucker et al., 1997). The peritraumatic response of being nervous, afraid, and upset by others predicted most of the distress at 6 months. After a mass shooting incident in Melbourne, Australia, 391 of a possible 838 trauma survivors were surveyed using the Impact of Event Scale and the Symptom Checklist 90 (Creamer et al., 1993). In comparison with a control group, survivors showed higher levels of intrusion and avoidance, as well as symptoms of depression, anxiety, poor concentration, and relationship problems. The subjective sense of vulnerability at the time of the shooting was a stronger predictor of PTSD outcome than the characteristics of exposure.

Longitudinal studies of civilian violence have shown that, in general, the highest rates of PTSD occur soon after exposure, with decreasing rates in morbidity over time, although a minority of cases do become chronic and severe (de Girolamo & McFarlane, 1996). Such long-term morbidity appears to have a greater association with exposure to intentional human violence in comparison with natural disasters (Green, 1996).

Exposure to War

Bombings of civilian targets in Britain during World War II did not appear to provoke widespread psychiatric disturbance in the population. An increase in "neurotic cases" was not detected (Lewis, 1942; Whitby, 1942), nor was there a substantial increase in psychiatric admissions during the war (Neustatter, 1946). However, some changes were documented in the rate of perforated peptic ulcers, which increased dramatically (Riley, 1942; Stewart & Winser, 1942), and particular forms of trauma, such as being buried under rubble for more than 1 hour after an air raid (Fraser & Phelps, 1942), did appear to be associated with psychiatric morbidity. But in general, reports from war zones have found little evidence of widespread psychiatric disturbances. For example, the race riots in Malaysia (Tan & Simons, 1973), the civil wars in Lebanon during 1975 and 1976 (Nasr, Racy, & Flaherty,

1983), and the ongoing political violence in Northern Ireland (Cairns & Wilson, 1993) do not appear to have provoked a uniform negative response in the general population. Although people directly exposed to terrorist attacks in Northern Ireland showed rates of PTSD of 23%, with high levels of comorbid depression (Loughrey, Curran, & Bell, 1993), responses in the general population were variable, with the most common reactions being mild and short-lived forms of stress (Cairns & Wilson, 1993).

The absence of severe, generalized psychiatric outcomes in war-affected societies is usually attributed to the cushioning effects of social solidarity and a sense of common purpose provoked by an identifiable external threat (Curran, 1988). Clearly, however, multiple methodological problems (sampling, group statistics obscuring individual variation in responses, unspecified diagnostic criteria, and few long-term follow-up studies) raise questions about the validity and generalizability of such findings.

More recent studies have demonstrated somewhat different results. A study of the civilian population of northeast Sri Lanka, which had been exposed to an ongoing secessionist war, showed that although local psychiatric admissions did not increase during the war, specific psychological syndromes appeared to be more prevalent, especially acute stress reactions, phobic disorders, anxiety and depressive states, and grief reactions (Somasundaram, 1993). In a related epidemiological study, Somasundaram and Sivayokan (1994) interviewed a random sample of 101 people living in the strife-affected town of Jaffna in northern Sri Lanka. More than 50% had experienced between five and nine war-related traumas, with 1% reporting exposure to torture. The most common psychiatric disorders and psychosocial difficulties were somatization (41%), PTSD (27%), anxiety disorder (26%), major depression (25%), hostility (19%), relationship problems (13%), alcohol and drug misuse (15%), and functional disability (18%). Therefore, these findings differ from earlier investigations among civilians living in a war zone by yielding much higher rates of frank psychiatric disturbance in the general population. However, these studies also differed in that they used more systematic and sophisticated sampling and diagnostic methods; in addition, conditions in the war zone in Sri Lanka were far more threatening than those in Northern Ireland or wartime Britain.

Studies of the psychiatric effects of genocidal wars such as those that have taken place in Bosnia and Africa are still under way. An early report on 25 Bosnian women who had been raped and impregnated (in addition to experiencing family deaths, dislocations, and beatings) indicated strong feelings of alienation from their unborn fetuses and, among those who carried a pregnancy to term, a desire to allow their babies to be adopted (Kozaric-Kovacic et al., 1995).

Displaced Populations Affected by War

A growing number of studies have been undertaken among refugee camp populations, asylum-seekers, refugee groups living in western countries, and refugee patients attending primary care and specialty clinics in western countries of resettlement. PTSD rates across these studies have varied, with the prevalence being lowest in epidemiological samples, moderate in convenience samples of community groups, and highest in psychiatric clinic populations. For example, an epidemiological study of Cambodian residents in a refugee camp found that 15% suffered from PTSD (Mollica et al., 1993), whereas the prevalence for PTSD in an unselected sample of Vietnamese refugees (n=145) entering Norway was 9% (Hauff & Vaglum, 1993). Lower rates (3.5%) were reported for Vietnamese refugees (n=209) attending a compulsory health screening service in San Francisco (Hinton et al., 1993). Such rates compare with PTSD prevalence figures of approximately 8% for peacekeepers in Somalia (Litz, Orsillo, Friedman, Ehlich, & Batres, 1997) and a lifetime prevalence of between 4% and 8% among the general U.S. population (Breslau & Davis, 1992; Kessler, Sonnega, Bromet, Hughes, & Nelson, 1995).

As noted earlier, somewhat higher rates of PTSD have been found when convenience methods of sampling have been used to access "hidden" populations. For example, 38% of asylum-seekers attending a welfare center in Sydney, Australia, received a diagnosis of PTSD according to the Composite International Diagnostic Interview for DSM-IV (Silove et al., 1997), and 23% of a snowball sample of Burmese political dissidents exiled in Thailand were assigned that diagnosis (Allden et al., 1996). War-affected populations attending clinics and hospitals have exhibited the highest rates of PTSD: 50% of sexually abused women attending a clinic in Zagreb (Kozaric-Kovacic et al., 1995), 40% of patients attending a clinic for immigrants and refugees in Stockholm (Ekblad & Roth, 1997), 65% of Bosnian refugees attending a clinic in the United States (Weine et al., 1995), and 48% of refugee patients attending a clinic in Oslo (Lavik, Hauff, Skrondal, & Solberg, 1996).

The prevalence of depressive disorders has been more variable across war-affected populations, but it is notable that in some studies, the numbers of those with depressive disorders have exceeded those with PTSD. For example, Mollica et al. (1993) found that 55% of Cambodians in a refugee camp suffered from depressive disorders according to western diagnostic criteria, while a larger number affirmed suffering from the "indigenous" form of depression. Hinton et al. (1993) also reported higher rates of major depression (5.5%) and dysthymia (6%) compared with PTSD (3.5%) in their sample of Vietnamese refugees attending a compulsory health screening program in California.

COMORBIDITY AND OTHER OUTCOMES

An experienced clinician working in a clinic for war-affected refugees commented,

> I find the current preoccupation with making a single diagnosis of PTSD unsatisfactory from a clinical point of view. Almost all my patients show a mixture of PTSD, depressive, and anxiety symptoms. Phobias are common, and many exhibit episodes of dissociation under stress, while almost all have somatoform symptoms. Clinically, the most important question is how severe and disabling the symptoms are and how well the person is coping with them. (Used with permission.)

Comorbidity of PTSD with other disorders, particularly depression, is common in all populations exposed to trauma (de Girolamo & McFarlane, 1996; Kessler et al., 1995), yet studies of war-related PTSD have paid insufficient attention to the etiology of such multiple diagnoses. In general, the focus of recent research on war survivors has been limited to a small number of diagnostic categories, usually PTSD, anxiety, and depression. Few studies have undertaken more comprehensive assessments that include other possible trauma-related diagnoses such as dissociative disorders, brief psychoses, specific somatoform disorders, personality change, or drug and alcohol dependence. Therefore, there is a risk that a preoccupation with only a few diagnoses, especially PTSD, may lead to a neglect of other possible psychiatric disorders that may have their roots in trauma exposure.

INFLUENCES ON PSYCHOPATHOLOGY

A 39-year-old asylum-seeker from East Timor was assessed at a trauma and torture service for panic attacks and symptoms of PTSD. She had arrived in Australia in the last month of pregnancy but had received no antenatal care. She had fled after her village was raided repeatedly by the military and her husband and two adolescent sons were taken away on suspicion that they were involved in the guerilla war. She had subsequently been told that all three had been interrogated and tortured. During the raids, huts were burned, people were arrested, and several villagers were beaten and raped. Since arriving in Australia, she faced multiple difficulties. She was living temporarily with cousins but had no financial resources. She could not afford to see a doctor and was unsure whether she was entitled to public health insurance. She had applied for asylum but had been told that her case might take years to decide. She experienced intense panic attacks prior to visiting her lawyer and whenever she was contacted by immigration officials. She was phobic about going out, fearing that every person in uniform she saw was either an enemy agent or an immigration officer searching for her. (Used with permission.)

The most striking finding across recent studies of refugees and other displaced populations, irrespective of the methodologies employed, is the confirmation that trauma exposure is the most consistent predictor of psychiatric disorder, particularly PTSD. Some studies have demonstrated dose–response relationships, with the number of traumas experienced predicting the severity of PTSD or PTSD symptoms. Consistent with research on torture survivors, as well as in the field of traumatology in general (Yehuda & McFarlane, 1995), evidence is accumulating that preexisting vulnerabilities, demographic factors, and the posttraumatic environment have an influence on the long-term psychiatric outcomes in war-affected communities. In some studies (e.g., Beiser et al., 1994; Chung & Kagawa-Singer, 1993; Hauff & Vaglum, 1993), female gender has appeared to be a risk factor for certain psychiatric disorders, but overall findings are not consistent. Few studies have recorded histories of psychiatric disorder in participants, but in those that have done so (e.g., Hauff & Vaglum, 1993), such prior vulnerabilities appear to increase the risk of developing PTSD. Internment in a refugee camp after escape from war or persecution has not been shown to be a predictor of long-term morbidity, with some studies (Abe et al., 1994; McKelvey & Webb, 1997) showing no differential effects on psychopathology for such experiences. These findings may reflect the vast differences in living conditions in different refugee camps. Some sites offer adequate levels of security, but in general, poor conditions may add to the traumas that inmates have previously suffered. The relationship of general physical injury and head injury to the risk of chronic PTSD has not been adequately studied, although a small investigation in Croatia (Delimar et al., 1995) has suggested that nondisabling injuries in war survivors—in this instance, combatants—may increase the risk of PTSD.

The socioeconomic status of resettled refugees appears to be a robust predictor of postmigration adaptation. In particular, unemployment, low family income, and poverty are emerging as important factors associated with persisting psychosocial impairment (Beiser et al., 1993; Chung & Kagawa-Singer, 1993; Lavik et al., 1996; Silove et al., 1997). Certain groups, such as asylum-seekers, continue to suffer ongoing insecurities and deprivations even after migrating to western countries (Silove et al., 1993). Traditional recipient countries have been implementing increasingly restrictive policies for granting refugee status, which often results in lengthy waiting periods for "onshore" asylum-seekers pursuing such claims. Apart from the ever-present threat of repatriation, asylum-seekers residing in western countries may face particular obstacles to accessing welfare and health services (Sinnerbrink, Silove, Manicavasagar, Steel, & Field, 1996). Postmigration stresses relating to residency insecurity and exclusion from essential services appear to be associated with heightened levels of PTSD, anxiety, and depressive symptoms in asylum-seekers (Silove et al., 1997).

Relatively little emphasis has been given to studying factors that may protect war-affected populations from experiencing severe psychiatric impairments, although there are a few exceptions. Allden et al. (1996) found that camaraderie and a belief in the Buddhist concept of self-confidence may act as protective factors that reduce levels of affective disturbance in dissident Burmese exiles. McKelvey, Mao, and Webb (1993) found that higher expectations of the migration process conferred a degree of protection against anxiety and depression in young adult Amerasians about to migrate to the United States from Vietnam.

RESEARCH RECOMMENDATIONS AND CONCLUSIONS

The review of studies on war survivors and civilians exposed to sporadic acts of mass violence suggests a number of directions for future research:

- More research is needed regarding measurement issues, especially the validation of accounts of trauma, and the standardization of measures of PTSD and related diagnoses. Further work is needed to establish the transcultural validity of diagnostic constructs such as PTSD. In particular, nonwestern cultures may have differing perspectives on both the nature and meaning of trauma and the symptoms that are considered to be characteristic of the PTSD complex. Thus, emic and etic constructs should be included in future studies of ethnically diverse communities that have been exposed to war or other forms of mass violence.

- A strong relationship between trauma and PTSD continues to emerge in almost all studies involving war-affected populations, with some investigations yielding a linear dose–response relationship. Nevertheless, the rates of PTSD vary substantially across studies, suggesting that multiple factors determine the onset and course of the disorder. Although logistically difficult to undertake, longitudinal studies are more likely to provide an accurate and comprehensive account of the pathogenesis and evolution of PTSD over time. In particular, further data are needed to strengthen the impression that survivors of single-event, civilian forms of trauma are more likely to recover from PTSD over time than those who are subjected to recurrent, intentional violence or abuse. Also, further information is needed about possible phenomenological differences in the psychic responses to intentional human violence, as compared with exposure to single-event, fateful traumas.

- Specification of the sampling frame and the characteristics of the sample is essential in undertaking studies of PTSD and other disorders in war-affected populations. Factors that are potentially relevant to psychiatric outcomes include whether survivors were victims of violence or were themselves perpetrators, what their legal status is (e.g., displaced person, asylum-seeker, refugee), and whether the survivors were tortured. Although rigorous epidemiological methods are appropriate in studying easily accessible populations, more flexible sampling techniques (such as the snowball technique) may be necessary in investigating "hidden" or dispersed groups.

- Rates of depression and other disorders (e.g., anxiety), although usually found to be high in affected populations, vary considerably across studies. The relationship of these disorders to trauma exposure remains less clear. Further work is needed to establish the pathogenic pathways and possible differential risk factor profiles that may lead to such diverse outcomes. In addition, the focus of research should not be limited to measures of PTSD, depression, and anxiety, but should include a wider array of psychiatric, psychological, and social indices such as grief, anger, guilt, shame, interpersonal difficulties, quality of life, and capacity to work. Broad indices, such as admission rates to psychiatric hospitals or overall rates of psychotropic drug usage, appear to be too blunt to provide a meaningful measure of communal distress in war-affected communities. Of interest, too, are those subgroups within traumatized populations that do not appear to manifest any psychiatric disturbances. Study of such groups may yield important data about resilience, coping, and endurance. Physical factors need to be studied more closely, both as direct causes of disability and as contributors to psychiatric disorder. War-affected populations may suffer high rates of physical injury, head injury, malnutrition, and chronic infectious diseases that directly affect the brain or add to the debility of functional psychological impairments.

- Risk factor research has tended to be guided in part by theoretical considerations. Of value to helping agencies, however, would be the identification of specific risk factors in the posttraumatic environment that are amenable to specific interventions. For example, strategies that maintain the integrity of the family unit may be a more powerful preventive intervention than direct psychological counseling in war-affected or refugee groups (Silove, 1996). Developing a composite index of risk to long-term psychiatric morbidity may also allow more rational use of scarce resources in targeting trauma survivors for intensive individual interventions.
- Patterns of group responses to mass trauma, both universal and culture-specific, warrant further investigation. Civil wars and other forms of mass conflict are so prevalent that they often prevent effective remediation on an individual level, particularly in developing countries. Western researchers often are accused of being overly atomistic, focusing on the individual without regard to the adaptation of the target community as a whole. Mental health professionals who have had the opportunity to attend communal ceremonies (e.g., weddings, religious festivals) held by refugee groups often comment about the contrast between the vibrancy of the group and the demoralization of individuals seen in the clinical setting. Thus, future research would profit from a focus on community mechanisms that either mitigate or exacerbate the experience of mass trauma. Rape and sexual abuse are of particular note in that regard, since much of the shame, guilt, and secrecy associated with long-term morbidity needs to be understood from the perspective of group mores and taboos.
- Ethical issues are paramount in conducting research on war-affected populations. Apart from confidentiality, researchers need to be mindful of the risk of retraumatization and carefully handle this potential problem. A useful theme of inquiry would be to conduct "research into research," that is, inquiries into the effect (positive or negative) of the research process on individual trauma survivors and their communities.

REFERENCES

Abe, J., Zane, N., & Chun, K. (1994). Differential responses to trauma: Migration-related discriminants of posttraumatic stress disorder among Southeast Asian refugees. *Journal of Community Psychology, 22*, 121–135.

Abenhaim, L., Dab, W., & Salmic, L. R. (1992). Study of civilian victims of terrorist attacks (France 1982–1987). *Journal of Clinical Epidemiology, 45*, 103–109.

Allden, K., Poole, C., Chantavanich, S., Ohmar, K., Aung, N., & Mollica, R. F. (1996). Burmese political dissidents in Thailand: Trauma and survival among young adults in exile. *American Journal of Public Health, 86*(11), 1561–1569.

American Psychiatric Association. (1980). *Diagnostic and statistical manual of mental disorders* (3rd ed.). Washington, DC: Author.

American Psychiatric Association. (1987). *Diagnostic and statistical manual of mental disorders* (3rd ed., rev.). Washington, DC: Author.

American Psychiatric Association. (1990). *Diagnostic and statistical manual of mental disorders* (4th ed.). Washington, DC: Author.

Basoglu, M., Paker, M., Osmen, E., Tasdemir, O., & Sahin, D. (1994). Factors related to long-term traumatic stress response in survivors of torture in Turkey. *Journal of the American Medical Association, 272*, 357–363.

Beiser, M., Cargo, M., & Woodbury, M. A. (1994). A comparison of psychiatric disorder in different cultures: Depressive typologies in Southeast Asian refugees and resident Canadians. *International Journal of Methods in Psychiatric Research, 4*, 157–172.

Beiser, M., & Fleming, J. A. (1986). Measuring psychiatric disorders among Southeast Asian refugees. *Psychological Medicine, 16*, 627–639.

Beiser, M., Johnson, P. J., & Turner, R. J. (1993). Unemployment, underemployment, and depressive affect among Southeast Asian refugees. *Psychological Medicine, 23*, 731–743.

Bracken, P. J., Giller, J. E., & Summerfield, D. (1995). Psychological responses to war and atrocity: The limitations of current concepts. *Social Science and Medicine, 40*(8), 1073–1082.

Breslau, N., & Davis, G. C. (1992). Posttraumatic stress disorder in an urban population of young adults: Risk factors for chronicity. *American Journal of Psychiatry, 149*(5), 671–675.

Brooks, N., & McKinley, W. (1992). Mental health consequences of the Lockerbie disaster. *Journal of Traumatic Stress, 5*, 527–543.

Cairns, E., & Wilson, R. (1993). Stress, coping, and political violence in Northern Ireland. In J. P. Wilson & B. Raphael (Eds.), *International handbook of traumatic stress syndromes* (pp. 365–376). New York: Plenum Press.

Chung, R. C., & Kagawa-Singer, M. (1993). Predictors of psychological distress among Southeast Asian refugees. *Social Science and Medicine, 36*(5), 631–639.

Creamer, M., Burgess, P. M., Buckingham, W. J., & Pattison, P. (1989). *The psychological aftermath of the Queen Street shooting.* Parkville, Victoria, Australia: Department of Psychology, University of Melbourne.

Creamer, M., Burgess, P., Buckingham, W., & Pattison, P. (1993). Posttrauma reactions following a multiple shooting. In J. P. Wilson & B. Raphael (Eds.), *International handbook of traumatic stress syndromes.* New York: Plenum Press.

Cremniter, D., Crocq, L., Louville, P., Batista, G., Grande, C., Lambert, Y., & Chemtob, C. M. (1997). Posttraumatic reactions of hostages after an aircraft hijacking. *Journal of Nervous and Mental Disease, 185*, 344–346.

Curran, P. S. (1988). Psychiatric aspects of terrorist violence: Northern Ireland, 1969–1987. *British Journal of Psychiatry, 153*, 470–475.

de Girolamo, G., & McFarlane, A. (1996). Epidemiology of posttraumatic stress disorder among victims of intentional violence: A review of the literature. In F. L. Mak & C. C. Nadelson (Eds.), *International review of psychiatry* (Vol. 2, pp. 93–119). Washington, DC: American Psychiatric Press.

Delimar, D., Sivik, T., Korenjak, P., & Delimar, N. (1995). The effect of different traumatic experiences on the development of posttraumatic stress disorder. *Military Medicine, 160*(12), 635–638.

Ekblad, S., & Roth, G. (1997). Diagnosing posttraumatic stress disorder in multicultural patients in a Stockholm psychiatric clinic. *Journal of Nervous and Mental Disease, 185*(2), 102–107.

El-Sarraj, E., Punamaki, R., Salmi, S., & Summerfield, D. (1996). Experiences of torture and ill-treatment and posttraumatic stress disorder symptoms among Palestinian political prisoners. *Journal of Traumatic Stress, 9*, 595–606.

Fraser, L. I., & Phelps, D. (1942). Psychiatric effects of severe personal experiences during bombing. *Proceedings of the Royal Society of Medicine, 36*, 119–123.

Green, B. L. (1996). Traumatic stress and disaster: Mental health effects and factors influencing adaptation. In F. L. Mak & C. C. Nadelson (Eds.), *International review of psychiatry* (Vol. 2, pp. 177–210). Washington, DC: American Psychiatric Press.

Hauff, E., & Vaglum, P. (1993). Vietnamese boat refugees: The influence of war and flight traumatization on mental health on arrival in the country of resettlement: A community cohort study of Vietnamese refugees in Norway. *Acta Psychiatrica Scandinavica, 88*, 162–168.

Hinton, W. L., Chen, Y. C. J., Du, N., Tran, C. G., Lu, F. G., Miranda, J., & Faust, S. (1993). DSM-IIIR disorders in Vietnamese refugees: Prevalence and correlates. *Journal of Nervous and Mental Disease, 181*, 113–122.

Kessler, R. C., Sonnega, A., Bromet, E., Hughes, M., & Nelson, C. B. (1995). Posttraumatic stress disorder in the National Comorbidity Survey. *Archives of General Psychiatry, 52*, 1048–1060.

Kinzie, J. D. (1993). Posttraumatic effects and their treatment among Southeast Asian refugees. In J. P. Wilson & B. Raphael (Eds.), *International handbook of traumatic stress syndromes*. New York: Plenum Press.

Kinzie, J. D., Manson, S. M., Vinh, D. T., Tolan, N. T., Anh, B., & Pho, T. N. (1982). Development and validation of a Vietnamese-language depression rating scale. *American Journal of Psychiatry, 139*, 1276–1281.

Kozaric-Kovacic, D., Folnegovic-Smalc, V., Skrinjaric, J., Szajnberg, N. M., & Marusic, A. (1995). Rape, torture, and traumatization of Bosnian and Croatian women: Psychological sequelae. *American Journal of Orthopsychiatry, 65*(3), 428–433.

Lavik, N. J., Hauff, E., Skrondal, A., & Solberg, O. (1996). Mental disorders among refugees and the impact of persecution and exile: Some findings from an outpatient population. *British Journal of Psychiatry, 169*, 726–732.

Lewis, A. (1942). Incidence of neurosis in England under war conditions. *Lancet, 2*, 175–183.

Litz, B. T., Orsillo, S. M., Friedman, M., Ehlich, P., & Batres, A. (1997). Posttraumatic stress disorder associated with peacekeeping duty in Somalia for U.S. military personnel. *American Journal of Psychiatry, 154*(2), 178–184.

Loughrey, G. C., Curran, P. S., & Bell, P. (1993). Posttraumatic stress disorder: Civil violence in Northern Ireland. In J. P. Wilson & B. Raphael (Eds.), *International handbook of traumatic stress syndromes* (pp. 377–383). New York: Plenum.

McFarlane, A. C. (1988). The longitudinal course of posttraumatic morbidity. The range of outcomes and their predictors. *Journal of Nervous and Mental Disease, 176*, 30–39.

McKelvey, R., Mao, A. R., & Webb, J. A. (1993). Premigratory expectations and mental health symptomatology in a group of Vietnamese Amerasian youth. *Journal of the American Academy of Child and Adolescent Psychiatry, 32*(2), 414–418.

McKelvey, R., & Webb, J. A. (1997). A prospective study of psychological distress related to refugee camp experience. *Australian and New Zealand Journal of Psychiatry, 31*(4), 549–554.

McKelvey, R., Webb, J. A., & Mao, A. R. (1993). Premigratory risk factors in Vietnamese Amerasians. *American Journal of Psychiatry, 150*(3), 470–473.

Mollica, R. F., & Caspi-Yavin, Y. (1991). Measuring torture-related symptoms: Psychological assessment. *Journal of Consulting and Clinical Psychology, 3*, 581–587.

Mollica, R. F., Donelan, K., Tor, S., Lavelle, J., Elias, C., Frankel, M., & Blendon, R. J. (1993). The effect of trauma and confinement on functional health and mental health status of Cambodians living in Thailand–Cambodia border camps. *Journal of the American Medical Association, 270*, 581–586.

Mollica, R., Wyshak, G., de Marneffe, D., Khuon, F., & Lavelle, J. (1987). Indo-Chinese versions of the Hopkins Symptom Checklist-25: A screening instrument for the psychiatric care of refugees. *American Journal of Psychiatry, 144*, 497–499.

Nasr, S., Racy, J., & Flaherty, J. A. (1983). Psychiatric effects of the civil war in Lebanon. *Psychiatric Journal of the University of Ottawa, 8*, 208–212.

Neustatter, W. L. (1946). 750 Psychoneurotics in 10 weeks fly bombing. *Journal of Nervous and Mental Disease, 92*, 110–117.

North, C. S., Smith, E. M., & Spitznagel, E. L. (1997). One-year follow-up of survivors of a mass shooting. *American Journal of Psychiatry, 154*, 1696–1702.

Ramsay, R., Gorst-Unsworth, C., & Turner, S. (1993). Psychiatric morbidity in survivors of organized violence including torture. *British Journal of Psychiatry, 162,* 55–59.

Riley, I. D. (1942). Perforated peptic ulcers in wartime. *Lancet, 2,* 485.

Schwartz, E. D., & Kowalski, J. M. (1991). Malignant memories: PTSD in children and adults after
a school shooting. *Journal of the American Academy of Child and Adolescent Psychiatry, 30,* 936–944.

Silove, D. (1996). Torture and refugee trauma: Implications for nosology and treatment of posttraumatic syndromes. In F. L. Mak & C. C. Nadelson (Eds.), *International review of psychiatry*
(Vol. 2, pp. 211–232). Washington, DC: American Psychiatric Press.

Silove, D., McIntosh, P., & Becker, R. (1993). Risk of retraumatization of asylum-seekers in Australia. *Australian and New Zealand Journal of Psychiatry, 27,* 606–612.

Silove, D., Sinnerbrink, I., Field, A., Manicavasagar, V., & Steel, Z. (1997). Anxiety, depression, and
posttraumatic stress disorder in asylum-seekers: Association with premigration trauma and
postmigration stressors. *British Journal of Psychiatry, 170,* 351–357.

Silove, D., Steel, Z., McGorry, P., & Mohan, P. (1998). Trauma exposure, postmigration stressors,
and symptoms of anxiety, depression, and posttraumatic stress in Tamil asylum-seekers: Comparisons with refugees and immigrants. *Acta Psychiatrica Scandinavica, 97*(3), 175–181.

Sinnerbrink, I., Silove, D., Manicavasagar, V., Steel, Z., & Field, A. (1996). Asylum-seekers: General
health status and problems with access to health care. *Medical Journal of Australia, 165*(11/12),
634–637.

Smith-Fawzi, M. C., Pham, T., Lin, L., Nguyen, T. V., Ngo, D., Murphy, E., & Mollica, R. F. (1997).
The validity of posttraumatic stress disorder among Vietnamese refugees. *Journal of Traumatic
Stress, 10*(1), 101–108.

Somasundaram, D. J. (1993). Psychiatric morbidity due to war in northern Sri Lanka. In J. P. Wilson
& B. Raphael (Eds.), *International handbook of traumatic stress syndromes* (pp. 333–348). New
York: Plenum Press.

Somasundaram, D. J., & Sivayokan, S. (1994). War trauma in a civilian population. *British Journal of
Psychiatry, 165,* 524–527.

Southwick, S. M., Morgan, C. A., III, Nicolau, A. L., & Charney, D. S. (1997). Consistency of memory
for combat-related traumatic events in veterans of Operation Desert Storm. *American Journal of
Psychiatry, 154*(2), 173–177.

Stewart, D. N., & Winser, D. M. (1942). Incidence of perforated peptic ulcers: Effects of heavy air
raids. *Lancet, 1,* 259–261.

Tan, E. S., & Simons, R. C. (1973). Psychiatric sequelae to a civil disturbance. *British Journal of
Psychiatry, 122,* 57–63.

Thompson, M., & McGorry, P. (1995). Psychological sequelae of torture and trauma in Chilean
and Salvadorean migrants: A pilot study. *Australian and New Zealand Journal of Psychiatry, 29,*
84–95.

Tucker, P., Dickson, W., Pfefferbaum, B., McDonald, N. B., & Allen, G. (1997). Traumatic reactions
as predictors of posttraumatic stress six months after the Oklahoma City bombing. *Psychiatric
Services, 48,* 1191–1194.

Weine, S. M., Becker, D. F., McGlashan, T. H., Laub, D., Lazrove, S., Vojvoda, D., & Hyman, L.
(1995). Psychiatric consequences of "ethnic cleansing": Clinical assessments and trauma testimonies of newly resettled Bosnian refugees. *American Journal of Psychiatry, 152*(4), 536–542.

Whitby, J. (1942). Neurosis in a London general practice during the second and third year of war.
Proceedings of the Royal Society of Medicine, 36, 123–128.

Yehuda, R., Keefe, R. S. E., Harvey, P. D., Levengood, R. A., Gerber, D. K., Geni, J., & Siever, L. J.
(1995). Learning and memory in combat veterans with posttraumatic stress disorder. *American
Journal of Psychiatry, 152,* 137–139.

Yehuda, R., & McFarlane, A. C. (1995). Conflict between current knowledge about posttraumatic
stress disorder and its original conceptual basis. *American Journal of Psychiatry, 152,* 1705–1713.

Zola, S. M. (1997). The neurobiology of recovered memory. *Journal of Neuropsychiatry and Clinical
Neuroscience, 9,* 449–459.

IV

Torture and the Impact of Social Violence

12

Rape and Sexual Assault

MARY P. KOSS and DEAN G. KILPATRICK

We had to be off the streets and in our homes before it got dark ... that was the law. If you weren't and the security police caught you, something terrible could happen. One day you would be here, the next day you could be disappeared. Since the sun was just beginning to set, I thought I was in no danger. I went to the neighborhood store to buy a few vegetables for dinner. I was in there no more than 3 minutes. Since it was still light, I didn't think I was in any danger. Shortly after I left, I heard the footsteps. I didn't turn around because I didn't want to give the impression that I was afraid. The faster I walked, the closer the footsteps seemed. I was almost home when two men in civilian clothes stepped in front of me and said I had to go with them. I told them that my mother and father were waiting for me, that I hadn't done anything wrong. The next thing I remember I was at the police station. I could hear screams and loud thumps ... the thumps sounded like a heavy blanket being beaten by a stick. "Would this happen to me?" I wondered. Then they took me into a small room and ordered me to remove my clothes. "Please," I pleaded with them, "I haven't done anything wrong." My pleas went unheard, and I was ordered again to remove my clothes ... but I didn't. Then one of the men started to tear at my clothes—he was the first one who raped me. I don't remember how many of them raped me; there were so many. In the morning, they told me I could go home, and they laughed. My clothes were torn and stained with blood. When I got home, my mother wept, but my father beat me. He said it was my fault; it was my fault that I was out at night. But how could it be my fault? It wasn't night, and what he didn't say was that he was the one who told me to stop at the store. I will never forgive him for blaming me. I cannot talk with my father. My mother tells me to forget about what happened, and the neighbors look away when I walk by. Do they blame me as well? Every day as I go to work, mother reminds me to be home before dark or I could get hurt again. How can she say that I was hurt? I was raped—doesn't she understand that this is

MARY P. KOSS • Arizona Prevention Center, University of Arizona College of Medicine, Tucson, Arizona 85719.   **DEAN G. KILPATRICK** • National Crime Victims Research and Treatment Center, Department of Psychiatry and Behavioral Sciences, Medical University of South Carolina, Charleston, South Carolina 29425.

The Mental Health Consequences of Torture, edited by Ellen Gerrity, Terence M. Keane, and Farris Tuma. Kluwer Academic/Plenum Publishers, New York, 2001.

not a cut that heals overnight? It is a wound inside of me—so, so deep. They took away my dignity. How am I supposed to get that back? It's been 10 years, and still I fear men as much as I did on the day that it happened. (Testimony from a survivor, used with permission.)

FOCUS OF SECTION

The focus of this section is on rape and sexual assault. The definition of rape is as follows: penetration of the mouth, anus, or vagina by the penis, fingers, or objects, forcibly without consent or nonforcibly if the victim is unable to consent. Two major classes of rape are identified: transgressive rape and tolerated rape. Transgressive rape is uncondoned, illicit genital contact that violates both the will of the victim and social norms (Rozee, 1993). This narrow category represents stereotypical forcible rape by a complete stranger. Even so, some national statutes restrict legal remedy only to those women with a respectable reputation and impose penalties for rape of children that phase out as womanhood is attained (Heise, Pitanguy, & Germain, 1993). Tolerated rapes are unwanted, yet do not violate norms for acceptable behavior held by self-isolated groups or subcultures, institutions, or nations (Rozee, 1993). Included in this diverse category are the following practices:

- Genital contact as part of cultural rituals, child rapes occurring under the guise of arranged marriage, rapes by acquaintances or dates, marital rape, punitive rape to control activists, gynecological rapes (including forced virginity examinations), rupture of the hymen, mutilation of female genitalia, and induced abortions (Amnesty International, 1992)
- Sexual torture, including sexual humiliation, threats, violence toward sexual organs, or sexual assault as part of discipline or interrogation by state security forces (Agger, 1989; Amnesty International, 1992; Aron, Corne, Fursland, & Zewler, 1991; Human Rights Watch, 1992a; Lunde & Ortmann, 1990, 1992)
- Forced prostitution, sexual slavery, and rape of refugees (Amnesty International, 1992; Friedman, 1992; Human Rights Watch, 1993b; United Nations High Commissioner for Refugees, 1986)
- Rape in war, including the deliberate degradation of women to break the spirit of the male enemy, as well as genocidal rape designed to destroy cultures and "cleanse" bloodlines by impregnating women or by raping them to death (Allen, 1996; Asia Watch, 1992; Harris, 1993; Human Rights Watch, 1993a; MacKinnon, 1994; Niarchos, 1995; Seifert, 1996; Stiglmayer, 1994; United Nations, 1993b; Valentich, 1994)

Several common threads occur among rapes under conditions of gross social breakdown. Under such conditions, perpetrators often claim they were ordered to rape, victims are imprisoned for long periods and raped repeatedly by groups of men, and victims are sexually abused with foreign objects, including broken bottles, clubs, and guns (Allen, 1996). MacKinnon has said, "These rapes are to everyday rape what the Holocaust was to everyday anti-Semitism. Without everyday anti-Semitism, a Holocaust is impossible, but anyone who has lived through a pogrom knows the difference" (1994, p. 188). The connection between rape atrocities and "everyday rapes" is that although both men and women can be raped, even in wartime, those who are raped are overwhelmingly women and girls (Schott, 1996), and the perpetrators are almost universally men. Neither youth nor pregnancy is a deterrent to rape (Goldfeld, Mollica, Pesavento, & Faraone, 1988). If biology were sufficient to explain rape, men and boys would be raped more often. Only widespread societal policies and attitudes casting women and girls into inferior status can account for the reality of how rape is used. The United Nations (U.N.) Commission on the Status of Women views rape as a form of gender-based abuse (Economic and Social Council, 1992). In January 1993, the U.N. resolved that rape is a violation of human rights (United Nations, 1993a). Rape in wartime has been forbidden by the Geneva Conventions since 1949 (for a review of rape in international law, see Meron, 1993).

SCOPE OF EXPOSURE

Depending on how it is defined and the cultural and geographic selection of cultures examined, some evidence of rape exists in virtually all human societies, including nonindustrial people (Koss, Heise, & Russo, 1994). Rape in war is documented throughout the historical record (Rozee, 1993; Seifert, 1996) and has been reported in almost every modern armed conflict (Amnesty International, 1992). More than half of those tortured have been subjected to some form of sexual torture (Basoglu, Paker, Paker, et al., 1994; Lunde & Ortmann, 1990, 1992). No reliable statistics describe the international scope of rape with any precision. The validity of crime statistics rests not only on the sophistication of criminal justice institutions, but also on citizens' attitudes toward police. It is unlikely that reliable statistics from societies at war or documents attesting to state-sponsored rape could exist. Furthermore, rape is one of the most underreported crimes, in both peacetime and wartime (Allen, 1996). As few as 10% to 20% of rapes are reported to law enforcement in the United States (Kilpatrick, Edmunds, & Seymour, 1992; for international crime statistics, see Rushton, 1995).

Crime victimization surveys attempt to identify the true scope of crime, but they are hampered by practical barriers (lack of expertise and resources) and methodological challenges (crossdefinition of sexual assault on which to ground the research, women's historical tendency to keep silent because of the stigmatization attached to rape, norms about discussing sexual matters, distrust of fellow citizens under conditions of social stress, and difficulty creating confidentiality in close-knit societies). Currently, a small database on rape prevalence, mostly developed in the United States, exists that has influenced the collection of victimization data worldwide (van Dijk & Mayhew, 1992). Many countries have changed their methodology in recent years to address criticisms of the measurement of rape (Bachman & Saltzman, 1995; Gartner & Doob, 1994; for a critical assessment of these changes, see Koss, Figueredo, Bell, Tharan, & Tromp, 1996). Victimization surveys can be designed to obtain either incidence (number of women victimized at least once in the previous year) or prevalence (percentage of the women who have been victimized during some long reference period up to their entire lifetime). Because of the long duration of the aftereffects of rape, prevalence data help gauge the cumulative societal burden of rape. In the United States, estimates of rape prevalence among adult women range between 14% and 25% in the majority of sources, with the 14% figure based on a national telephone survey being widely accepted as a reliable, but conservative, estimate (Koss, 1993). Selected data from international nongovernmental organizations suggest that, as in the United States, the majority of rape perpetrators are men known to the victim who prey not on adult women, but on female adolescents and children (Koss, Heise, et al., 1994). Across diverse continents and hemispheres, between one and two thirds of those raped are girls who are 15 years old or younger.

IMPACT

It has been said that the rape is "forcefully inserting land mines of emotional upheaval" into the bodies of victims (Winkler & Wininger, 1994). A large empirical literature documents the psychological aftermath of rape (Crowell & Burgess, 1996; Koss, Goodman, et al., 1994). Given the nature of rape, it is understandable that immediate distress results; what is surprising is the longevity of the effects. Approximately one fourth of women who are several years beyond rape continue to experience negative effects. However, there is considerable heterogeneity in recovery rates: Some women do very well; others remain symptomatic for long periods (Hanson, 1990; Koss, Figueredo, & Boeschen, 1997; Koss, Figueredo, Boeschen, & Coan, in press).

POSTTRAUMATIC STRESS DISORDER

Rape and physical assault are associated with the highest rates of posttraumatic stress disorder (PTSD) among women when compared with other civilian traumas (Davis & Breslau, 1994; Norris, 1992; Resnick, Kilpatrick, Dansky, Saunders, & Best, 1993). Because of its high prevalence compared with other extreme events, the largest single group of PTSD sufferers is attributed to rape (Foa, Olasov, & Steketee, 1987). In a prospective study of hospital-referred rape victims, 94% met PTSD criteria at the initial assessment conducted a mean of 12 days after the assault; 46% still met the criteria 3 months later (Rothbaum, Foa, Riggs, Murdock, & Walsh, 1992). The lifetime prevalence of rape-related PTSD in a U.S. national sample was 32%; criteria for current PTSD were met by 12% of rape survivors (Kilpatrick et al., 1992). These data are based on a reliable assessment of both rape victimization and PTSD symptoms. Many of the studies assessed an individual's lifetime history of multiple traumas. This practice is recommended because it avoids the mistake of ascribing a symptom picture to one event when other plausible alternative events exist. In the presence of a multiple trauma history, achieving precision in associating PTSD symptoms to a single trauma is problematic.

OTHER PSYCHOLOGICAL OUTCOMES

Even when evaluated many years later, rape survivors are more likely to receive several psychiatric diagnoses, including major depression, alcohol abuse or dependence, drug abuse or dependence, generalized anxiety, obsessive–compulsive disorder, and PTSD (Burnam et al., 1988; Kilpatrick, Acierno, Resnick, Saunders, & Best, 1997; Kilpatrick et al., 1985; Liebschultz, Mulvey, & Samet, 1997; Winfield, George, Schwartz, & Blazer, 1990; for data on adolescents, see Boney-McCoy & Finkelhor, 1995). In one community sample, 19% of rape victims had attempted suicide compared with 2% of nonvictims (Kilpatrick et al., 1985). Thirteen percent of rape victims suffer from a major depressive disorder sometime in their life, compared with 5% of nonvictims (Burnam et al., 1988; Sorenson & Golding, 1990).

NEUROBIOLOGICAL FINDINGS

Women with a history of past sexual assault have lower mean acute cortisol levels after a revictimization by rape compared with women who had never been assaulted before (Resnick, Yehuda, Pitman, & Foy, 1995). Other rape research addressing neurobiological theory has focused on the memory characteristics that are influenced by intense emotional arousal during encoding. Higher arousal is known to lead to long-lasting memories with more central detail compared with memories formed under neutral emotions (Koss et al., 1996). However, findings from three large samples using standardized memory assessment have demonstrated that rape memories, compared with memories for nonrape negative events and with positive memories, are more affectively intense and negative, while simultaneously being more vague and hazy and providing less sensory detail and less evidence of reexperiencing the physical and emotional states associated with the event (Koss et al., 1996, 1997). More detailed rape memories may have been encoded, but they are not recalled this way, suggesting that cognitive mechanisms may regulate the intensity of reexperienced memory. One empirically tested theoretical model demonstrated that the effect of rape on PTSD is fully accounted for by its influences on memory reexperiencing and social cognitive mediators, with the strongest prediction accruing from causal attributions and beliefs (Koss et al., 1997).

COGNITIVE OUTCOMES

Rape confronts survivors with the overwhelming challenge of coping with intense psychological distress *and* reconstructing a world of meaning (Leibowitz, 1993). Although self-blame theory suggests that those who blame their own actions for traumatic victimization are better adjusted than those who blame unalterable features of themselves, among rape survivors, all forms of self-blame predict greater distress (Abbey, 1987; Frazier, 1990; Frazier, Klein, & Seales, 1996; Frazier & Schauben, 1994; Katz & Burt, 1988; Koss et al., 1997; Meyer & Taylor, 1986; Wyatt, Notgrass, & Newcomb, 1990). Negative changes in the areas of safety, esteem, and trust lead to greater PTSD severity and may persist for at least 18 months following rape (Goodman & Dutton, 1996; Koss et al., 1997, in press; Murphy et al., 1988; Norris & Kaniasty, 1991). One belief—perceived control over negative events—was as important as subjective life threat and objective level of brutality in predicting symptom severity (Kushner, Riggs, Foa, & Miller, 1992).

Laboratory studies suggest that rape creates cognitive schemas that operate at some level of arousal at all times, leading to sensitivity to threat cues, among other effects (Cassiday, McNally, & Zeitlin, 1992; Foa, Feske, Murdock, Kozak, & McCarthy, 1991; Zeitlin & McNally, 1991). Coping strategies most helpful in the immediate postrape period are emotion focused (thinking positively, expressing feelings), not problem focused, and are directed toward "approach" (seeking social support, getting counseling, and keeping busy) rather than "avoidance" (staying home, withdrawing) (Frazier & Burnett, 1994). A long-term connection between greater psychological distress and disengagement methods of coping has been reported (Frazier, 1990; Frazier & Schauben, 1994; Santello & Leitenberg, 1993; Valentiner, Foa, Riggs, & Gershuny, 1996). Others have suggested that using positive distancing, or blocking, can be adaptive in recovery from rape because this method lessens the intensity of memories. In addition, when coupled with other cognitive coping techniques such as minimization and selectivity, distancing facilitates the positive illusions that maintain mental health (Koss et al., 1997, in press; Taylor, 1983; Taylor & Brown, 1988). Under the best of circumstances, surviving rape can lead to a more personally meaningful, better articulated, and more flexible belief system (Burt & Katz, 1987), and some experts argue that the place to begin treatment of rape and other violent trauma is with its metaphysical and spiritual effects (Garbarino, 1996). Although a core of cognitive outcomes of sexual assault may be universal, many postrape cognitions are very likely to be influenced by cultural and spiritual belief systems that have not yet been examined. As a result, conclusions about cognitive outcomes cannot yet be considered generalizable.

PHYSICAL HEALTH

Under civilian conditions, between one half and two thirds of rape victims sustain no physical injuries, and only a small percentage (4%) sustain serious injuries (Kilpatrick et al., 1992). Genital injuries are more likely in the elderly victim

(Muram, Miller, & Cutler, 1992). Rape in detention and during war can result in serious internal injuries and tissue changes, but reliable data are unavailable (Goldfeld et al., 1988; Rabbe, 1992; Swiss & Giller, 1993). Sexually transmitted disease incidence is between 3.6% and 30% of survivors (Beebe, 1991; Jenny et al., 1990; Lacey, 1990; Murphy, 1990). The rate of human immunodeficiency virus (HIV) transmission due to rape is unknown but is of concern to a sizable proportion of rape victims (Baker, Burgess, Brickman, & Davis, 1990). Pregnancy is estimated to result from approximately 5% of rapes (Holmes, Resnick, Kilpatrick, & Best, 1996; Koss, Koss, & Woodruff, 1991). Among survivors of genocidal rape in one study who gave birth to live children, all abandoned them in the hospital (Kozaric-Kovacic, Folnegovic-Smalc, Skrinjaric, Szajnberg, & Marusic, 1995).

Rape also has chronic health effects. Self-report and interview-administered symptom checklists routinely reveal that victims of rape or sexual assault report more symptoms than nonvictimized women (Golding, 1994; Kimerling & Calhoun, 1994; Koss et al., 1991). Victims also perceived their health less favorably and were more likely to engage in health hazards such as smoking, chemical use, and failure to wear seat belts while driving. Rape victims, when compared with nonvictimized women, were more likely to report both medically explained (30% versus 16%) and medically unexplained symptoms (11% versus 5%) (Golding, 1994). Therefore, it is not surprising that rape victims also received more medical care than nonvictims (Kimerling & Calhoun, 1994; Koss et al., 1991). Women in primary care populations with a history of severe sexual and physical assault had nearly twice as many documented physician visits a year as nonvictimized women (6.9 versus 3.5). Medical utilization across 5 years increased between 31% and 56% in the second year following traumatization, depending on the severity of the assault and controlling for the possibility that victims had been high utilizers prior to attack (Acierno, Resnick, & Kilpatrick, 1997). A number of chronic conditions are diagnosed disproportionately among rape victims, including chronic pelvic pain, gastrointestinal disorders, headaches, chronic pain, psychogenic seizures, and premenstrual symptoms (Dunn & Gilchrist, 1993; Heise et al., 1993; Koss & Heslet, 1992; Leserman & Drossman, 1995). Somatic symptoms that are approximately twice as frequent among sexual assault survivors include vomiting, diarrhea, food intolerances, pain during urination, other pain, double vision, seizure or convulsions, paralysis, urinary retention, burning pain in sexual organs, and excessive menstrual bleeding (Golding, 1994). Persons with serious substance abuse problems and high-risk sexual behaviors are also characterized by elevated prevalence of sexual victimization (Dansky, Brady, Saladin, & Killeen, 1996; Kilpatrick et al., 1997; Liebschultz et al., 1997; Paone, Chavkin, Willets, Friedman, & Des Jarlais, 1992; Zierler et al., 1991). At the present stage of development in this research area, less than optimal measurement of both sexual assault and physical health outcomes often occurs, and reliance on self-report for both independent and dependent variables is the norm. In addition, many studies have failed to assess other relevant background characteristics, such as adverse childhood environments, that may contribute to the health effects that are ascribed solely to sexual assault. Longitudinal designs and statistical modeling of temporal sequences can help delineate the relative contributions of personal characteristics, trauma history, and characteristics of the index event in the causation of health outcomes. Nevertheless, the science is sufficiently developed for the American Medical Association to adopt a policy that urges physicians to undertake routine screening for victimization by violence at the entry points to the health care system, validate disclosures of victimization, and develop the ability to link patients to trauma-specific resources in the community (Council on Scientific Affairs, 1992).

ECONOMIC IMPACT

The average rape in the United States is estimated to cost $5,100 in tangible, out-of-pocket expenses and $87,000 when a monetary value is attached to emotional distress and lost quality of life, making it the most costly crime in aggregate (Miller, Cohen, & Wiersema, 1994). The global health consequences of rape have been quantified by the World Bank (Heise et al., 1993) to guide investments in health interventions. Every year lost due to premature death was counted as one disability adjusted life year (DALY), and every year spent sick or incapacitated as a fraction of a DALY. Rape and domestic assault were included in these worldwide calculations because they are risk factors for the major causes of morbidity and mortality. Results showed that gender-based victimization accounted for almost 20% of healthy years of life lost to women aged 15 to 44 years in established market economies and 5% in demographically developing countries where maternal mortality and poverty-related diseases are uncontrolled. On a global basis, the health burden from gender-based victimization (9.5 million DALYs) was comparable to that posed by other diseases or risk factors high on the world health agenda, such as HIV infection (10.6 million DALYs), tuberculosis (10.9 million DALYs), sepsis during childbirth (10 million DALYs), all cancers (9.0 million DALYs), and cardiovascular disease (10.5 million DALYs).

SOCIAL FUNCTIONING

The social functioning of rape survivors is documented by a literature that contains both prospective and retrospective studies and is characterized by standardized assessments of social behavior. The findings suggest that survivors continue to fulfill their nuclear and extended family roles but may have impaired functioning for up to 8 months postrape (Resick, Calhoun, Atkeson, & Ellis, 1981). Although intuition might suggest it would be higher, raped women are just 1.2 times more likely than nonvictims to have sexual problems (Letourneau, Resnick, Kilpatrick, Saunders, & Best, 1996). For those affected, however, the results are long lasting. Thirty percent of rape victims reported that their sexual functioning had not returned to normal as long as 6 years postassault (Burgess & Holmstrom, 1979).

Social support may moderate the effect of rape. Victims who received support from friends and family showed better adjustment than those who lacked it (Atkeson, Calhoun, Resick, & Ellis, 1982; Ruch & Chandler, 1983; Sales, Baum, & Shore, 1984). Unsupportive behavior in particular predicted poorer social adjustment (Davis, Brickman, & Baker, 1991; Ullman, 1996).

RISK AND PROTECTIVE FACTORS

Four bodies of literature exist relevant to risk and protective factors for rape: (a) causal factors that lead perpetrators to rape, (b) vulnerability factors that increase the likelihood that a woman will become the target of a rapist, (c) avoidance behaviors that are associated with incidents that failed to progress beyond "attempted rape," and (d) risk factors that predict the severity of emotional distress of rape victims. Causal factors of rape are outside the scope of this section (for reviews, see Crowell & Burgess, 1996; Koss, Goodman et al., 1994). Regarding vulnerability factors, the scientific consensus is that the most powerful predictor of rape is female gender. Beyond gender, previous victimization is the most powerful predictor, but even optimal combinations of different vulnerability factors fail to achieve prediction accuracy that is clinically significant over chance (Abbey, Ross, McDuffie, & McAuslan, 1996; Koss & Dinero, 1989). The large rape avoidance literature summarizes the characteristics that distinguish rape attempts from completed rapes (Ullman & Knight, 1992). Generally, these studies conclude that all victim behaviors are of lesser significance than offender characteristics in determining the outcome of a sexual assault.

Finally, the variables that predict the severity of reactions to rape have been extensively studied. The major predictors of the presence of PTSD are experiencing life threat, physical injury, and rape (Girelli, Resick, Marhoefer-Dvorak, & Hutter, 1986; Kilpatrick et al., 1989). Victims whose incident included these elements were 8.5 times more likely than other crime victims to experience PTSD. Rape continued to predict the presence of PTSD symptoms even after controlling for violence and dangerousness. The addition of social cognitive mediators to the prediction of PTSD fully accounted for rape's unique capacity to induce PTSD (Koss et al., 1997).

Additional factors that may be associated with higher levels of general psychological distress include younger age (Burnam et al., 1988) and membership in a cultural group that links rape to intense, irremediable shame (Lefley, Scott, Llabre, & Hicks, 1993; Ruch, Gartrell, Amedeo, & Coyne, 1991; Ruch & Leon, 1983; Sorenson & Siegel, 1992; also see Wyatt, 1992, for an African-American perspective). Reactions to rape within a culture may be tied to the stance toward rape that characterizes the predominant religions in an area, even when survivors are not active practitioners (Lykes, Brabeck, Ferns, & Radan, 1993; Mollica & Son, 1989).

Empirical comparisons of those previously victimized with first-time rape victims have found the former to be less disturbed (Ruch & Leon, 1983), more disturbed (Kilpatrick, Saunders, Veronen, Best, & Von, 1987; Ruch, Amedeo, Leon, & Gartrell, 1991; Sorenson & Golding, 1990), or equally disturbed (Frank

& Anderson, 1987; Frank, Turner, & Stewart, 1980; Marhoefer-Dvorak, Resick, Hutter, & Girelli, 1987; McCahill, Meyer, & Fishman, 1979). Differences in the studies that contribute to the variance in results include (a) how disturbance is measured, (b) the point in time when measurements are made, and (c) the adequacy of the design and statistical analyses for separating symptoms that predated the index assault from symptoms that arose in response to it. However, it is undisputed that ongoing and repetitive violence is highly deleterious to psychological adjustment (Follingstad, Brennan, Hause, Polek, & Rutledge, 1991; Gelles & Harrop, 1989).

Acquaintance rapes are equally as devastating to the victim as stranger rapes, as measured by standard measures of psychopathology (Katz, 1991; Koss, Dinero, Seibel, & Cox, 1988; for an exception, see Ullman & Siegel, 1993). But women who know their offender are much less likely to report their rape to police or to seek victim assistance services (Golding, Siegel, Sorenson, Burnam, & Stein, 1989; Stewart et al., 1987). Many women who are raped hesitate for a variety of reasons to call themselves rape victims. Examination of acknowledged versus unacknowledged rape status has shown that the former had more PTSD than the latter, but both groups exceeded levels in nonvictimized women (Layman, Gidycz, & Lynn, 1996). Furthermore, the characteristic effects of rape on memory are seen regardless of a woman's cognitive label for the trauma (Koss et al., 1996).

Research on torture survivors reveals that people are subjected to multiple forms of maltreatment numerous times over the period of incarceration (Basoglu, Paker, Erdogan, Tasdemir, & Sahin, 1994). Among the groups that have been studied systematically to date, rape has been infrequent. However, this picture will almost certainly change as torture is studied more broadly. Whether rape atrocities have an additional traumatic effect over and above that attributable to other forms of torture has not been examined. Although this might not be the case uniformly, some women may be additively affected by rape because of (a) its unique stigma, (b) their cultural or religious group's belief that the damage is irremediable, and (c) lack of support that stems from culturally based prohibitions on discussion of such private matters.

RESEARCH RECOMMENDATIONS

A number of published research agendas address rape directly or indirectly as a component of violence against women or violence in the family. Examples include the violence against women section of the women's mental health research agenda (Koss, 1990), the call for action of the American Psychological Association Task Force on Male Violence Against Women (Koss, Goodman, et al., 1994), the recommendations for crosscultural and global research on these issues (Koss, Heise, & Russo, 1994), the recommendations for the research infrastructure of the National Research Council Panel on Violence Against Women (Crowell & Burgess, 1996), the recommendations for psychological research of the American Psychological Association Presidential Task Force on Violence and the Family (American

Psychological Association, 1996b), and the research agenda for psychosocial and behavioral factors in women's health (American Psychological Association, 1996a). It is impossible within the present space constraints to adequately review all these recommendations. What is remarkable in examining them is the convergence in perspectives among these multiple sources. Recommendations with multiple endorsements include the following:

- Gather nationally representative data on sexual victimization, providing scientific oversight within each nation on the quality of governmentally sanctioned statistics on rape.
- Create a lexicon of terminology so that the literature from diverse societies can be correlated.
- Develop basic epidemiological data.
- Develop a new instrument that addresses undeveloped areas such as cognitive impacts.
- Systematically evaluate interventions.
- Provide funding mechanisms that foster new research partnerships among academic researchers and community providers to increase both the technical quality and practical significance of the research effort.

However, one theme that was echoed universally was the need for more ecological and ethnographic research that describes interpretations and meanings of rape across diverse groups. This research should include studies of the social networks through which people deal with sexual violence as a basis for formulating culturally appropriate responses to rape. Finally, this research needs to examine how cultures and social institutions shape recovery.

The symptoms of PTSD have been found universally to follow extreme trauma, and some aspects of the human response to trauma are hard-wired by biology. Nevertheless, knowledge of (a) subjective understandings of sexual assault in various contexts, (b) cultural explanations for the origins and meaning of symptoms, and (c) beliefs about effective methods for treating distress must shape a society's response to rape.

REFERENCES

Abbey, A. (1987). Perceptions of personal avoidability versus responsibility: How do they differ? *Basic and Applied Social Psychology, 8*, 3–19.

Abbey, A., Ross, L. T., McDuffie, D., & McAuslan, P. (1996). Alcohol and dating risk factors for sexual assault among college women. *Psychology of Women Quarterly, 20*, 147–169.

Acierno, R., Resnick, H. S., & Kilpatrick, D. G. (1997). Health impact of interpersonal violence. Section 1: Prevalence rates, case identification, and risk factors for sexual assault, physical assault, and domestic violence in men and women. *Behavioral Medicine, 23*(2), 53–64.

Agger, I. (1989). Sexual torture of political prisoners: An overview. *Journal of Traumatic Stress, 2*, 305–318.

Allen, B. (1996). *Rape/war: The hidden genocide in Bosnia-Herzegovina and Croatia.* Minneapolis, MN: University of Minnesota Press.

American Psychological Association. (1996a). *Research agenda for psychosocial and behavioral factors in women's health. Recommendations from the advisory committee of the Psychological and Behavioral Factors in Women's Health: Creating an Agenda for the 21st Century Conference.* Washington, DC: Author.

American Psychological Association. (1996b). *Violence and the family: Report of the American Psychological Association Presidential Task Force on Violence and the Family.* Washington, DC: Author.

Amnesty International. (1992). *Rape and sexual abuse: Torture and ill-treatment of women in detention.* New York: Author.

Aron, A., Corne, S., Fursland, A., & Zewler, B. (1991). The gender-specific terror of El Salvador and Guatemala: Posttraumatic stress disorder in Central American refugee women. *Women's Studies International Forum, 14,* 37–47.

Asia Watch. (1992). *Burma: Rape, forced labor, and religious persecution in Northern Arakan.* Washington, DC: Author.

Atkeson, B., Calhoun, K. S., Resick, P. A., & Ellis, E. (1982). Victims of rape: Repeated assessment of depressive symptoms. *Journal of Consulting and Clinical Psychology, 50,* 96–102.

Bachman, R., & Saltzman, L. W. (1995). *Violence against women: Estimates from the redesigned survey* (Bureau of Justice Statistics Special Report NCJ-154348). Washington, DC: U.S. Department of Justice, Bureau of Justice Statistics.

Baker, T. C., Burgess, A. W., Brickman, E., & Davis, R. C. (1990). Rape victims' concerns about possible exposure to HIV infection. *Journal of Interpersonal Violence, 5,* 49–60.

Basoglu, M., Paker, M., Erdogan, O., Tasdemir, O., & Sahin, D. (1994). Factors related to long-term traumatic stress responses in survivors of torture in Turkey. *Journal of the American Medical Association, 272*(5), 357–363.

Basoglu, M., Paker, M., Paker, O., Ozmen, E., Marks, I., Incesu, C., Sahin, D., & Sanmurat, N. (1994). Psychological effects of torture: A comparison of tortured with matched nontortured political activists in Turkey. *American Journal of Psychiatry, 151,* 76–81.

Beebe, D. K. (1991). Emergency management of the adult female rape victim. *American Family Physician, 43,* 2041–2046.

Boney-McCoy, S., & Finkelhor, D. (1995). Psychosocial sequelae of violent victimization in a national youth sample. *Journal of Consulting and Clinical Psychology, 63,* 726–736.

Burgess, A. W., & Holmstrom, L. L. (1979). Rape: Sexual disruption and recovery. *American Journal of Orthopsychiatry, 49,* 648–657.

Burnam, M. A., Stein, J. A., Golding, J. M., Siegel, J. M., Sorenson, S. B., Forsythe, A. B., & Telles, C. A. (1988). Sexual assault and mental disorders in a community population. *Journal of Consulting and Clinical Psychology, 56,* 843–850.

Burt, M. R., & Katz, B. (1987). Dimensions of recovery from rape: Focus on growth outcomes. *Journal of Interpersonal Violence, 2,* 57–81.

Cassiday, K., McNally, R., & Zeitlin, S. (1992). Cognitive processing of trauma cues in rape victims with posttraumatic stress disorder. *Cognitive Therapy and Research, 16,* 283–295.

Council on Scientific Affairs. (1992). Violence against women: Relevance for medical practitioners. *Journal of the American Medical Association, 267*(23), 3184–3189.

Crowell, N. A., & Burgess, A. W. (Eds.). (1996). *Understanding violence against women.* Washington, DC: National Academy Press.

Dansky, B. S., Brady, K. T., Saladin, M. E., & Killeen, T. (1996). Victimization and PTSD in individuals with substance use disorders: Gender and racial differences. *American Journal of Drug and Alcohol Abuse, 22,* 75–93.

Davis, G. C., & Breslau, N. (1994). Posttraumatic stress disorder in victims of civilian trauma and criminal violence. *Psychiatric Clinics of North America, 17,* 289–299.

Davis, R. C., Brickman, E., & Baker, T. (1991). Supportive and unsupportive responses of others to rape victims: Effects on concurrent victim adjustment. *American Journal of Community Psychology, 19,* 443–451.

Dunn, S. P., & Gilchrist, V. J. (1993). Sexual assault. *Primary Care, 20,* 359–373.

Economic and Social Council. (1992). *Report of the Working Group on Violence Against Women* (E/CN.6/WG.21/1992/L.3). Vienna: United Nations.

Foa, E., Feske, U., Murdock, T., Kozak, M., & McCarthy, P. (1991). Processing of threat-related information in rape victims. *Journal of Abnormal Psychology, 100,* 156–162.

Foa, E. B., Olasov, B., & Steketee, G. (1987). *Treatment of rape victims.* Paper presented at the conference, "State-of-the-Art in Sexual Assault," Charleston, SC.

Follingstad, D. R., Brennan, A. F., Hause, E. S., Polek, D. S., & Rutledge, L. L. (1991). Factors moderating physical and psychological symptoms of battered women. *Journal of Family Violence, 6,* 81–95.

Frank, E., & Anderson, B. P. (1987). Psychiatric disorders in rape victims: Past history and current symptomatology. *Comprehensive Psychiatry, 28,* 77–82.

Frank, E., Turner, S. M., & Stewart, B. D. (1980). Initial response to rape: The impact of factors within the rape situation. *Journal of Behavioral Assessment, 2,* 39–53.

Frazier, P. A. (1990). Victim attributions and postrape trauma. *Journal of Personality and Social Psychology, 59,* 298–304.

Frazier, P. A., & Burnett, J. W. (1994). Immediate coping strategies among rape victims. *Journal of Counseling and Development, 72*(6), 633–639.

Frazier, P., Klein, C., & Seales, L. (1996). *A longitudinal study of causal attributions, perceived control, coping strategies, and postrape symptoms.* Manuscript submitted for publication.

Frazier, P., & Schauben, L. (1994). Causal attributions and recovery from rape and other stressful life events. *Journal of Social and Clinical Psychology, 14,* 1–14.

Friedman, A. (1992). Rape and domestic violence: The experience of refugee women. In *Understanding refugees: From the inside out* (pp. 65–77). New York: Hawthorne Press.

Garbarino, J. (1996). The spiritual challenge of violent trauma. *American Journal of Orthopsychiatry, 66,* 162–163.

Gartner, R., & Doob, A. N. (1994). Trends in criminal victimization: 1988–1993. *Juristat Service Bulletin, 14*(13), 1–19.

Gelles, R. J., & Harrop, J. W. (1989). Violence, battering, and psychological distress among women. *Journal of Interpersonal Violence, 4,* 400–420.

Girelli, S. A., Resick, P. A., Marhoefer-Dvorak, S., & Hutter, C. K. (1986). Subjective distress and violence during rape: Their effects on long-term fear. *Violence and Victims, 1,* 35–45.

Goldfeld, A. E., Mollica, R. F., Pesavento, B. H., & Faraone, S. V. (1988). The physical and psychological sequelae of torture: Symptomatology and diagnosis. *Journal of the American Medical Association, 259*(18), 2725–2729.

Golding, J. M. (1994). Sexual assault history and physical health in randomly selected Los Angeles women. *Health Psychology, 13,* 130–138.

Golding, J. M., Siegel, J. M., Sorenson, S. B., Burnam, M. A., & Stein, J. A. (1989). Social support sources following sexual assault. *Journal of Community Psychology, 17*(1), 92–107.

Goodman, L. A., & Dutton, M. A. (1996). The relationship between victimization and cognitive schemata among episodically homeless, seriously mentally ill women. *Violence and Victims, 11,* 159–174.

Hanson, R. K. (1990). The psychological impact of sexual assault on women and children: A review. *Annals of Sex Research, 3,* 187–232.

Harris, R. (1993). The "child of the barbarian": Rape and nationalism in France during the First World War. *Past and Present, 141,* 170–207.

Heise, L., Pitanguy, J., & Germain, A. (1993). *Violence against women: The hidden health burden* (Discussion paper prepared for the World Bank). Washington, DC: World Bank.

Holmes, M. M., Resnick, H. S., Kilpatrick, D. G., & Best, C. L. (1996). Rape-related pregnancy: Estimates and descriptive characteristics from a national sample of women. *American Journal of Obstetrics and Gynecology, 175,* 320–325.

Human Rights Watch. (1992a). *Double jeopardy: Police abuse of women in Pakistan.* New York: Author.

Human Rights Watch. (1992b). *Untold terror: Violence against women [in Peru].* New York: Author.

Human Rights Watch. (1993a). *War crimes in Bosnia-Hercegovina: Volume II*. New York: Author.
Human Rights Watch. (1993b). *Widespread rape of Somali women refugees in NE Kenya*. New York: Author.
Jenny, C., Hooton, T. M., Bowers, A., Copass, M. K., Krieger, J. N., Hiller, S. L., Kiviat, N., & Corey, L. (1990). Sexually transmitted diseases in victims of rape. *New England Journal of Medicine, 322*, 713–716.
Katz, B. L. (1991). The effects of acquaintance rape on the female victim. In A. Parrot & L. Bechhofer (Eds.), *Acquaintance rape: The hidden crime* (pp. 251–269). New York: Wiley.
Katz, B., & Burt, M. (1988). Self-blame in recovery from rape: Help or hindrance? In A. Burgess (Ed.), *Rape and sexual assault II* (pp. 151–169). New York: Garland.
Kilpatrick, D. G., Acierno, R., Resnick, H. S., Saunders, B. E., & Best, C. L. (1997). A two-year longitudinal analysis of the relationships between violent assault and substance use in women. *Journal of Consulting and Clinical Psychology, 65*(5), 834–847.
Kilpatrick, D. G., Best, C. L., Veronen, L. J., Amick, A. E., Villeponteaux, L. A., & Ruff, G. A. (1985). Mental health correlates of criminal victimization: A random community survey. *Journal of Consulting and Clinical Psychology, 53*(6), 866–873.
Kilpatrick, D. G., Edmunds, C., & Seymour, A. E. (1992). *Rape in America: A report to the nation*. Arlington, VA: National Victim Center, and Charleston, SC: Crime Victims Research and Treatment Center.
Kilpatrick, D. G., Saunders, B., Amick-McMullan, A. E., Best, C. L., Veronen, L. J., & Resnick, H. (1989). Victim and crime factors associated with the development of posttraumatic stress disorder. *Behavior Therapy, 20*, 199–214.
Kilpatrick, D. G., Saunders, B. E., Veronen, L. J., Best, C. L., & Von, J. M. (1987). Criminal victimization: Lifetime prevalence, reporting to police, and psychological impact. *Crime and Delinquency, 33*, 479–489.
Kimerling, R., & Calhoun, K. S. (1994). Somatic symptoms, social support, and treatment seeking among sexual assault victims. *Journal of Consulting and Clinical Psychology, 62*, 333–340.
Koss, M. P. (1990). The women's mental health research agenda: Violence against women. *American Psychologist, 45*(3), 374–380.
Koss, M. P. (1993). Detecting the scope of rape: A review of prevalence research methods. *Journal of Interpersonal Violence, 8*(2), 198–222.
Koss, M. P., & Dinero, T. E. (1989). Discriminant analysis of risk factors for sexual victimization among a national sample of college women. *Journal of Consulting and Clinical Psychology, 57*(2), 242–250.
Koss, M. P., Dinero, T. E., Seibel, C. A., & Cox, S. L. (1988). Stranger and acquaintance rape: Are there differences in the victim's experience? *Psychology of Women Quarterly, 12*(1), 1–24.
Koss, M. P., Figueredo, A. J., Bell, I., Tharan, M., & Tromp, S. (1996). Traumatic memory characteristics: A cross-validated mediational model of response to rape among employed women. *Journal of Abnormal Psychology, 105*(3), 421–432.
Koss, M., Figueredo, A. J., & Boeschen, L. (1997, August). *Filling in the black box between rape and PTSD*. Presentation at the American Psychological Association annual meeting, Boston, MA.
Koss, M. P., Figueredo, A. J., Boeschen, L. E., & Coan, J. A. (in press). Experiential avoidance and posttraumatic stress disorder: A cognitive mediational model of rape recovery. In J. J. Freyd & A. P. DePrince (Eds.), *Trauma and memory*. Lexington, MA: Heath.
Koss, M. P., Goodman, L., Browne, A., Fitzgerald, L., Keita, G. P., & Russo, N. F. (1994). *No safe haven: Violence against women at home, work, and in the community*. Washington, DC: American Psychological Association Press.
Koss, M. P., Heise, L., & Russo, N. F. (1994). The global health burden of rape. *Psychology of Women Quarterly, 18*(4), 509–537.
Koss, M. P., & Heslet, L. (1992). Somatic consequences of violence against women. *Archives of Family Medicine, 1*(1), 53–59.

Koss, M. P., Koss, P. G., & Woodruff, W. J. (1991). Deleterious effects of criminal victimization on women's health and medical utilization. *Archives of Internal Medicine, 151*(2), 342–347.

Kozaric-Kovacic, D., Folnegovic-Smalc, V., Skrinjaric, J., Szajnberg, N., & Marusic, A. (1995). Rape, torture, and traumatization of Bosnian and Croatian women: Psychological sequelae. *American Journal of Orthopsychiatry, 65*(3), 428–433.

Kushner, M. G., Riggs, D. S., Foa, E. B., & Miller, S. M. (1992). Perceived controllability and the development of posttraumatic stress disorder (PTSD) in crime victims. *Behavior Research and Therapy, 31*(1), 193–199.

Lacey, H. B. (1990). Sexually transmitted diseases and rape: The experience of a sexual assault centre. *International Journal of STD and AIDS, 1,* 405–409.

Layman, M. J., Gidycz, C. A., & Lynn, S. J. (1996). Unacknowledged versus acknowledged rape victims: Situational factors and posttraumatic stress. *Journal of Abnormal Psychology, 105,* 124–131.

Lefley, H. P., Scott, C. S., Llabre, M., & Hicks, D. (1993). Cultural beliefs about rape and victims' response in three ethnic groups. *American Journal of Orthopsychiatry, 63,* 623–632.

Leibowitz, L. (1993). Treatment of rape trauma: Integrating trauma-focused therapy with feminism. *Journal of Training and Practice in Professional Psychology, 7,* 81–99.

Leserman, J., & Drossman, D. A. (1995). Sexual and physical abuse history and medical practice. *General Hospital Psychiatry, 17*(2), 71–74.

Letourneau, E. J., Resnick, H. S., Kilpatrick, D. G., Saunders, B. E., & Best, C. L. (1996). Comorbidity of sexual problems and posttraumatic stress disorder in female crime victims. *Behavior Therapy, 27,* 321–336.

Liebschultz, J. M., Mulvey, K. P., & Samet, J. H. (1997). Victimization among substance-abusing women. *Archives of Internal Medicine, 157,* 1093–1097.

Lunde, I., & Ortmann, J. (1990). Prevalence and sequelae of sexual torture. *Lancet, 336*(8710), 289–291.

Lunde, I., & Ortmann, J. (1992). Sexual torture and the treatment of its consequences. In M. Basoglu (Ed.), *Torture and its consequences: Current treatment approaches* (pp. 310–327). New York: Cambridge University Press.

Lykes, M. B., Brabeck, M. M., Ferns, T., & Radan, A. (1993). Human rights and mental health among Latin American women in situations of state-sponsored violence. *Psychology of Women Quarterly, 17,* 525–544.

MacKinnon, C. A. (1994). Rape, genocide, and women's human rights. In A. Stiglmayer (Ed.), *Rape: The war against women in Bosnia-Herzegovina* (pp. 183–196). Lincoln, NE: University of Nebraska Press.

Marhoefer-Dvorak, S., Resick, P. A., Hutter, C. K., & Girelli, S. A. (1987). Single versus multiple incident rape victims: A comparison of psychological reactions to rape. *Journal of Interpersonal Violence, 3,* 145–160.

McCahill, T. W., Meyer, L. C., & Fishman, A. M. (1979). *The aftermath of rape.* Lexington, MA: Heath.

Meron, T. (1993). Rape as a crime under international humanitarian law. *American Journal of International Law, 87,* 424–428.

Meyer, C. B., & Taylor, S. E. (1986). Adjustment of rape. *Journal of Personality and Social Psychology, 50,* 1226–1234.

Miller, T. R., Cohen, M. A., & Wiersema, B. (1994). *Crime in the United States: Victim costs and consequences* (NCJ Report No. 155281). Washington, DC: U.S. Department of Justice, Bureau of Justice Statistics.

Mollica, R., & Son, L. (1989). Cultural dimensions in the evaluation and treatment of sexual trauma: An overview. *Psychiatric Clinics of North America, 12,* 363–379.

Muram, D., Miller, K., & Cutler, A. (1992). Sexual assault of the elderly victim. *Journal of Interpersonal Violence, 7,* 70–77.

Murphy, S. M. (1990). Rape, sexually transmitted diseases, and human immunodeficiency virus infection. *International Journal of STD and AIDS, 1,* 79–82.

Murphy, S. M., Amick-McMullan, S., Kilpatrick, D. G., Haskett, M. E., Veronen, L. J., Best, C. L., & Saunders, B. E. (1988). Rape victims' self-esteem: A longitudinal analysis. *Journal of Interpersonal Violence, 3,* 355–370.

Niarchos, C. N. (1995). Women, war, and rape: Challenges facing the international tribunal for the former Yugoslavia. *Human Rights Quarterly, 17,* 649–690.

Norris, F. H. (1992). Epidemiology of trauma: Frequency and impact of different potentially traumatic events on different demographic groups. *Journal of Consulting and Clinical Psychology, 60*(3), 409–418.

Norris, F. H., & Kaniasty, K. (1991). The psychological experience of crime: A test of the mediating role of beliefs in explaining the distress of victims. *Journal of Social and Clinical Psychology, 10,* 239–261.

Paone, D., Chavkin, W., Willets, I., Friedman, P., & Des Jarlais, D. (1992). The impact of sexual abuse: Implications for drug treatment. *Journal of Women's Health, 1,* 149–153.

Rabbe, A. (1992). Gynaecological sequelae of torture. *Torture, 1,* 36–37.

Resick, P. A., Calhoun, K. S., Atkeson, B. M., & Ellis, E. M. (1981). Social adjustment in victims of sexual assault. *Journal of Consulting and Clinical Psychology, 49,* 705–712.

Resnick, H. S., Kilpatrick, D. G., Dansky, B. S., Saunders, B. E., & Best, C. L. (1993). Prevalence of civilian trauma and posttraumatic stress disorder in a representative national sample of women. *Journal of Consulting and Clinical Psychology, 61,* 984–991.

Resnick, H. S., Yehuda, R., Pitman, R. K., & Foy, D. W. (1995). Effect of previous trauma on acute plasma cortisol level following rape. *American Journal of Psychiatry, 152,* 1675–1677.

Rothbaum, B. O., Foa, E. B., Riggs, D. S., Murdock, T., & Walsh, W. (1992). A prospective examination of posttraumatic stress disorder in rape victims. *Journal of Traumatic Stress, 5,* 455–475.

Rozee, P. D. (1993). Forbidden or forgiven?: Rape in cross-cultural perspective. *Psychology of Women Quarterly, 17,* 499–514.

Ruch, L. O., Amedeo, S. R., Leon, J. J., & Gartrell, J. W. (1991). Repeated sexual victimization and trauma change during the acute phase of the sexual assault trauma syndrome. *Women and Health, 17,* 1–19.

Ruch, L. O., & Chandler, S. M. (1983). Sexual assault trauma during the acute phase: An exploratory model and multivariate analysis. *Journal of Health and Social Behavior, 24,* 174–185.

Ruch, L. O., Gartrell, J. W., Amedeo, S., & Coyne, B. J. (1991). The sexual assault symptom scale: Measuring self-reported sexual assault trauma in the emergency room. *Psychological Assessment, 3,* 3–8.

Ruch, L. O., & Leon, J. J. (1983). Sexual assault trauma and trauma change. *Women and Health, 8,* 5–21.

Rushton, J. P. (1995). Rape and crime: International data for 1989–1990. *Psychological Reports, 76,* 307–312.

Sales, E., Baum, M., & Shore, B. (1984). Victim readjustment following assault. *Journal of Social Issues, 37,* 5–27.

Santello, M. D., & Leitenberg, H. (1993). Sexual aggression by an acquaintance: Methods of coping and later psychological adjustment. *Violence and Victims, 8,* 91–104.

Schott, R. M. (1996). Gender and "postmodern war." *Hypatia, 11*(4), 19–30.

Seifert, R. (1996). The second front: The logic of sexual violence in wars. *Women's Studies International Forum, 19,* 35–43.

Sorenson, S. B., & Golding, J. M. (1990). Depressive sequelae of recent criminal victimization. *Journal of Traumatic Stress, 3,* 337–350.

Sorenson, S. B., & Siegel, J. M. (1992). Gender, ethnicity, and sexual assault: Findings from a Los Angeles study. *Journal of Social Issues, 48,* 93–104.

Stewart, B. D., Hughes, C., Frank, E., Anderson, B., Kendall, K., & West, D. (1987). The aftermath of rape: Profiles of immediate and delayed treatment seekers. *Journal of Nervous and Mental Disease, 175,* 90–94.

Stiglmayer, A. (Ed.). (1994). *Mass rape and the war against women in Bosnia-Herzegovina.* Lincoln, NE: University of Nebraska Press.

Swiss, S., & Giller, J. E. (1993). Rape as a crime of war: A medical perspective. *Journal of the American Medical Association, 270*(5), 612–615.

Taylor, S. E. (1983). Adjustment to threatening events: A theory of cognitive adaptation. *American Psychologist, 38,* 1161–1173.

Taylor, S. E., & Brown, J. D. (1988). Illusion and well-being: A social-psychological perspective on mental health. *Psychological Bulletin, 103,* 193–210.

Ullman, S. E. (1996). Social reactions, coping strategies, and self-blame attributions in adjustment to sexual assault. *Psychology of Women Quarterly, 20,* 505–526.

Ullman, S. E., & Knight, R. A. (1992). Fighting back: Women's resistance to rape. *Journal of Interpersonal Violence, 7,* 31–43.

Ullman, S. E., & Siegel, J. M. (1993). Victim–offender relationship and sexual assault. *Violence and Victims, 8*(2), 121–134.

United Nations. (1993a). *Declaration on the elimination of violence against women.* Resolution 481104. December 20, 1993.

United Nations. (1993b). *Rape and the abuse of women in the territory of former Yugoslavia* (U.N. document E/CN.4/1993/L.21). Geneva, Switzerland: Author.

United Nations High Commissioner for Refugees. (1986). *Services for Vietnamese refugees who have suffered from violence at sea: An evaluation of the project in Thailand and Malaysia.* Geneva, Switzerland: Author.

Valentich, M. (1994). Rape revisited: Sexual violence against women in the former Yugoslavia. *Canadian Journal of Human Sexuality, 3,* 53–64.

Valentiner, D. P., Foa, E. B., Riggs, D. S., & Gershuny, B. S. (1996). Coping strategies and posttraumatic stress disorder in female victims of sexual and nonsexual assault. *Journal of Abnormal Psychology, 105*(3), 455–458.

van Dijk, J., & Mayhew, P. (1992). *Criminal victimization in the industrial world.* The Hague, The Netherlands: Ministry of Justice.

Winfield, I., George, L. K., Schwartz, M., & Blazer, D. G. (1990). Sexual assault and psychiatric disorders among a community sample of women. *American Journal of Psychiatry, 147,* 335–341.

Winkler, C., & Wininger, K. (1994). Rape trauma: Contexts of meaning. In T. J. Csordas (Ed.), *Embodiment and experience: The existential ground of culture and self* (pp. 248–268). New York: Cambridge University Press.

Wyatt, G. E. (1992). The sociocultural context of African American and White American women's rape. *Journal of Social Issues, 48,* 77–92.

Wyatt, G. E., Notgrass, C. M., & Newcomb, M. (1990). Internal and external mediators of women's rape experiences. *Psychology of Women Quarterly, 14,* 153–157.

Zeitlin, S., & McNally, R. (1991). Implicit and explicit memory bias for threat in posttraumatic stress disorder. *Behaviour and Research Therapy, 29*(5), 451–457.

Zierler, S., Feingold, L., Laufer, D., Velentgas, P., Kantorwitz-Gordon, S. B., & Mayer, K. (1991). Abuse and subsequent risk of HIV infection. *American Journal of Public Health, 81,* 572–575.

13

Homicide and Physical Assault

DEAN G. KILPATRICK and MARY P. KOSS

Violent physical assault and the murder of a family member or close friend are traumatic events that can produce posttraumatic stress disorder (PTSD) or other mental health problems. Understanding the scope and effect of violent physical assaults and homicide is relevant to the topic of torture and its consequences in two ways: First, these types of events are elements of the torture experience itself for torture survivors, many of whom have been physically attacked as a part of the torture or have lost a family member or friend who was murdered as part of government-sanctioned political repression. Second, individuals in many nations are at risk of losing a family member or friend to homicide or of becoming victims of violent crimes involving physical assault. Such experiences, regardless of whether they occur before or after a torture experience, might be expected to influence the extent to which torture survivors develop problems or recover from the experience.

For the purposes of this review, criminal homicide is defined as "causing the death of another person without legal justification or excuse" (Rand, Klaus, & Taylor, 1983). Legally justified forms of homicide include military combat, self-defense, and capital punishment. Assault is defined as "unlawful intentional inflicting, or the attempted inflicting, of injury upon the person of another" (Klaus et al., 1988, p. 1). Aggravated assaults involve the use of a weapon and substantial physical injury or threat of the same. Aggravated assault can also be committed without a weapon. Simple assaults produce less injury and do not involve use of a weapon. Unless otherwise noted, this report will address aggravated assaults because they are at the most violent end of the physical assault spectrum.

DEAN G. KILPATRICK • National Crime Victims Research and Treatment Center, Department of Psychiatry and Behavioral Sciences, Medical University of South Carolina, Charleston, South Carolina 29425.   MARY P. KOSS • Arizona Prevention Center, University of Arizona College of Medicine, Tucson, Arizona 85719.

The Mental Health Consequences of Torture, edited by Ellen Gerrity, Terence M. Keane, and Farris Tuma. Kluwer Academic/Plenum Publishers, New York, 2001.

Serious physical assaults and homicides often occur in the context of domestic violence, which is a major problem in the United States and probably other countries as well (Browne, 1993; Crowell & Burgess, 1996; Garner & Fagan, 1997; Gelles & Straus, 1988). Domestic violence, particularly that of the most serious nature, generally takes a much heavier toll on women than on men (Crowell & Burgess, 1996). Domestic violence is discussed in chapter 15 in this volume.

SCOPE OF EXPOSURE

Comparing rates of physical assault across nations is difficult because legal definitions of crime differ. In addition, there is limited access to information about physical assaults that are not reported to police. If the legal definition of physical assault differs in two countries or if the proportion of cases reported to police in each country differs, then comparisons based on cases reported to police are likely to be inaccurate (Hanson, Kilpatrick, Falsetti, & Resnick, 1995). This is less of a problem for criminal homicide, which is legally defined more similarly across jurisdictions. Also, homicides are generally reported to authorities.

In the United States, governmental data on the number of criminal homicides occurring each year are provided in the Federal Bureau of Investigation Uniform Crime Reports (UCR), which record the number of homicides reported to police in local jurisdictions. The number of criminal homicides has exceeded 20,000 per year since 1990. For example, the number of criminal homicides recorded in the UCR for the years 1990, 1991, 1992, 1993, and 1994 were 23,400; 24,700; 23,760; 24,530; and 23,305, respectively. Unfortunately, no governmental data are available on the number of indirect victims of homicide that are created by the deaths of family members or close friends.

Data on the number of physical assaults in the United States are provided by two governmental sources: the UCR and the National Crime Victimization Survey (NCVS). For the years 1990, 1991, 1992, and 1993, the UCR indicates that there were 1,054,860; 1,092,740; 1,126,970; and 1,135,100 assaults reported to police in the United States. The NCVS is a victimization survey conducted with a sample of approximately 100,000 respondents aged 12 years and older from a probability sample of approximately 50,000 households. Respondents are interviewed about crimes that occurred during a 6-month bounded interview period, including crimes that were not reported to police. The NCVS underwent a major redesign in 1992 to improve its ability to detect cases of sexual assault and domestic violence. Estimates for 1990 and 1991 were obtained using the old NCVS, and the 1992 and 1993 estimates were obtained using the revised NCVS. For 1990, 1991, 1992, and 1993, the NCVS estimates of assaults were 6,007,000; 6,436,000; 10,840,000; and 11,236,000, respectively. The large increase in assaults after the redesign suggests that the changes appear to have been at least somewhat successful in improving the NCVS's sensitivity in detecting assaults.

Some comparative data are available about homicide rates in different countries. Reiss and Roth (1993) described such comparisons based on homicide data reported to the World Health Organization between 1981 and 1986. Comparisons were made of homicide deaths per 100,000 population. Reiss and Roth found that the homicide mortality rate in the United States of 8.3 per 100,000 was much higher than the rate in any European nation. For example, the rate in Spain was 4.3 per 100,000, and the rates for Italy, Denmark, Portugal, Austria, Sweden, France, West Germany, Great Britain, and Norway were all less than 2.0 per 100,000. The Bahamas and Ecuador were the only countries in which the homicide rate exceeded that of the United States, but rates in several Central and South American countries (e.g., Costa Rica, Argentina, Guatemala, and Chile) were higher than in most European nations.

As previously noted, comparisons of crimes other than homicide in different countries are more difficult because of differing definitions and reporting rates. However, de Girolamo and McFarlane (1996) recently described work done by van Dijk and Mayhew (1993) in which victimization surveys were conducted in 20 countries. Respondents were asked about physical assaults or threat of physical assaults occurring within the year before the survey, so past-year prevalence data were recorded (de Girolamo & McFarlane, 1996). The average percentage having experienced such an assault in all countries was 3.0%. Past-year prevalence rates were highest in New Zealand (5.7%), the United States (5.0%), Australia (5.0%), and Canada (4.4%) and lowest in Japan (0.6%), Italy (0.8%), Switzerland (1.2%), Scotland (1.8%), and Northern Ireland (1.8%).

A major limitation of all these governmentally based crime statistics is that they measure only homicides and assaults that occurred recently, usually within the past year. Clearly, the effects of homicide on its indirect victims and the effects of physical assault might be expected to last longer than 1 year. Therefore, it is also important to obtain information about the proportion of the population that has ever experienced an assault or the homicide death of a relative or close friend.

With respect to homicide, only one study has examined the lifetime prevalence of indirect victimization due to homicide in a nationally representative sample of adults. Amick-McMullan, Kilpatrick, and Resnick (1991) screened a national probability sample of 12,500 adults in the United States and found that 3.8% of adults had experienced the homicide death of an immediate family member (1.6%), other relative (1.5%), or close friend (0.7%).

Lifetime prevalence data on physical assaults are available from several sources. Norris (1992) reported that the lifetime prevalence of physical assault was 18.7% for male and 11.7% for female respondents in four cities in the southeastern United States. Breslau, Davis, Andreski, and Peterson (1991) found that 8.3% of their sample of young adults from the Detroit area had been victims of physical assault. Resnick, Kilpatrick, Dansky, Saunders, and Best (1993) found that 10.3% of a national household probability sample of adult women in the United States had been victims of aggravated assault. Kilpatrick and Saunders (1997) interviewed a national household probability sample of adolescents between the ages of 12 and 17 years and found that 17.4% had been victims of physical assault. Prevalence was higher among male adolescents (21.3% versus 13.4% for female adolescents). Kessler, Sonnega, Bromet, Hughes, and Nelson (1995) conducted a national survey of adolescents and adults (age 15 to 54 years) and found that 6.9% of women and 11.1% of men reported having been physically attacked. Also, 6.8% of women and 19.0% of men had been threatened by a weapon. Thus, the findings from all these studies consistently demonstrate that a substantial proportion of adolescents and adults in the United States have experienced physical assault.

IMPACT

Posttraumatic Stress Disorder

Establishing the extent to which homicide and physical assault per se increase the risk of PTSD or other types of mental health problems is complicated by the fact that the traumatic event history of many individuals is complex. For example, Resnick et al. (1993) found that more than two thirds of a national probability sample of adult women had experienced at least one potentially traumatic event; 35.6% had experienced a crime, and about half (48.2%) of those who had experienced a crime had experienced only a single incident of a single type of crime. If someone also has experienced other potentially traumatic events, it is difficult to evaluate the unique increase in risk of PTSD or other mental health problems associated with a physical assault or homicide.

Within general population samples, homicide has been shown to produce PTSD in family members and close friends. Amick-McMullan et al. (1991) found that 19.1% of family members and friends of homicide victims had met the revised third edition *Diagnostic and Statistical Manual of Mental Disorders* (DSM-III-R; American Psychiatric Association, 1987) criteria for PTSD sometime following the homicide and that 5.2% had current PTSD. At the time of assessment, the mean length of time since the homicide was 16.6 years. Likelihood of developing PTSD was not significantly related to whether the homicide occurred when the respondent was a child, adolescent, or adult.

Resnick et al. (1993) found that of aggravated assault victims in the National Women's Study who developed PTSD, 17.8% had current PTSD (i.e., met DSM-III-R criteria within the 6 months prior to assessment). Kilpatrick, Resnick, and Saunders (1997) found that 23.4% of physical assault victims among a national probability household sample of adolescents developed PTSD as measured using fourth edition DSM (DSM-IV; American Psychiatric Association, 1994) criteria, and 14.8% had current PTSD.

In unpublished data from the National Survey of Adolescents, Kilpatrick, Resnick, and Saunders (1997) reported that 23.4% of adolescent physical assault victims had lifetime PTSD and that 14.8% of these victims had current PTSD. Other unpublished data from the National Survey of Adolescents indicate that the number of physical assaults an adolescent had experienced significantly increased the risk of PTSD after controlling for the effects of demographics, family history, and exposure to other types of violence (Kilpatrick, Saunders, Resnick, & Best, 1997).

Kessler et al. (1995) used the following procedure to determine whether given events increased risk of PTSD: If respondents had experienced only one traumatic event, then PTSD was assessed in relation to that event. If they had experienced more than one event, respondents were asked to pick the event that was the "most upsetting," and PTSD was assessed in relation to that event. Among men, rates of PTSD were 22.3% for those with physical abuse as the index traumatic event and 1.8% among those who were physically attacked. Among women, 48.5% of those with physical abuse, 32.6% of those threatened with a weapon, and 21.3% of those physically attacked as the index event had PTSD.

As might be expected, rates of PTSD appear to be higher among surviving family members of homicide victims and physical assault victims who are involved with the criminal justice system or who are seeking services than among general population samples used in epidemiological studies. For example, Freedy, Resnick, Kilpatrick, Dansky, and Tidwell (1994) examined rates of PTSD among a sample of crime victims who had reported crimes to police. Among relatives of homicide victims, 71.0% had lifetime PTSD, and 59.4% of aggravated assault victims had lifetime PTSD. Freedy et al. (1994) hypothesized that these higher rates of PTSD might be attributable to more violent cases being more likely to be reported to police or to aggravation of symptoms produced by interacting with the criminal justice system. Likewise, several studies indicated that samples of battered women from shelters show high rates of PTSD (e.g., Astin, Ogland-Hand, Coleman, & Foy, 1995; Weaver & Clum, 1995).

In summary, the evidence is strong that PTSD is a common outcome for victims of homicide deaths of relatives and for physical assault victims.

Other Psychological Disorders or Outcomes

The bulk of research on other psychological disorders and outcomes involves studies of sexual assault victims, not physical assault victims and relatives of homicide victims. However, some excellent reviews on the effects of crime in general exist (e.g., Frieze, Hyman, & Greenberg, 1987; Hanson et al., 1995; Resick, 1993; Weaver & Clum, 1995). These reviews suggest that a host of crime-related problems may occur, such as major depression, substance abuse or dependence, sexual dysfunction, suicidal ideation, suicide attempts, and changes in lifestyle and behavior.

Space limitations do not permit a comprehensive review of findings in this area, so illustrative findings from the most methodologically sound studies will be reviewed. It is also important to consider the Kessler et al. (1995) finding that PTSD was highly comorbid with a number of other diagnoses. This finding suggests that potentially traumatic events, such as crime, can probably increase the risk of a host of other DSM disorders and that this increased risk may be at least partially mediated by PTSD.

Data from the National Women's Study indicated that more than half of aggravated assault victims (54.7%) and 41.4% of relatives and close friends of homicide victims met diagnostic criteria for a major depressive episode some time during their life (Hanson et al., 1995). Rates for these groups were substantially higher than for women who had never been victims of crime. Likewise, Duncan, Saunders, Kilpatrick, Hanson, and Resnick (1996) examined women from the National Women's Study who had been victims of aggravated assault before age 18 years and found the odds of a lifetime major depressive episode to be three times greater among child victims of aggravated assault than among nonvictims. Odds for a current major depressive episode were almost four times greater for victims (14.4% versus 3.6%).

Kilpatrick et al. (1985) examined rates of suicidal ideation and suicide attempts in a household probability sample of 2,004 adult women in Charleston County, South Carolina. The proportion of aggravated assault victims who said they had thought seriously about committing suicide was significantly higher compared with women who had never been victims of sexual assault, robbery, or aggravated assault (14.9% versus 6.8%). However, there was no significant difference in the proportion of the two groups who made actual suicide attempts (4.3% versus 2.2%).

Data from several lines of research suggest that there is a relationship between physical assault and substance use, abuse, and dependence disorders. Several studies indicate that a substantial proportion of treatment-seeking women have a history of physical or sexual assault (Dansky et al., 1995; B. A. Miller, Downs, Gondoli, & Keil, 1987; Polusny & Follette, 1995). Another line of research demonstrates that a substantial association exists between a history of substance use disorders and a history of violent assault (Breslau et al., 1991; Burnam et al., 1988; Cottler, Compton, Mager, Spitznagel, & Janca, 1992; Duncan et al., 1996; Kessler et al., 1995; Kilpatrick, Acierno, Resnick, Saunders, & Best, 1997). Kilpatrick, Acierno, et al. (1997) identified and tested three hypotheses using longitudinal data from the National Women's Study: (a) substance use leads to assault, (b) assault leads to substance use, and (c) substance use and assault have a reciprocal relationship. At each of two assessments conducted 2 years apart, 3,006 women were asked about lifetime and new cases of aggravated assault and rape, as well as about alcohol and drug use. Wave 1 use of drugs, but not abuse of alcohol, increased the odds of new assault in the 2-year follow-up period. However, after a new assault, the odds of both drug use and alcohol abuse increased substantially, even among women with no previous substance use or assault history. These findings support two hypotheses: (a) "assault leads to substance use," specifically alcohol, and (b) "substance use and assault have a reciprocal relationship" for drug use.

Other retrospective data from Wave 1 of the National Women's Study compared rates of substance use among women who were victims of childhood aggravated assault with those who were not (Duncan et al., 1996). Victims were significantly more likely than nonvictims to have used prescription drugs in a nonprescribed manner and to have used marijuana and hard drugs. They were also significantly more likely to be current users of marijuana (15.9% versus 3.4%) and cocaine (3.4% versus 0.7%). Victims reported having started alcohol use almost 3 years before nonvictims (17.0 years versus 19.9 years) and having more days drunk within the past year (7.0 days versus 2.2 days). Victims were more likely than nonvictims to have experienced a number of substance-abuse-related problems, including legal problems, work problems, and problems with family members or friends. Victims were also more likely to have driven while intoxicated and to have had alcohol-related accidents at home or while driving.

Unpublished data from the National Survey of Adolescents examined the relationship between victimization history and past-year substance abuse or dependence among a national household probability sample of 12- to 17-year-olds (Kilpatrick, Saunders, Resnick, & Acierno, 1997). Past-year substance abuse or dependence measured using DSM-IV criteria for alcohol or drugs was significantly higher among physical assault victims than among nonvictims (19.6% versus 4.2%). Victims of physical assault had twice the odds of past-year substance abuse or dependence as nonvictims of physical assault after controlling for the effects of age, gender, race, sexual assault, witnessing violence, and PTSD. Of victims who had used substances, only 34.3% said their first substance use occurred in a year before the year in which they were first victimized, and 20.8% said that their first victimization and first drug use occurred during the same year.

Neurobiological Findings

To the best of the authors' knowledge, there have been no studies specifically focusing on neurobiological changes associated with physical assault or indirect victimization due to homicide. However, one would expect that such studies would produce findings similar to research with other types of trauma victims.

Cognitive Outcomes

Limited information is available about cognitive outcomes among surviving family members of homicide victims. Kilpatrick, Amick, and Resnick (1990) gathered data about some relevant outcomes among a national sample of surviving family members. More than one third (36%) of family members of criminal homicide victims stated that they were much more careful about their personal safety than they had been before the homicide death, and three fourths of family members of alcohol-related vehicular homicide victims (74.7%) said they took some precautions to protect themselves from crime. The most frequently mentioned precautions were keeping doors or windows locked (26.2%) and carrying a gun (11.7%). A small proportion (16.4%) reported that they had seriously considered seeking revenge by attempting to harm the perpetrator in some way.

There was clear evidence that the vast majority of surviving family members had engaged in an attributional search for the meaning of their relative's homicide death. Less than 1 family member in 10 (9.3%) said they had never asked themselves why the death occurred or had never found themselves searching for some reason, meaning, or other way to make sense of the death. About 1 family member in 5 said that they were still searching for meaning "always" or "frequently" at the time they were assessed.

Physical Health

A comprehensive review of the effect of interpersonal violence on health was recently published in a series of three articles (Acierno, Resnick, & Kilpatrick, 1997; Kilpatrick, Resnick, & Acierno, 1997; Resnick, Acierno, & Kilpatrick, 1997). A hypothetical model that attempted to explain the many ways that a violent assault might increase the risk of health problems was presented in the Resnick et al. (1997) article.

In brief, Resnick et al. (1997) identified a number of potential mechanisms by which violent assault could increase the risk of health problems, ranging from producing acute physical injuries to increasing generalized stress. Increased stress may result in impaired functioning of the immune, endocrine, or autonomic systems leading to increased risk of mental health problems, such as PTSD or depression. These problems have been shown to negatively affect health status. Other potential risk factors for health problems are risky health behaviors and inappropriate health care utilization.

Patients treated for violence-related physical injuries in emergency departments were studied in 91 hospitals throughout the United States. Results showed that 1.4 million people were treated during 1994 for such injuries (Rand, 1997). Ninety-four percent of these violence-related injury victims received their injuries as part of an assault as opposed to some other type of crime. Approximately 7% of victims had to be hospitalized for further treatment.

A history of physical or sexual assault has been found to increase the risk of irritable bowel syndrome (Irwin et al., 1996; Leserman et al., 1996) and sexual dysfunction (Letourneau, Resnick, Kilpatrick, Saunders, & Best, 1996).

As noted by Resnick et al. (1997), a host of behaviors can affect health status and are related to a history of physical and sexual abuse. These behaviors include substance use and abuse, tobacco use, health care neglect, risky sexual behavior, and eating disorders. Substance use and abuse among violence victims has been reviewed. Tobacco use is the largest contributor to mortality in the United States, accounting for approximately 400,000 deaths each year (McGinnis & Foege, 1993). Tobacco-related health costs and costs associated with tobacco-related reductions in worker productivity have been estimated at $65 billion each year (Department of Health and Human Services, 1990). In addition to two studies that found increased rates of smoking among veterans with PTSD (Beckman et al., 1995; Shalev, Bleich, & Ursano, 1990), data from the National Women's Study indicate that a history of physical or sexual assault increased the risk of current tobacco use by a factor of two after controlling for the effects of race, education, prior PTSD, and prior depression (Acierno, Kilpatrick, Resnick, Saunders, & Best, 1996). This same study found that PTSD and depression also increased rates of tobacco use, and women with PTSD smoked greater quantities of cigarettes than women without PTSD.

Sexual and physical assault have also been shown to increase HIV-risk behaviors (Harlow, Quina, Morokoff, Rose, & Grimley, 1993; Resnick, Kilpatrick, Seals, Acierno, & Nayak, 1996), as well as the risk for bulimia nervosa (Dansky, Brewerton, Kilpatrick, & O'Neil, 1997) and low body weight (Laws & Golding, 1996). In several of these studies, the risk of health problems appeared to be at least partially mediated by PTSD, thus indicating the need to include measurement of PTSD in future studies.

Economic Impact

A recent study by Miller, Cohen, and Wiersema (1994) attempted to estimate the annual economic costs of crime in the United States. Each homicide was estimated to have an economic cost of $2.94 million. Of this amount, tangible costs (e.g., productivity losses and medical bills) were $1.03 million, and intangible costs (e.g., emotional pain and suffering estimates derived from judgments in civil litigation) were $1.91 million. For physical assaults, estimated costs were $9,350 per assault, with $1,550 constituting tangible costs and $7,800 being intangible costs.

Social and Societal Impact

Fear of crime takes a major toll on society at large (Kilpatrick, Seymour, & Boyle, 1991). In a study of a national probability sample of adults in the United States, a substantial proportion of respondents said they were fearful of being attacked or robbed at home, in their neighborhood, and when traveling. Fear of crime was higher among women than among men. Because of fear of crime, many respondents said they limit places they go shopping (32%) and the time or places they will work (22%). More women than men reported restricting aspects of their lifestyle and behavior based on fear of crime.

RISK FACTORS

As is described elsewhere (Acierno et al., 1997; Hanson et al., 1995), relatively little research has focused on risk and protective factors for PTSD and other problems specifically among surviving family members and physical assault victims. However, two types of risk have been investigated: (a) the risk for becoming a victim of this type of crime and (b) the risk of developing PTSD and other problems following exposure to these types of events. Hanson et al. (1995) argued that it is important to distinguish among three different types of assaults: (a) those perpetrated by intimate partners, such as husbands or boyfriends; (b) those perpetrated by acquaintances, such as family members, friends, or neighbors; and (c) those perpetrated by strangers. This distinction is important for two reasons. First, it is possible that different factors would increase the risk for each of these types of assault. Second, virtually no research has included all of these types of assault, so what findings are available are not yet comprehensive as to overall risk factors for assault.

With these qualifications, several factors appear to increase the risk of violent crime in general (Acierno et al., 1997; Hanson et al., 1995; Reiss & Roth, 1993). With the exception of sexual assault and domestic violence, men have higher rates of assault than women and a lifetime risk of homicide that is three to four times greater than the risk for women. Risk of assault and homicide is inversely related to age, with adolescents and young adults having the highest rates. Most studies indicate that African-Americans and Hispanics have higher rates of assault than other racial or ethnic groups in the United States, and African-Americans are approximately six times as likely as Whites to be homicide victims. Findings are mixed with respect to household income as a risk factor. Demographic variables are often confounded because young people are generally poorer than older people, most women are poorer than most men, and the mean income of most African-Americans is less than that of most Whites.

Positive victimization history also increases risk of assault (e.g., Kilpatrick, Acierno, et al., 1997; Kilpatrick, Resnick, Saunders, & Best, 1998; Koss & Dinero, 1989; Zawitz, 1988). Kilpatrick et al. (1998) found that the odds of new rapes or aggravated assaults in the 2-year follow-up period of the National Women's Study were increased 2.3 times for victims of one prior assault, 5.3 times for victims of two prior assaults, and 13.2 times for victims of three or more prior assaults, when compared with women with no prior assaults. Substance abuse, particularly of illicit drugs, clearly increases the risk of assault (Cottler et al., 1992). Longitudinal data from the National Women's Study indicated that increased risk of new aggravated assault or rape occurred among drug users, but not among women who exclusively abused alcohol (Kilpatrick, Acierno, et al., 1997).

None of these risk factors can produce an assault unless a potential assailant has access to a potential victim. It is important to remember that predatory assailants, not victims, cause assaults, irrespective of any risk factors the victims might possess.

Hanson et al. (1995) identified individual, family, and community factors related to the development of violence-related mental health problems, such as PTSD and depression. As was the case for the risk of exposure to violence, the risk of developing PTSD appears to vary according to demographic characteristics such as age and race. Historical factors such as past victimization and subject factors such as psychopathology are also associated with the risk of PTSD following trauma (Hanson et al., 1995). Moreover, contextual aspects of torture or other violent trauma, including quantitative characteristics such as the degree of injury suffered and qualitative characteristics such as the level of perceived life threat experienced by the victim, also play a role in developing PTSD.

Age is inversely related to risk of PTSD following trauma (Kilpatrick et al., 1989). In an age- and gender-balanced study, Norris (1992) found a PTSD rate of 3.35% among older adults, which was less than half that of younger adults. An age-related downward trend for PTSD incidence was also noted by Kessler et al. (1995), although the age range in this sample was limited to 15 to 54 years. Data on the effects of race on PTSD are inconsistent. Norris (1992), Kilpatrick et al. (1989), and Breslau et al. (1991) found no differences in the rates of PTSD across African-American and White participants who had been exposed to trauma. Similarly, after controlling for age, gender, cocaine use, and depression, Cottler et al. (1992) noted that race did not predict PTSD. However, in their analyses of noncriminal trauma (e.g., natural disaster) Green et al. (1990) noted increased rates of PTSD in African-Americans. Kilpatrick et al. (1998) have shown that repeated trauma exposure also increases the risk of PTSD. Their study found that 3.2% of women with no prior history of assault had PTSD, compared with 19.4% of women with one assault in the previous 2 years, and 18.3% of women who were assaulted in the previous 2 years and also before that time. By contrast, fully 52.9% of women with two prior assaults and a new assault presented with current PTSD.

Characteristics of assaultive violence may also play a part in developing PTSD. Kilpatrick et al. (1989) and Resnick et al. (1993) examined rates of lifetime PTSD in female crime victims who were classified into distinct groups on the basis of perceived life threat and injury during crime. Among victims who experienced life threat but not injury, prevalence of PTSD ranged from 20.6% to 26.6%; among those with injury only, the rate varied from 25% to 30.6%. However, women who experienced both life threat and injury as a result of their victimization were found to have a rate of PTSD ranging from 30.8% to 45.2%. By comparison, the rate of crime-related PTSD in victims with neither life threat nor injury was 19.0% (Resnick et al., 1993). Overall, Kilpatrick et al. (1989) found that female rape victims who experienced both physical injury and perceived life threat were 8.5 times more likely to develop PTSD than crime victims who did not experience these events.

In addition, data indicate that the homicide of a family member is a potential risk factor for PTSD in family survivors. Kilpatrick et al. (1990) reported that about 25% of family members of recent homicide victims have PTSD. Factors that increased the risk of PTSD in survivors of homicide victims included the following:

- Degree of relationship to the victim (with more immediate relationships carrying greater risk—parents, spouses, and siblings were at highest risk)
- A greater or more pervasive fear of crime or accidents in general
- Feelings or thoughts related to taking revenge against the perpetrator
- History of suicidal ideation or attempts
- Presence of diffuse symptoms of psychological distress

Additional factors that may be positively related to developing posttrauma psychopathology include intensity of anxiety and distress experienced during trauma, extent of dissociation during trauma, and limited education or low socioeconomic status (Breslau et al., 1991; Freedy et al., 1994; Norris, 1992). By contrast, stable sources of social support appear to buffer the development of posttraumatic problems in psychological functioning (Burgess & Holmstrom, 1974).

As is evident from the above review, variables that increase the risk of PTSD have only begun to be identified. To date, the interactions between trauma type, age, race, and gender on PTSD remain unknown, and few multivariate analyses of the risk factors for PTSD and crime-related PTSD have been conducted. Such analyses are essential to determining the actual risk of PTSD associated with each factor. What is clear, however, is that perceived life threat, physical injury, and homicide of family members—events and characteristics associated with torture—substantially increase the risk of PTSD.

REFERENCES

Acierno, R., Kilpatrick, D. G., Resnick, H. S., Saunders, B. E., & Best, C. L. (1996). Violent assault, posttraumatic stress disorder, and depression: Risk factors for cigarette use among adult women. *Behavior Modification, 20*(4), 363–384.

Acierno, R., Resnick, H. S., & Kilpatrick, D. G. (1997). Health impact of interpersonal violence. Section I: Prevalence rates, case identification, and risk factors for sexual assault, physical assault, and domestic violence in men and women. *Behavior Medicine, 23*(2), 53–64.

American Psychiatric Association. (1987). *Diagnostic and statistical manual of mental disorders* (3rd ed., rev.). Washington, DC: Author.

American Psychiatric Association. (1990). *Diagnostic and statistical manual of mental disorders* (4th ed.). Washington, DC: Author.

Amick-McMullan, A., Kilpatrick, D. G., & Resnick, H. S. (1991). Homicide as a risk factor for PTSD among surviving family members. *Behavior Modification, 15*(4), 545–559.

Astin, M. C., Ogland-Hand, S. M., Coleman, E. M., & Foy, D. W. (1995). Posttraumatic stress disorder in battered women: Comparisons with maritally distressed controls. *Journal of Consulting and Clinical Psychology, 63,* 308–312.

Beckman, J. C., Rodman, A. A., Shipley, R. H., Hertzberg, M., et al. (1995). Smoking in Vietnam combat veterans with posttraumatic stress disorder. *Journal of Traumatic Stress, 8*(3), 461–472.

Breslau, N., Davis, G. C., Andreski, P., & Peterson, E. (1991). Traumatic events and posttraumatic stress disorder in an urban population of young adults. *Archives of General Psychiatry, 48,* 216–222.

Browne, A. (1993). Violence against women by male partners: Prevalence, incidence, and policy implications. *American Psychologist, 48,* 1077–1087.

Burgess, A. W., & Holmstrom, L. (1974). Rape trauma syndrome. *American Journal of Psychiatry, 131*(9), 981–986.

Burnam, M. A., Stein, J. A., Golding, J. M., Siegel, J. M., Sorenson, S. B., Forsythe, A. B., & Telles, C. A. (1988). Sexual assault and mental disorders in a community population. *Journal of Consulting and Clinical Psychology, 56,* 843–850.

Cottler, L. B., Compton, W. M., Mager, D., Spitznagel, E. L., & Janca, A. (1992). Posttraumatic stress disorder among substance users from the general population. *American Journal of Psychiatry, 149*(5), 664–670.

Crowell, N. A., & Burgess, A. W. (Eds.). (1996). *Understanding violence against women.* Washington, DC: National Academy Press.

Dansky, B. S., Brewerton, T. D., Kilpatrick, D. G., & O'Neil, P. M. (1997). The National Women's Study: Relationship of crime victimization and PTSD to bulimia nervosa. *International Journal of Eating Disorders, 21*(3), 213–228.

Dansky, B. S., Saladin, M. E., Kilpatrick, D. G., Brady, K. T., Resnick, H. S., Killeen, T., & Becker, S. (1995). Prevalence of victimization and PTSD among women with substance use disorders: Comparison of telephone and in-person assessment samples. *International Journal of the Addictions, 30*(9), 1079–1099.

de Girolamo, G., & McFarlane, A. C. (1996). The epidemiology of PTSD: A comprehensive review of the international literature. In A. J. Marsella, M. J. Friedman, E. T. Gerrity, & R. M. Scurfield (Eds.), *Ethnocultural aspects of posttraumatic stress disorder: Issues, research, and clinical applications* (pp. 33–85). Washington, DC: American Psychological Association.

Department of Health and Human Services. (1990). *Healthy people 2000: National health promotion and disease prevention objectives* (PHS 91-50213). Washington, DC: U.S. Government Printing Office.

Duncan, R. D., Saunders, B. E., Kilpatrick, D. G., Hanson, R. F., & Resnick, H. S. (1996). Childhood physical assault as a risk factor for PTSD, depression, and substance abuse: Findings from a national survey. *American Journal of Orthopsychiatry, 66*(3), 437–448.

Federal Bureau of Investigation. (1991). *Uniform crime reports for the United States: 1990.* Washington, DC: U.S. Government Printing Office.

Federal Bureau of Investigation. (1992). *Uniform crime reports for the United States: 1991.* Washington, DC: U.S. Government Printing Office.

Federal Bureau of Investigation. (1993). *Uniform crime reports for the United States: 1992.* Washington, DC: U.S. Government Printing Office.

Federal Bureau of Investigation. (1994). *Uniform crime reports for the United States: 1993.* Washington, DC: U.S. Government Printing Office.

Federal Bureau of Investigation. (1995). *Uniform crime reports for the United States: 1994.* Washington, DC: U.S. Government Printing Office.

Freedy, J. R., Resnick, H. S., Kilpatrick, D. G., Dansky, B. S., & Tidwell, R. P. (1994). The psychological adjustment of recent crime victims in the criminal justice system. *Journal of Interpersonal Violence, 9*(4), 450–468.

Frieze, I. H., Hyman, S., & Greenberg, M. S. (1987). Describing the crime victim: Psychological reactions to victimization. *Professional Psychology, 18*(4), 299–315.

Garner, J., & Fagan, J. (1997). Victims of domestic violence. In R. C. Davis, A. J. Lurigio, & W. G. Skogan (Eds.), *Victims of crime* (pp. 53–85). Thousand Oaks, CA: Sage.

Gelles, R. J., & Straus, M. A. (1988). *Intimate violence.* New York: Simon & Schuster.

Green, B. L., Lindy, J., Grace, M., Gleser, G., Leonard, A., Korol, M., & Winger, C. (1990). Buffalo Creek survivors in the second decade: Stability of stress symptoms. *American Journal of Orthopsychiatry, 60,* 43–54.

Hanson, R. F., Kilpatrick, D. G., Falsetti, S. A., & Resnick, H. S. (1995). Violent crime and mental health. In J. R. Freedy & S. E. Hobfoll (Eds.), *Traumatic stress: From theory to practice* (pp. 129–162). New York: Plenum Press.

Harlow, L. L., Quina, K., Morokoff, P. J., Rose, J. S., & Grimley, D. M. (1993). HIV risk in women: A multifaceted model. *Journal of Applied Behavioral Research, 1,* 3–38.

Irwin, C., Falsetti, S. A., Lydiard, R. B., Ballenger, J. C., Brock, C. D., & Brener, W. (1996). Comorbidity of posttraumatic stress disorder and irritable bowel syndrome. *Journal of Clinical Psychiatry, 57*(12), 576–578.

Kessler, R. C., Sonnega, A., Bromet, E., Hughes, M., & Nelson, C. B. (1995). Posttraumatic stress disorder in the National Comorbidity Survey. *Archives of General Psychiatry, 52,* 1048–1060.

Kilpatrick, D. G., Acierno, R., Resnick, H. S., Saunders, B. E., & Best, C. L. (1997). A two-year longitudinal analysis of the relationship between violent assault and substance use in women. *Journal of Consulting and Clinical Psychology, 65*(5), 834–847.

Kilpatrick, D. G., Amick, A., & Resnick, H. S. (1990). *The impact of homicide on surviving family members.* NIJ Grant No. 87-IJ-CX-0017, submitted to the National Institute of Justice, U.S. Department of Justice.

Kilpatrick, D. G., Best, C. L., Veronen, L. J., Amick, A. E., Villeponteaux, L. A., & Ruff, G. A. (1985). Mental health correlates of criminal victimization: A random community survey. *Journal of Consulting and Clinical Psychology, 53*(6), 866–873.

Kilpatrick, D. G., Resnick, H. S., & Acierno, R. (1997). Health impact of interpersonal violence. Section III: Implications for clinical practice and public policy. *Behavior Medicine, 23*(2), 79–85.

Kilpatrick, D. G., Resnick, H. S., & Saunders, B. E. (1997, October). *Criminal victimization and posttraumatic stress disorder.* Paper presented at the 12th Annual Tokyo Institute of Psychiatry International Symposium, Tokyo, Japan.

Kilpatrick, D. G., Resnick, H. S., Saunders, B. E., & Best, C. L. (1998). *Rape, other violence against women, and posttraumatic stress disorder* (pp. 161–176). New York: Oxford University Press.

Kilpatrick, D. G., & Saunders, B. E. (1997). *The prevalence and consequences of child victimization* (Report No. FS000179, Research in Progress Seminar Series). Washington, DC: U.S. Department of Justice, Office of Justice Programs, National Institute of Justice.

Kilpatrick, D. G., Saunders, B. E., Amick-McMullan, A., Best, C. L., Veronen, L. J., & Resnick, H. S. (1989). Victim and crime factors associated with the development of crime-related posttraumatic stress disorder. *Behavior Therapy, 20,* 199–214.

Kilpatrick, D. G., Saunders, B. E., Resnick, H. S., & Acierno, R. E. (1997, February). *Patterns of substance abuse and victimization: How do male and female adolescents differ?* Paper presented at the 87th Annual Meeting of the American Psychopathological Association, New York, NY.

Kilpatrick, D. G., Saunders, B. E., Resnick, H. S., & Best, C. L. (1997, August). *Patterns of violence exposure and PTSD within a national sample of adolescents.* Paper presented at the 105th Annual Convention of the American Psychological Association, Chicago, IL.

Kilpatrick, D. G., Seymour, A. K., & Boyle, J. (1991). *America speaks out: Citizens' attitudes about victims' rights and violence.* Arlington, VA: National Center for Victims of Crime.

Klaus, P. A., Kaplan, C. G., Rand, M. R., Taylor, B. M., Zawitz, M. W., & Smith, S. E. (1988). *The criminal event* (Report No. NCJ-105506, 2nd ed.). Washington, DC: U.S. Department of Justice, Bureau of Justice Statistics, National Institute of Justice.

Koss, M. P., & Dinero T. E. (1989). Discriminant analysis of risk factors for sexual victimization among a national sample of college women. *Journal of Consulting and Clinical Psychology, 57,* 242–250.

Laws, A., & Golding, J. M. (1996). Sexual assault history and eating disorder symptoms among White, Hispanic, and African-American women and men. *American Journal of Public Health, 86*(4), 579–581.

Leserman, J., Drossman, D. A., Zhiming, L., Toomey, T. C., Nachman, G., & Glogan, L. (1996). Sexual and physical abuse history in gastroenterology practice: How types of abuse impact health status. *Psychosomatic Medicine, 58,* 4–15.

Letourneau, J. E., Resnick, H. S., Kilpatrick, D. G., Saunders, B. E., & Best, C. L. (1996). Comorbidity of sexual problems and PTSD in female crime victims. *Behavior Therapy, 27,* 321–336.

McGinnis, M., & Foege, W. H. (1993). Actual causes of death in the United States. *Journal of the American Medical Association, 270,* 2207–2212.

Miller, B. A., Downs, W. R., Gondoli, D. M., & Keil, A. (1987). The role of childhood sexual abuse in the development of alcoholism in women. *Violence and Victims, 2*(3), 157–172.

Miller, T. R., Cohen, M. A., & Wiersema, B. (1994). *Crime in the United States: Victim costs and consequences* (NCJ Report No. 155281). Washington, DC: U.S. Department of Justice, Bureau of Justice Statistics.

Norris, F. (1992). Epidemiology of trauma: Frequency and impact of different potentially traumatic events on different demographic events. *Journal of Consulting and Clinical Psychology, 60,* 409–418.

Polusny, M.A., & Follette, V. M. (1995). Long-term correlates of child sexual abuse: Theory and review of the empirical literature. *Applied and Preventive Psychology, 4,* 143–166.

Rand, M. R. (1997). *Violence-related injuries treated in hospital emergency departments* (NCJ Report No. 156921). Washington, DC: Bureau of Justice Statistics Special Report, U.S. Department of Justice, Office of Justice Programs.

Rand, M. R., Klaus, P. A., & Taylor, B. M. (1983). The criminal event. In M. W. Zawitz (Ed.), *U.S. Department of Justice, Report to the nation on crime and justice* (pp. 1–16). Washington, DC: U.S. Department of Justice, Bureau of Justice Statistics.

Reiss, A. J., & Roth, J. A. (1993). *Understanding and preventing violence.* Washington, DC: National Academy Press.

Resick, P. A. (1993). The psychological impact of rape. *Journal of Interpersonal Violence, 8,* 223–255.

Resnick, H. S., Acierno, R., & Kilpatrick, D. G. (1997). Health impact of interpersonal violence. Section II: Medical and mental health outcomes. *Behavior Medicine, 23*(2), 65–78.

Resnick, H. S., Kilpatrick, D. G., Dansky, B. S., Saunders, B. E., & Best, C. L. (1993). Prevalence of civilian trauma and posttraumatic stress disorder in a representative national sample of women. *Journal of Consulting and Clinical Psychology, 61,* 984–991.

Resnick, H. S., Kilpatrick, D. G., Seals, B., Acierno, R., & Nayak, M. (1996, November). *Rape and HIV risk: Implications for prevention.* Presented at the annual meeting of the Society for Traumatic Stress Studies, San Francisco, CA.

Shalev, A., Bleich, A., & Ursano, R. J. (1990). Posttraumatic stress disorder: Somatic comorbidity and effort tolerance. *Psychosomatics, 31,* 197–203.

van Dijk, J. J., & Mayhew, P. (1993). Criminal victimization in the industrialized world: Key findings of the 1989 and 1992 international crime surveys. In A. Alvazzi del Frate, U. Zvekic, & J. J. van Dijk (Eds.), *Understanding crime: Experiences of crime and crime control* (pp. 1–5). Rome, Italy: United Nations Interregional Crime and Justice Research Institute.

Weaver, T. L., & Clum, G. A. (1995). Psychological distress associated with interpersonal violence: A meta-analysis. *Clinical Psychology Review, 15*(2), 115–140.

Zawitz, M. W. (Ed.). (1988). *Report to the nation on crime and justice* (2nd ed.). Washington, DC: U.S. Department of Justice.

14

Children, Adolescents, and Families Exposed to Torture and Related Trauma

ROBERT S. PYNOOS, J. DAVID KINZIE,
and MALCOLM GORDON

The child and adolescent population of South Africa will be the first generation to enter into adulthood in the postapartheid period. The academic achievement and economic productivity of these young people, as well as the stability they bring to marriage and family life, their views of their social institutions, and their role in society, are all vital to the future of this region. Thus, their recovery from the years of political violence and apartheid, together with their adaptive response to the challenges of the adverse social conditions of the postapartheid era, is essential for the well-being of South Africa. (Used with permission.)

INTRODUCTION

Prior research among adolescent populations exposed to chronic political violence and oppression or prolonged inadequate postdisaster community recovery indicates that without proper therapeutic attention and commitment of societal resources, this age group can become a "lost generation." Adolescents are at significant risk for compromised academic performance and occupational

ROBERT S. PYNOOS • UCLA Trauma Psychiatry Service, Department of Psychiatry, University of California at Los Angeles, Los Angeles, California 90095.   J. DAVID KINZIE • Department of Psychiatry, Oregon Health Sciences University, Portland, Oregon 97201.   MALCOLM GORDON • National Institute of Mental Health, Neuroscience Center Building, Bethesda, Maryland 20892.

The Mental Health Consequences of Torture, edited by Ellen Gerrity, Terence M. Keane, and Farris Tuma. Kluwer Academic/Plenum Publishers, New York, 2001.

achievement, impaired physical and mental health, and disrupted social and moral development. As a result, society can suffer from the prolonged consequences of increased gang affiliation, peer assaults, criminal violence, substance abuse, unstable marriages with increased domestic violence, and sexual or physical abuse of children. In circumstances where young people have been trained in armed and unarmed resistance, efforts to "demobilize" them and reintegrate them into the community can be considered an important aspect of broader public efforts to assist their recovery and that of their families. Experience indicates that these broader efforts are likely to be more successful if they include outreach programs that provide remedial education opportunities, job training, and organized prosocial activities. The national and international work of the Trauma Psychiatry Program at the University of California at Los Angeles has repeatedly shown how societies can easily overlook the necessity of providing adequate mental health and social programs for the most seriously affected children and adolescents, leaving them vulnerable to the effects of unremediated chronic posttraumatic stress symptoms, depression, and disturbed grief reactions.

Over the past 20 years, there has been a substantial increase in knowledge about children, adolescents, and their families who have been exposed to traumatic situations. Epidemiological and clinical research, along with a wealth of clinical experience, have heightened our appreciation of the range and prevalence of traumatic circumstances to which children and adolescents are exposed; the nature and course of psychological, physical, social, and developmental consequences; the important factors that influence vulnerability, adjustment, and recovery; and effective methods of prevention and intervention.

RANGE AND PREVALENCE OF TRAUMA EXPOSURE IN CHILDREN AND ADOLESCENTS

The alarming prevalence of children and adolescents exposed to trauma has been documented by studies from around the world of catastrophic disasters, war, political and state-sponsored violence, terrorism, community violence, interpersonal and intrafamilial violence, and serious transportation or other types of accidents. Recent studies have cited the frequent serial or sequential nature of traumatic exposures in childhood, the latter commonly occurring in the context of political violence (Gibson, 1989; Keilson, 1980; Swartz & Levett, 1989). Many children in war zones or in politically sanctioned violent or repressive environments may also endure other types of traumas or victimization when these chronic societal conditions give rise to high rates of interpersonal and family violence (Bawa, 1995). Such experiences of interpersonal violence can be expected to increase as a result of the effects of unremediated posttraumatic stress reactions and social stress or social disruption on caretakers, children, and peer groups. Studies documenting the adverse short- and long-term consequences among children, adolescents, and their families have underscored the critical need for community, state, and international public mental health efforts to provide appropriate child and family services, rehabilitation, and restitution.

The range of traumatic exposures is age related. Younger children are extremely vulnerable to such traumatic experiences as violently imposed separation from parents and siblings, abduction, and the traumatic disappearance or death of primary caretakers. Imposed poor nutrition and lack of adequate hygiene and medical treatment constitute physical traumatization that may compromise brain development and future health status and could result in physical disabilities or mortality.

Over the past 20 years, we have become increasingly aware of the extent to which preschool and school-aged children are witnesses to violence, injury, and traumatic death, including the witnessing of the torture, rape, beating, or killing of a parent, sibling, or other relative or caretaker. Assailants may be indifferent to child witnesses or may intentionally make the child a witness to further degrade the adult victim and purposely traumatize the child. Adolescents are at increased risk of being placed in direct life-threat by being targeted for internment, torture, rape, injury, or death, as occurred during the 1990 Iraqi occupation of Kuwait. Adolescents are also more likely to engage in, or be conscripted into, activities that place them at serious risk of traumatic exposures or violent encounters. In addition, older children and adolescents attempt rescues, give first aid, and carry the wounded and dead, thereby increasing their exposure to grotesque and mutilating injury and death (Stuvland, 1993; UNICEF, 1995). Because of the growing importance of peer affiliations, adolescents are especially at risk of experiencing direct life-threat while witnessing the injury, political arrest, beating, rape, torture, or death of a friend. Among other studies (Kirsten, Holzer, Koch, & Severin, 1980), recent population-based studies from Kuwait (Eisa & Nofel, 1993) and the former Yugoslavia region (UNICEF, 1995) have documented that school-age children and adolescents are tortured. Such actions may be carried out with the primary intent of compromising the psychological and physical integrity of the next generation.

Even though improvements to instrumentation are now being made to more specifically characterize violent exposures, Straker (1992), among others, has cautioned against the tendency to generalize across quite disparate experiences of violence in various cultures and to "decontextualize" the description and meaning of the violence. She provided a descriptive clinical account of activist youths in the South African Leandra township, highlighting the ways in which their horrific exposure to violence was rooted in apartheid policies that included police brutality, arrest and detainment, slaying, and vigilante terrorism. The sequential nature of these exposures is illustrated in her case studies, including how the escalation of violent struggle resulted in adolescents being witnesses to and perpetrators of new forms of violence, for example, "necklacing." More long-term longitudinal studies are needed to understand the serial effects of postapartheid exposures to urban crime, domestic violence and abuse, and injurious accidents.

NATURE AND COURSE OF PSYCHOLOGICAL, PHYSICAL, SOCIAL, AND DEVELOPMENTAL CONSEQUENCES

Clinical Conditions

It is now widely accepted that the degree of the original traumatic exposure(s) (i.e., dose of exposure) is strongly predictive of the subsequent severity and chronicity of posttraumatic stress reactions. Political or community violence characteristically exposes children and adolescents to sequential traumatization, which compounds their traumatic reactions (Boothby, 1994; Kilpatrick, Saunders, Resnick, & Smith, 1995). The United Nations Children's Fund (UNICEF) study of children exposed to a wide spectrum of war-related traumatic experiences in the former Yugoslavia region has provided clear evidence that children and adolescents who have been tortured report the most severe and persistent levels of comorbid posttraumatic stress disorder (PTSD) and depression (UNICEF, 1995).

Studies of children and adolescents exposed to extreme forms of violence report high levels of persistent hypervigilance, sleep disturbance (including parasomnias), and exaggerated startle (Eth & Pynoos, 1994; Kirsten et al., 1980). A recent report indicates that physical abuse is associated with enduring sleep disturbance (Glod, Teicher, Martin, Hartman, & Harakal, 1997), a problem that requires clinical attention among children who have been tortured or physically beaten while interned. Among children exposed to a sniper attack at school, those with chronic sleep disturbances reported serious difficulties with daytime learning (Pynoos et al., 1987). Disturbances in arousal are of special concern because they may lead to alterations in the normal maturation of biological systems. Recent biological studies among children and adolescents with chronic PTSD have found alterations in peripheral autonomic functioning (Perry, 1994; Perry & Pate, 1994), in the modulation of the startle reflex (Ornitz & Pynoos, 1989), and in baseline and responsiveness of stress and neurohormones (De Bellis et al., 1994; Goenjian et al., 1996); also, reduced hippocampal volume was detected among women victimized by childhood sexual abuse (Stein, Koverola, Hanna, Torchia, & McClarty, 1997).

Studies of children and adolescents exposed to extreme life-threat and traumatic bereavement have often documented comorbid psychiatric conditions, especially concurrent chronic PTSD and depression. Both chronic intrusive posttraumatic symptoms (Goenjian et al., 1996) and current stresses and adversities (Sack, Clarke, & Seeley, 1996) contribute to the risk of comorbid depression. The death of family members or friends under traumatic circumstances can seriously complicate childhood bereavement by keeping the child and family focused on the circumstances of the death and surrounding issues of human accountability (Clark, Pynoos, & Goebel, 1996). PTSD, grief, depression, traumatic reminders, and secondary stresses and adversities constitute a pernicious interactive matrix that strongly affects the recovery of children from violence and disaster (Goenjian et al., 1995).

There can be a tonic and phasic nature to symptom presentation, with exacerbation or rekindling of symptoms in response to traumatic reminders, even years after the experiences, to intercurrent traumas or under conditions of current stress. The Cambodian refugee studies have shown how PTSD symptoms, especially those that are intrusive, tend to wax and wane over time and therefore require serial evaluations for proper assessment (Kinzie, Sack, Angell, Clarke, & Binn, 1989).

Our understanding of the consequences of traumatic exposures among children and adolescents is moving toward an approach that recognizes well-defined symptoms and clinical syndromes, as well as disturbances in normal biological and developmental maturation (Pynoos, Steinberg, & Wraith, 1995). Within the past several years, systematic clinical and community-based studies have conclusively documented that school-age children and adolescents experience the full range of posttraumatic stress symptoms. In addition, dissociative reactions are commonly found among children and adolescents who have been subjected to violation of their bodily integrity (Putnam & Trickett, 1993). Longitudinal studies of Cambodian child survivors of the Pol Pot regime (Kinzie et al., 1989; Kinzie, Sack, Angell, Manson, & Rath, 1986; Sabin, Sack, Clarke, Meas, & Richart, 1996) and child survivors of the 1988 catastrophic earthquake in Armenia (Goenjian et al., 1995, 1997; Pynoos et al., 1993) have shown that posttraumatic distress persists for many years. As Sack, Seeley, and Clarke (1997) have noted, the crosscultural findings support the conclusion that PTSD "surmounts barriers of culture and language."

Psychological, Social, and Behavioral Consequences

Preschool children may exhibit persistent symptoms of separation anxiety and disturbances in attachment. School-age children may manifest extremes of internalizing or externalizing behaviors, or both, including inhibitions and withdrawal, disruptive behavior, and attentional disturbances. Adolescents are likely to exhibit comorbid conditions similar to those of adults, including PTSD, depression, substance abuse, and antisocial behavior. However, as the Cambodian refugee studies have indicated, the rates of substance abuse and antisocial behavior may depend on cultural and socioenvironmental factors (Sack, Angell, Kinzie, & Rath, 1986). Somatic complaints in all age groups may be a prominent feature of the symptom profile and prompt increased utilization of physical health care services. Persistent somatic symptoms may be mediated by the degree of communication with family members and close friends about the prior traumatic experiences (Pennebaker & Susman, 1988). Among South African youths, including Leandra township activists, Straker (1992) and Dawes (1989) have reported significant depression, anxiety, PTSD, and psychosomatic symptoms at levels that impaired function in everyday life.

In addition to posttraumatic stress symptoms, depression, and somatic symptoms, there can also be associated features such as guilt and revenge fantasies that mediate distress and behavior. Our studies (Pynoos et al., 1993) and those of Yule (1992) among school-age children and adolescents have repeatedly demonstrated a positive correlation of distress with guilt over a sense of ineffectiveness or cowardliness and the belief that an act of commission or omission caused injury, imprisonment, or death to a friend or family member. In addition, a child's sense of ineffectiveness in the face of catastrophic violence to a family member or friend can result in preoccupation with revenge fantasies, which are debilitating to impulse control. Preoccupation with revenge fantasies can lead to severe acting-out behavior or inhibitions that affect initiative in daily life. Adolescents are at special risk of acting out their rage and revenge through direct action (van der Kolk, 1985).

Developmental Consequences

Traumatic sequelae for children and adolescents extend beyond those captured by the symptom profile. The developmental impact affects many domains, where disturbances carry independent risk of later psychopathology and functional impairment. The two potential major effects on development are (a) disruption of successful negotiation of current developmental tasks, resulting in developmental delays or lacunae, and (b) delayed developmental effects, when issues associated with trauma experienced at earlier ages become salient at later developmental stages, for example, prepubertal sexual assaults can become salient around sexual identity issues during adolescence.

The combination of wartime traumatic experiences and postwar adversities can have a strong detrimental effect on adolescent motivation, ambition, and adaptation, which may compromise the accomplishment of developmental tasks essential to the transition to adulthood. For example, in the first years after the occupation, Kuwait experienced an unprecedented drop in enrollment in institutions of higher education and increased rates of reckless driving that resulted in adolescent and young adult deaths. Some traumatized and grieving adolescents may embark on a period of postwar acting-out behavior in the form of school truancy, precocious sexual activity, substance abuse, delinquency, or self-endangering reenactment behavior. Others may become much more passive and withdrawn and may avoid engaging in necessary developmental tasks; they may also retain restricted views of their own future that adversely alter their developmental trajectory. In the literature on children's exposure to political violence, Cairns (1996) recently argued that, in addition to areas of stress and coping, adequate attention needs to be given to levels of aggression, moral development, and political socialization, as well as to the complex interaction of these vectors.

Recent studies have suggested that alterations in moral development and conscience functioning may result from traumatic experiences and the disruption of the social ecology that occurs after years of political violence and apartheid and prolonged inadequate postdisaster community recovery (Goenjian et al., 1999; Straker, 1993; Tudin, Straker, & Mendolsohn, 1994). These studies suggest that while certain accelerations in moral judgment may be beneficial in nature, continuing posttraumatic stress symptoms and adversities may lead to disturbances in conscience functioning that are strongly influenced by negative self-attributions and negative expectations about others, the world, and the social contract.

FACTORS THAT INFLUENCE VULNERABILITY, ADJUSTMENT, AND RECOVERY

The degree of persistent posttraumatic distress is mediated by a number of child-intrinsic factors, including current developmental competencies, temperament, self-esteem, locus of control, history of previous trauma, psychopathology, and adaptational successes to adversities, as well as the child's ability to make cognitive discriminations and to tolerate psychological and physiological symptoms or reactivity to reminders. The adverse influence of prior traumatic experiences has been reported among Palestinian and Lebanese children exposed to chronic political violence (Garbarino, Kostelny, & Dubrow, 1991). As reported in adult studies, commitment to the social ideology of the threatened or repressed group can serve as a protective factor, at least during the time of the political violence (Baker, 1990). However, in her descriptive study of South African activist youths, Straker (1992) argued that short-term adaptations can also significantly limit long-term development.

Neither a child's traumatic experiences, subsequent posttraumatic distress, nor course of recovery can be separated from consideration of the effects on the family. These effects include sustained disruptions of the family (Stuvland, 1993); deterioration in family functioning, including depression in mothers of infants and toddlers (Raundalen, 1993); and demoralization of parents (Punamaki, 1987). These factors can undermine early positive parent–child attachment and parental capacity to buffer the effects of trauma and stress on their children (Laor et al., 1997). In circumstances where family members are together during traumatic situations, the subjective experiences are greatly intensified by the overwhelming meaning of the threat, not only to the child and parent but also to the family unit. Within a family, levels of parent and child distress in response to shared traumatic experiences interact to impair the recovery of the family. In addition, parental symptoms and responsiveness influence the children's course of recovery. Dawes (1989) reported a strong association between PTSD in mothers following political violence and symptoms of psychological distress in their children. Studies have documented that maternal trauma-related avoidance (Laor et al., 1997; Stuber, Nader, Yasuda, Pynoos, & Cohen, 1991) and overt anxious responses by parents to traumatic reminders and fears of recurrence (Green et al., 1991) increase young children's posttraumatic distress. Reestablishment of relationships with other surviving family members after prolonged massive trauma is associated with improved PTSD outcome for children and adolescents (Kinzie et al., 1986). Montgomery (1996) observed that keeping refugee families intact throughout the process of seeking political asylum and eventual resettlement significantly modifies children's anxieties. Zur (1990), in a UNICEF-sponsored study of Guatemalan children, reported on the importance of extended family networks to buffer the loss of parents in civil war.

Montgomery (1996) also reported that 50% of the children of Middle Eastern refugee families seeking political asylum in Denmark are living with a parent who survived various forms of torture. She commented that the more frequent use of corporal punishment by these parents during the resettlement period had an adverse effect on their children's anxiety. Other reports suggest that a major long-term consequence of the torture of a parent is a disruption of efforts to reorganize the family because of the parent's trauma-related inability to cope with generational confrontation (Comite di Defensa da los Derechos del Pueblo, 1989). Loughrey, Bell, Kee, Roddy, and Curran (1988) reported that symptoms of hyperarousal, including startle reactions and sleep disturbances, were pervasive among survivors of civil and terrorist violence in Northern Ireland. Marital disharmony and suicidal behavior were highly associated with chronic PTSD. These latter parental factors are well known to contribute significantly to the risk of childhood psychopathology. Pynoos and Nader (1988) observed that mothers who have been raped may continue to exhibit exaggerated startle responses to the unexpected approaches of their own children. Such responses can profoundly interfere with supportive parent–child interactions and elicit negative self-attributions in the child. An important conclusion to be drawn from findings on the effect of parental trauma on children is that mental health interventions for traumatized parents should include strategies to repair disturbances in the family milieu.

ASSESSMENT AND INTERVENTION

There are special considerations in the assessment of children and adolescents exposed to trauma. Numerous studies over the past decade have confirmed the ability of school-age children and adolescents to provide reliable and valid self-report regarding the nature of their traumatic experiences and current levels of distress. A comprehensive assessment should include a structured screening for context-specific and culturally informed traumatic (violent) experiences and documentation of objective features and subjective appraisals and responses. Sequential or serial traumatization can be approached through a rank ordering by the child or adolescent of his or her worst experiences and worst moments. Several parameters of distress should be evaluated with age-appropriate instruments to assess posttraumatic stress, grief, and depressive reactions, and, according to age, separation anxiety in younger children and attentional or behavioral disturbances in older children and adolescents.

Where it is feasible to do so, children's self-reports should be complemented with additional information from other informants, including parents, teachers, and other caretakers. In addition, since many children and adolescents are traumatized by witnessing acts of violence committed against their parents or siblings, evaluation of family members is essential. A comprehensive evaluation requires assessment of the nature and frequency of traumatic reminders and level of psychological and physiological reactivity; secondary stresses and adversities; intervening trauma, loss, medical illness and treatment; and developmental consequences in the areas of family, peer, and academic functioning. In adolescents, the evaluation might also include age-appropriate screening questions in regard to substance abuse, reckless behavior, and delinquency. In cases of child torture, beating, injury, or rape, a comprehensive medical examination with appropriate specialized consultation is required, similar in scope to that recommended for adult survivors (Vesti & Kastrup, 1995).

Research and clinical experiences with comprehensive child mental health programs in postwar, political violence, or catastrophic disaster situations provide support for a three-tier approach to intervention (Pynoos, Goenjian, & Steinberg, 1998). The first tier provides general support to a wide population of children through their schools, community agencies, and religious institutions. These efforts can be directed at the anxieties and fears exhibited by many children as a result of their common experiences. This first tier also provides psychoeducational forums, including classroom activities and discussions and teacher and parent meetings intended to enhance school and family milieu, foster mechanisms of peer support and conflict resolution, and initiate mentorship and supplemental afterschool programs. The second-tier interventions are specifically directed toward children and adolescents with severe levels of personal traumatic exposure and continuing posttraumatic distress, grief, and depression. A third tier provides appropriate referral to child mental health services for children identified as requiring evaluation and treatment for a broader range of child and adolescent psychiatric disorders.

Advances in the treatment of traumatized children and adolescents have paralleled those for adult trauma victims. In terms of the second-tier intervention, there is accumulating empirical evidence that trauma- and grief-focused psychotherapy and selected pharmacologic interventions can be effective in alleviating PTSD symptoms and in addressing comorbid depression (Goenjian et al., 1997; March, Amaya-Jackson, & Pynoos, 1997; Murphy, Pynoos, & James, 1997; Yule & Canterbury, 1994). This approach can be applied across a spectrum of intervention settings, including individual, group, family, or classroom, employing the selective and integrated use of psychoeducation, developmental psychodynamic psychotherapy (Pynoos & Nader, 1989), cognitive–behavioral therapy (Saigh, Yules, & Inamdar, 1996), educational assistance, physical rehabilitation, and remedial interventions to address developmental disruptions (Marmar, Foy, Kagan, & Pynoos, 1994). For very young children, working with the parents' reactions and enhancing their responsiveness to their child's posttrauma distress and reaction to reminders can be a primary approach to assisting their child's recovery.

Central features of trauma- and grief-focused therapy include (a) reconstructing traumatic events in an appropriately timed, developmentally sensitive, and culturally informed manner, paying special attention to worst moments, thoughts of intervention or protective action, and management of intense negative emotions; (b) enhancing recognition, cognitive discrimination, and recovery from reactivity to traumatic reminders; (c) improving problem-solving and coping skills in regard to secondary stresses and adversities; (d) facilitating age, family, and culturally appropriate bereavement, less encumbered by traumatic preoccupations and images; and (e) promoting normal developmental progression by resuming disrupted or lost opportunities and initiating age-appropriate prosocial activities and future planning. Medications have been reported to selectively ameliorate

arousal symptoms, including sleep disturbance and autonomic reactivity to reminders (Famularo, Kinscherff, & Fenton, 1988; Harmon & Riggs, 1996; Marmar et al.,
1994). Additional focused interventions may be required to treat other comorbid
conditions that persist, including depression, panic disorder, and substance abuse.
Furthermore, the treatment of medical conditions and adequate physical rehabilitation for trauma-related injuries are essential to the mental health recovery of
children and adolescents. Finally, a developmental approach to intervention should
include planned interventions at later developmental transitions, anticipated future reminders, subsequent adversities, and experiential and maturational reap-
praisals to facilitate additional adaptation and recovery.

Clinical and administrative experience from national and international efforts strongly indicates that in societies where school systems are stable, schools
constitute an effective and efficient clinical setting in which to provide mental
health assistance to children and their families after disaster, war, or political violence. The recovery of children and adolescents requires an expanded intervention framework that includes additional educational resources for remediation of
trauma-related interferences with learning and interruptions in schooling. The
developmental disturbances often require providing mentorship opportunities and
constructive afterschool recreation, social, work, spiritual, and community activities. Engaging with representatives of social agencies and institutions may be important in repairing breaches in children's or adolescents' belief in the social
contract. Neither the therapeutic nor the social interventions are to be overlooked
in efforts to prevent adolescents exposed to chronic violence from becoming a
"lost generation."

In addition, when traumatic experiences and losses are due to human agency,
there is a necessary link between judicial accountability and trauma resolution
among children and adolescents (Pynoos & Eth, 1986). Whereas specific posttrauma
symptoms can reappear at critical junctures during judicial hearings, other symptoms, including nightmares and preoccupations with revenge, can be observed to
remediate with proper judicial accountability. Care must be taken to minimize
unnecessary exposure to unknown or unexperienced traumatic details that may
generate renewed or new posttraumatic reactions and symptoms (Nader, Pynoos,
Fairbanks, Al-Ajeel, & Al-Asfour, 1993). There are many case examples and bio-
graphical accounts of children who were preoccupied throughout adulthood with
unanswered questions about perpetration of violence against family members. The
availability of information can be especially important in young adulthood, when
increased cognitive capacities can be brought to bear on working through prior
traumas and the violent loss of family members.

In the aftermath of major political violence and catastrophic disaster, secondary adversities are often pervasive and strongly contribute to chronicity of child
and parent posttraumatic distress and secondary comorbidity, especially depression. Such adversities include family relocation, physical disability, parental unemployment, economic hardship, overcrowding or lack of housing, shortages of
needed goods and services, and disruption of community and social ecology, even
social disintegration. These conditions can breed a continued culture of violence

characterized by increases in domestic violence, violent crime, gang-related violence among the unemployed and disenfranchised youth, and other forms of unlawful behavior, for example, black marketeering. Remediation of these adverse conditions is essential to establishing a societal milieu that promotes the recovery of children, adolescents, and their families and facilitates the critical transition from adolescence to productive young adulthood and responsible parenthood.

CONCLUSION

Recent international studies have documented the frequent traumatic exposures that occur in childhood, often in the context of political violence (Gibson, 1989; Keilson, 1980; Swartz & Levett, 1989). Population-based studies from Kuwait (Eisa & Nofel, 1993) and the former Yugoslavia region (UNICEF, 1995) have documented that school-age children and adolescents are tortured and that such experiences can result in severe and persistent levels of comorbid PTSD and depression.

There is clear evidence that younger children are extremely vulnerable to traumatic experiences such as violently imposed separation from parents and siblings, abduction, and the traumatic disappearance or death of primary caretakers. Children and adolescents exposed to these and other forms of violence often exhibit high levels of persistent hypervigilance, sleep disturbance, exaggerated startle, difficulties with learning, symptoms of separation anxiety, and disturbances in attachment. The occurrence of such difficulties during critical periods of development can have profound implications for future health status.

The degree of posttraumatic distress in children and adolescents exposed to extreme forms of violence appears to be mediated by a number of individual and family factors (e.g., current developmental competencies, temperament, self-esteem, locus of control, history of previous trauma, social support, intactness of families) that may help guide interventions. Public mental health and social programs to assist the recovery of young people and their families exposed to traumatic situations, particularly those involving youth in armed conflict, are likely to be more successful if they include community outreach efforts to provide remedial education opportunities, job training, and organized prosocial activities.

In societies where school systems are relatively stable, schools constitute an effective and efficient setting in which to provide mental health assistance to children and their families in the aftermath of disaster, war, or political violence.

REFERENCES

Baker, A. M. (1990). The psychological impact of the intifada on Palestinian children in the occupied West Bank and Gaza: An exploratory study. *American Journal of Orthopsychiatry, 60*, 496–505.

Bawa, U. (1995). Organized violence in apartheid South Africa: Children as victims and perpetrators. In Foundation for Children (Ed.), *Children: War and persecution, Proceedings of the Congress, Hamburg, September 26–29, 1993* (pp. 182–190). Osnabrück, Germany: Secolo.

Boothby, N. (1994). Trauma and violence among refugee children. In A. J. Marsella, T. P. Bornemann, E. Solvig, & J. Orley (Eds.), *Amidst peril and pain: The mental health and well-being of the world's refugees*. Washington, DC: American Psychological Association Press.

Cairns, E. (1996). *Children and political violence*. Oxford, England: Blackwell.

Clark, D. C., Pynoos, R. S., & Goebel, A. E. (1996). Mechanisms and processes of adolescent bereavement. In R. J. Haggerty, L. R. Sherrod, N. Garmezy, & M. Rutter (Eds.), *Stress, risk, and resilience in children and adolescents: Processes, mechanisms, and interventions* (pp. 100–146). New York: Cambridge University Press.

Comite di Defensa da los Derechos del Pueblo. (1989). The effects of torture and political repression in a sample of Chilean families. *Social Science in Medicine, 28,* 735–740.

Dawes, A. (1989). The effects of political violence on socio-moral reasoning and conduct. In A. Dawes & D. Donald (Eds.), *Childhood and adversity: Psychological perspectives from South African research* (pp. 200–219). Cape Town, South Africa: Philip.

De Bellis, M. D., Chrousos, G. P., Dorn, L. D., Burke, L., Helmers, K., Kling, M. A., Trickett, P. K., & Putnam, F. W. (1994). Hypothalamic–pituitary–adrenal axis dysregulation in sexually abused girls. *Journal of Clinical Endocrinology and Metabolism, 78,* 249–255.

Eisa, J., & Nofel, E. (1993). *Screening for war exposure and posttraumatic stress disorder among children in Kuwait. Age 7–17. Preliminary report*. Ministry of Education, Kuwait [in Arabic].

Eth, S., & Pynoos, R. S. (1994). Children who witness the homicide of a parent. *Psychiatry, 57,* 287–305.

Famularo, R., Kinscherff, R., & Fenton, T. (1988). Propranolol treatment for childhood posttraumatic stress disorder, acute type. *American Journal of Diseases of Children, 142,* 1244–1247.

Garbarino, J., Kostelny, K., & Dubrow, N. (1991). What children can tell us about living in danger. *American Psychologist, 46*(4), 376–383.

Gibson, K. (1989). Children in political violence. *Social Science in Medicine, 28,* 659–667.

Glod, C. A., Teicher, M. H., Martin, H., Hartman, C., & Harakal, T. (1997). Increased nocturnal activity and impaired sleep maintenance in abused children. *Journal of the American Academy of Child and Adolescent Psychiatry, 36*(9), 1236–1243.

Goenjian, A. K., Pynoos, R. S., Karayan, I., Minassian, D., Najarian, L. M., Steinberg, A. M., & Fairbanks, L. A. (1997). Outcome of psychotherapy among pre-adolescents after the 1988 earthquake in Armenia. *American Journal of Psychiatry, 154,* 536–542.

Goenjian, A. K., Pynoos, R. S., Steinberg, A. M., Najarian, L. M., Asarnow, J. R., Karayan, I., Ghurabi, M., & Fairbanks, L. A. (1995). Psychiatric co-morbidity in children after the 1988 earthquake in Armenia. *Journal of the American Academy of Child and Adolescent Psychiatry, 34*(9), 1174–1184.

Goenjian, A. K., Stilwell, B. M., Steinberg, A. M., Fairbanks, L. A., Galvin, M., Karayan, I., & Pynoos, R. S. (1999). Moral development and psychopathological interference with conscience functioning in adolescents after trauma. *Journal of the American Academy of Child and Adolescent Psychiatry, 38*(4), 376–384.

Goenjian, A. K., Yehuda, R., Pynoos, R. S., Steinberg, A. M., Tashjian, M., Yang, R. K., Najarian, L. M., & Fairbanks, L. A. (1996). Basal cortisol and dexamethasone suppression of cortisol and MHPG among adolescents after the 1988 earthquake in Armenia. *American Journal of Psychiatry, 153,* 929–934.

Green, B. L., Korol, M., Grace, M. C., Vary, M. G., Leonard, A. C., Gleser, G. C., & Smitson-Cohen, S. (1991). Children and disaster: Age, gender, and parental effects on PTSD symptoms. *Journal of the American Academy of Child and Adolescent Psychiatry, 30*(6), 945–951.

Harmon, R. J., & Riggs, P. D. (1996). Clonidine for posttraumatic stress disorder in preschool children. *Journal of the American Academy of Child and Adolescent Psychiatry, 35*(9), 1247–1249.

Keilson, H. (1980). Sequential traumatization of children. *Danish Medical Bulletin, 27,* 235–237.

Kilpatrick, D. G., Saunders, B. E., Resnick, H. S., & Smith, D. W. (1995). *The national survey of adolescents: Preliminary findings on lifetime prevalence of traumatic events and mental health correlates*. Charleston, SC: National Crime Victims Research and Treatment Center, Medical University of South Carolina.

Kinzie, J. D., Sack, W., Angell, R., Clarke, G., & Binn, R. (1989). A three-year follow-up of Cambodian young people traumatized as children. *Journal of the American Academy of Child and Adolescent Psychiatry, 28*(4), 501–504.

Kinzie, J. D., Sack, W. H., Angell, R. H., Manson, S., & Rath, B. (1986). The psychiatric effects of massive trauma on Cambodian children: I. The children. *Journal of the American Academy of Child and Adolescent Psychiatry, 25*(3), 370–376.

Kirsten, J. C., Holzer, I. M., Koch, L., & Severin, B. (1980). Children and torture. *Danish Medical Bulletin, 27*, 238–239.

Laor, N., Wolmer, L., Mayes., L. C., Gershon, A., Weizman, R., & Cohn, D. J. (1997). Israel preschool children under Scuds: A 30-month follow-up. *Journal of the American Academy of Child and Adolescent Psychiatry, 36*(3), 349–356.

Loughrey, G. C., Bell, P., Kee, P., Roddy, R. J., & Curran, P. S. (1988). Post-traumatic stress disorder and civil violence in Northern Ireland. *British Journal of Psychiatry, 153*, 554–560.

March, J. S., Amaya-Jackson, L., & Pynoos, R. S. (1997). Pediatric posttraumatic stress disorder. In J. M. Weiner (Ed.), *Textbook of child and adolescent psychiatry* (2nd ed.). Washington, DC: American Psychiatric Press.

Marmar, C. R., Foy, D., Kagan, B., & Pynoos, R. S. (1994). An integrated approach for treating posttraumatic stress. In R. S. Pynoos (Ed.), *Posttraumatic stress disorder: A clinical review* (pp. 99–132). Lutherville, MD: Sidran Press.

Montgomery, E. (1998). Refugee children from the Middle East. *Scandinavian Journal of Social Medicine, 54*(Suppl.): 1–152.

Murphy, L., Pynoos, R. S., & James, C. B. (1997). The trauma/grief focused group psychotherapy module of an elementary school-based violence prevention/intervention program. In J. D. Osofsky (Ed.), *Children in a violent society* (pp. 223–255). New York: Guilford Press.

Nader, K., Pynoos, R. S., Fairbanks, L. A., Al-Ajeel, M., & Al-Asfour, A. (1993). A preliminary study of PTSD and grief among the children of Kuwait following the Gulf crisis. *British Journal of Clinical Psychology, 32*, 407–416.

Ornitz, E. M., & Pynoos, R. S. (1989). Startle modulation in children with posttraumatic stress disorder. *American Journal of Psychiatry, 146*, 866–870.

Pennebaker, J. W., & Susman, J. R. (1988). Disclosure of traumas and psychosomatic processes. *Social Science and Medicine, 26*(3), 327–332.

Perry, B. D. (1994). Neurobiological sequelae of childhood trauma: Posttraumatic stress disorders in children. In M. Murberg (Ed.), *Catecholamine function in posttraumatic stress disorder: Emerging concepts, progress in psychiatry* (pp. 233–255). Washington, DC: American Psychiatric Press.

Perry, B. D., & Pate, J. E. (1994). Neurodevelopment and the psychobiological roots of posttraumatic stress disorder. In L. F. Koziol & C. E. Stout (Eds.), *The neuropsychology of mental disorders: A practical guide* (pp. 129–146). Springfield, IL: Thomas.

Punamaki, R. (1987). Psychological stress responses of Palestinian mothers and children in conditions of military occupation and political violence. *Quarterly Newsletter of the Laboratory of Comparative Human Cognition, 9*, 76–84.

Putnam, F. W., & Trickett, P. K. (1993). Child sexual abuse: A model of chronic trauma. *Psychiatry, 56*, 82–95.

Pynoos, R. S., & Eth, S. (1986). Special intervention programs for child witnesses to violence. In M. Lystad (Ed.), *Violence in the home: Interdisciplinary perspectives* (pp. 193–216). New York: Brunner/Mazel.

Pynoos, R. S., Frederick, C., Nader, K., Arroyo, W., Steinberg, A. M., Eth, S., Nunez, F., & Fairbanks, L. (1987). Life threat and posttraumatic stress in school-age children. *Archives of General Psychiatry, 44*, 1057–1063.

Pynoos, R. S., Goenjian, A. K., & Steinberg, A. M. (1998). A public mental health approach to the postdisaster treatment of children and adolescents. *Child and Adolescent Psychiatric Clinics of North America, 7*(1), 195–210.

Pynoos, R., Goenjian, A. K., Tashjian, M., Karakashian, M., Manjikian, R., Manoukian, G., Steinberg, A. M., & Fairbanks, L. (1993). Posttraumatic stress reactions in children after the 1988 Armenian earthquake. *British Journal of Psychiatry, 163,* 239–247.

Pynoos, R. S., & Nader, K. (1988). Children who witness the sexual assaults of their mothers. *Journal of the American Academy of Child and Adolescent Psychiatry, 27*(5), 567–572.

Pynoos, R. S., & Nader, K. (1989). Children's memory and proximity to violence. *Journal of the American Academy of Child and Adolescent Psychiatry, 28*(2), 236–241.

Pynoos, R. S., Steinberg, A. M., & Wraith, R. (1995). A developmental model of childhood traumatic stress. In D. Cicchetti & D. J. Cohen (Eds.), *Manual of developmental psychopathology: Vol. 2. Risk, disorder, and adaptation* (pp. 72–95). New York: Wiley.

Raundalen, M. (1993, June). *Family and war: Some observations and suggestions for further research.* Paper presented at the Third European Conference on Traumatic Stress, Bergen, Norway.

Sabin, D., Sack, W. H., Clarke, C. N., Meas, N., & Richart, I. (1996). The Khmer Adolescent Project: 3. A study of the trauma from Thailand Site Two Refugee Camp. *Journal of the American Academy of Child and Adolescent Psychiatry, 35*(3), 384–391.

Sack, W. H., Angell, R. H., Kinzie, J. D., & Rath, B. (1986). The psychiatric effects of massive trauma on Cambodian children: II. The family, the home, and the school. *Journal of the American Academy of Child and Adolescent Psychiatry, 25*(3), 377–383.

Sack, W. H., Clarke, G. N., & Seeley, J. (1996). Multiple forms of stress in Cambodian adolescent refugees. *Child Development, 67*(11), 107–116.

Sack, W. H., Seeley, J. R., & Clarke, G. N. (1997). Does PTSD transcend cultural barriers: A look from the Khmer Adolescent Refugee Project. *Journal of the American Academy of Child and Adolescent Psychiatry, 36*(1), 49–54.

Saigh, P. A., Yule, W., & Inamdar, S. C. (1996). Imaginal flooding of traumatized children and adolescents. *Journal of School Psychology, 34*: 163–183.

Stein, M. B., Koverola, C., Hanna, C., Torchia, M. G., & McClarty, B. (1997). Hippocampal volume in women victimized by childhood sexual abuse. *Psychology and Medicine, 27*(4), 951–959.

Straker, G. (1992). *Faces in the revolution: The psychological effects of violence on township youth in South Africa.* Athens, OH: Ohio University Press.

Straker, G. (1993). The effects of diverse forms of political violence on adolescent emotional and moral concerns. In Foundation for Children (Ed.), *Children: War and persecution, Proceedings of the Congress, Hamburg, September 26–29, 1993* (pp. 182–190). Osnabrück, Germany: Secolo.

Stuber, M. L., Nader, K., Yasuda, P., Pynoos, R. S., & Cohen, S. (1991). Stress responses after pediatric bone marrow transplantation: Preliminary results of a prospective longitudinal study. *Journal of the American Academy of Child and Adolescent Psychiatry, 30*(6), 952–957.

Stuvland, R. (1993). *Psychological and educational help to school-children affected by war: Results from a screening of children in Croatia.* Zagreb, Croatia: Ministry of Education, Government of Croatia, in cooperation with UNICEF Zagreb.

Stuvland, R., & Barath, A. (1993). The "case" of former Yugoslavia. In Foundation for Children (Ed.), *Children: War and persecution, Proceedings of the Congress, Hamburg, September 26–29, 1993* (pp. 182–190). Osnabrück, Germany: Secolo.

Swartz, L., & Levett, A. (1989). Political repression and children in South Africa: The social construction of damaging effects. *Social Science in Medicine, 28,* 741–750.

Tudin, P., Straker, G., & Mendolsohn, M. (1994). Social and political complexity and moral development. *South African Journal of Psychology, 24*(3), 163–168.

UNICEF. (1995). *War-time survey of exposure, posttraumatic stress reactions, and depression among children and adolescents.* Report of UNICEF Psychological Program for the ex-Yugoslavia region.

van der Kolk, B. A. (1985). Adolescent vulnerability to post-traumatic stress. *Psychiatry, 48,* 365–370.

Vesti, P., & Kastrup, M. (1995). Refugee status, torture, and adjustment. In J. R. Freedy & S. E. Hobfoll (Eds.), *Traumatic stress: From theory to practice.* New York: Plenum Press.

Yule, W. (1992). Post-traumatic stress disorder in child survivors of shipping disasters: The sinking of the Jupiter. *Psychotherapy and Psychosomatics, 57*, 200–205.

Yule, W., & Canterbury, R. (1994). The treatment of posttraumatic stress disorder in children and adolescents. *International Review of Psychiatry, 6*, 141–151.

15

Domestic Violence in Families Exposed to Torture and Related Violence and Trauma

MALCOLM GORDON

In general, research on domestic violence in families with members who have experienced severe trauma is not comprehensive enough to fully describe the relationship between such trauma and domestic violence. More research on this topic is needed. Such domestic violence could occur in new families formed by trauma victims following their traumatic experiences or in established families in which some or all members have experienced severe trauma. The continuing effects of the trauma might also play a role in the initiation, continuation, or escalation of victimization or perpetration of domestic violence.

To a large extent, domestic violence in tortured and extremely traumatized populations is a hidden problem. This situation exists because clinical and research studies focus primarily on *individual* traumatic experience rather than on trauma in families. Moreover, prohibitions within traumatized families against disclosing family problems because of cultural norms, language difficulties, and residency and status problems (e.g., fear of compromising refugee or asylum status or welfare eligibility) may also keep family violence concealed. Nonetheless, findings relevant to this issue can be derived from small-scale studies, clinical reports, and the large body of literature on the effects of torture and trauma on individual and family functioning.

Much of this related literature focuses on pathology and dysfunction in trauma survivors. However, such research has also shown the extraordinary capacity of some individuals to function humanely and competently despite experiencing

MALCOLM GORDON • National Institute of Mental Health, Neuroscience Center Building, Bethesda, Maryland 20892.

The Mental Health Consequences of Torture, edited by Ellen Gerrity, Terence M. Keane, and Farris Tuma. Kluwer Academic/Plenum Publishers, New York, 2001.

almost unimaginable trauma and loss and significant physical and psychological effects of their traumatic experiences. For example, Kahana, Harel, and Kahana (1988) discussed both the positive and the negative adaptation of a sample of Holocaust survivors, including low divorce rates and long-term marriages. However, although severe domestic violence may affect only a small minority of traumatized families, studies indicate that trauma survivors have heightened vulnerabilities for relationship problems in their families, including domestic violence, as a result of the effects of their traumatic experiences.

This chapter on domestic violence and trauma will focus primarily on spouse (or intimate partner) abuse, with a more limited discussion of the effect of traumatic experiences on other family members, especially children. A considerable body of research exists on domestic violence, primarily with North American and European samples. This research has established some important general conclusions (e.g., Crowell & Burgess, 1996).

Families vary greatly in the types, severity, frequency, and situational context of physical aggression. Some couples engage in infrequent and mild or moderate aggressive acts; other couples experience relatively frequent and severe physical aggression. With some couples, only one partner, usually the male, assaults the other; other couples engage in reciprocal aggression. Similarly, the motivations of victims to continue in violent relationships can vary, such as emotional attachment to or dependence on the perpetrator, fear for safety of self or children, lack of economic or social resources to establish an independent household, or familial or societal disapproval of marital disruption. Societies vary greatly in the prevalence and severity of domestic violence, but usually only small minorities of couples engage in chronic and severe violence.

Severe domestic violence often involves verbal and physical humiliation and degradation of the victim, chronic threats, and intimidation and other forms of psychological abuse. Episodes of domestic violence may be rationalized in various ways (e.g., allegations of infidelity, failure to perform household duties), but these episodes are usually motivated by underlying hostility toward the victim or an attempt to dominate the victim.

Individual, interpersonal, social group, societal, and cultural factors interact as risk factors for the occurrence of domestic violence. Perpetrator characteristics that function as risk factors for domestic violence include individual biological factors (e.g., impulsive aggression, organic brain dysfunction), individual psychological factors (e.g., jealousy, hostility, psychopathy), and individual experiential factors (e.g., a history of aggressive behavior, a history of childhood maltreatment, drug or alcohol intoxication). Researchers have been less able to identify characteristics of victims that place them at risk for domestic violence. Prior physical or sexual victimization in childhood or adulthood may be a risk factor for domestic violence. Also, inasmuch as physically abusive relationships are frequently terminated because of the abuse, chronically abusive relationships usually involve a victim who is economically, socially, or emotionally dependent on the perpetrator; is afraid of severe abuse or death if attempts are made to terminate the relationship; or faces significant social or legal barriers against terminating the relationship. Relationship factors that may be involved in marital violence include differences or deficiencies in couple communication, conflict resolution, emotional expression, or attitudes about important family issues (e.g., child rearing or sexual expectations). Social factors include societal support for physical "discipline" of family members, legal and social barriers against terminating abusive relationships, and encouragement of abuse by extended family members or peers.

The course of domestic violence in relationships can vary over time. In some couples, the severity of violent acts can escalate; in other couples, violence may be episodic and associated with social, economic, or interpersonal stressors or with alcohol or substance abuse. Some couples may desist in physical violence with age or longevity but may continue to engage in or substitute emotionally abusive and coercive behavior for physical aggression. Domestic violence is strongly associated with dissatisfaction with the intimate relationship, and physically abusive relationships are at high risk for termination.

Emotional and sexual abuse is frequently associated with physical assault, especially in more seriously abusive relationships. Spousal violence and child abuse frequently co-occur within the same family and intergenerationally (i.e., parents who were victims of abuse in childhood are more likely to abuse their own children or not to protect their children from abuse than nonabused parents, although most abused children do not grow up to be abusive parents). Moreover, children almost always witness or are aware of spousal violence and are seriously negatively affected by exposure to spousal violence.

Most torture victims and victims of war-zone trauma come from nonwestern countries, and the societal and cultural context of domestic violence is especially important. The amount of literature on domestic violence in other societies and cultures is growing (e.g., Counts, Brown, & Campbell, 1992; Levinson, 1989; Wilson & Raphael, 1993). Domestic violence associated with torture, war, ethnic or political warfare, and oppression is superimposed on the underlying norms of domestic violence in the society and the culture.

The societal and cultural context of domestic violence is important in a number of ways.

- Societies differ in the types of dominant familial structures (e.g., nuclear families or extended, multigenerational families). Differences in family structure can play a role in, for example, the frequency, severity, and rationale for domestic violence and in who may "normatively" assault, "discipline," or protect a wife or other family member (see, for example, Fernandez's 1997 discussion of the role of older females in the domestic beating of young wives in India).
- Societies also differ in expectations and valuations of marital and family roles. Many western societies value a romantic attachment between marital partners with relatively equal decision-making power and a nurturant relationship between parents and their children. However, in many societies, other expectations and values are the basis of marital and parent–child relationships (e.g., to cement alliances between familial clans, to

guarantee continuation of familial lineage, or to provide additional workers for family income or subsistence) (see, for example, Tseng & Hsu, 1991).

• Societies and cultures can differ in prescriptions of normative or accepted aggression and nonnormative aggression between spouses and between parents and children. A survey of ethnographic studies estimated that some form of spousal violence, almost always wife beating, occurred in more than 80% of societies, and physical aggression against children occurred in more than 75% of societies. Most societies sanction use of physical "punishment" of both wives and children for real or perceived violations of socially defined role and behavioral standards, for example, confirmed or alleged infidelity, disagreements about sex, insubordination or disobedience, or alleged or confirmed failure of the wife or a child to meet household responsibilities. Societies also differ in the criteria for unjustified or excessive spousal or child aggression, in the likelihood that the community will intervene in such cases, and in the available avenues open to the wife or child for termination of physical violence (divorce, separation into shelter by relatives, or arrest or other sanctions against the perpetrator) (see, for example, Zimmerman's 1994 discussion of the overwhelming priority placed on reconciliation of marital conflict in Cambodia and the resultant severe barrier to divorce for abused Cambodian women).

• Domestic violence is strongly related to the general level of acceptance of interpersonal violence in a society. Domestic violence is also associated with social strain and disorganization in a society, which is often associated with weakening or disruption of traditional cultural norms on interpersonal behavior in families, as, for example, when traditional rural tribal or clan societies are disrupted by migration to urban areas or by prolonged communal violence. In addition, as societies experience transitions between traditional cultural notions concerning physical aggression between spouses and between parents and children and western notions of gender equality and welfare of children, this transition can lead to intergenerational conflict about family-role expectations. Thus, legal sanctions against family violence are increasing throughout the world as a result of the influence of western media, education, and the advocacy of women's and children's rights by national and international women's groups (see, for example, the discussion by Choi and Edelson, 1995, of the changing perception of societal intervention in domestic violence in Singapore). Domestic violence appears to be somewhat more related to gender inequality in a society, especially economic inequality between men and women, than to differences in social status or decision-making power (Korbin, 1991; Levinson, 1989).

The remainder of this chapter will address three questions relevant to domestic violence in families that have experienced torture, detention, war, ethnic or political warfare and oppression, and refugee displacement: (a) Does exposure to torture detention; war-zone, political, and ethnic violence; and refugee resettlement increase the likelihood or severity of domestic violence? (b) Are the characteristics of domestic violence different in families that have experienced severe trauma? (c) Should approaches to treatment and prevention of domestic violence be different for families that have experienced trauma? Most individuals who have experienced torture, serious war-zone trauma, or refugee flight and resettlement have endured wide variations in the length, types, and severity of experience of torture and war-zone trauma. Thus, a torture survivor may be either a combatant or member of an oppressed political or ethnic group, may be a noncombatant in an area that supports a political or armed resistance, or may be a member of a general population randomly selected to serve as a deterrent to dissent. Moreover, detention and torture often co-occur with various other forms of trauma and deprivation, especially physical and sexual trauma; hunger and deprivation; and loss of family members, friends, and community. Thus, in one study of a clinical sample group of Cambodian women, 12 of the 14 women were widows; they had an average of 2 children, had spent an average of 4 years in a refugee resettlement camp before emigrating, and had experienced an average of more than six traumatic losses and six other traumas, including torture, rape, seeing the massacre or torture of others, and starvation (Herbst, 1992). Torture survivors and their families may also have experienced prolonged imprisonment, death and injury of other family members, chronic fear and danger of rearrest or other harassment if they remain in their homeland, internal or refugee resettlement, immigration and adjustment stress in a different society, and social deprivation and uncertainty as to refugee or asylum status in a foreign host country (Herbst, 1992; Lavik, Hauff, Skrondal, & Solberg, 1996; Sinnerbrink, Silove, Field, Steel, & Manicavasagar, 1997). Trauma survivors can also vary greatly in the acute and chronic effects of trauma.

Trauma can affect people in a number of ways: (a) increasing psychological (e.g., flashbacks) and physical (e.g., sequelae from head injuries) symptoms; (b) diminishing psychological (e.g., difficulties concentrating or remembering) or psychosocial functioning (e.g., avoidance of social interaction, inability to work); and (c) disrupting or degrading a basic conceptualization of self-worth and of connections to the social world (e.g., hopelessness, demoralization, cynicism) (see, for example, Turner & Gorst-Unsworth, 1993).

The complexity of these varying patterns of trauma exposure and effects means that making generalizations or prediction of the effects on particular individuals is very difficult. Nevertheless, these varying experiential and co-occurring traumatic experiences play a significant role in the likelihood and types of interpersonal problems and domestic violence in families that have experienced torture or war-zone trauma (Cunningham & Silove, 1993).

DOES EXPOSURE TO TORTURE DETENTION; WAR-ZONE, POLITICAL, AND ETHNIC VIOLENCE; AND REFUGEE RESETTLEMENT INCREASE THE LIKELIHOOD OR SEVERITY OF DOMESTIC VIOLENCE?

It is not entirely clear whether and how stress or trauma increases the likelihood of domestic violence. Research on trauma and domestic violence has focused primarily on relationship conflict and aggression in families of combat veterans, returned prisoners of war (POWs), and refugees. The domestic violence in families has been associated with two hypothesized (probably overlapping) mediators: (a) relationship conflict and (b) anger, rage, and aggression (Cascardi & Vivian, 1995; Eckhardt, Babour, & Stuart, 1997; Rodriguez & Green, 1997). These two mediators may be heightened in traumatized individuals or families and make such families vulnerable to the initiation, continuance, or increase in the severity of spousal and child abuse.

Relationship Conflict and Aggression

In general, research studies support an association of war experiences or prolonged detention with problems with marital relationships and marital dissolution. In societies that value an emotional and sexual attachment between marital partners, the effects of trauma may affect primarily the emotional relationship between partners; in societies that value role performance of marital partners, trauma may affect primarily family and social role functioning.

A large national study of Vietnam veterans reported more than 40% had divorced or never married, approximately one third reported moderate to serious problems in their current intimate relationship, and approximately one half of the veterans who had children reported moderate to serious parenting difficulties. Approximately 10% of the sample had engaged in multiple acts of physical aggression or threats of aggression against their partner in the prior year (Jordan et al., 1992). A study of American Vietnam POWs, most of whom had been tortured, reported that 30% divorced during their first year postreturn compared with only 10% in a matched comparison group; approximately 50% of the POWs were divorced after 5 years (Hunter, 1986, 1993). Byrne and Riggs (1996) directly tested the relationship of trauma symptoms, war experiences, and partner aggression. In a sample of 50 male Vietnam veterans and their partners, they found high levels of relationship aggression (physical aggression, verbal aggression, and psychological abuse) and relationship dissatisfaction. Relationship aggression was more related to trauma symptoms than to war exposure and seemed to be mediated by relationship conflict.

Increased marital and family conflict in families of survivors of torture and related trauma may be a result of (a) the direct effects of trauma-coping behavior and symptoms on interpersonal relationships, (b) the inability of trauma survivors to function in expected family and social roles because of physical or psychological disability resulting from traumatic experiences, and (c) conflicts associated with changes in gender and family roles during and following prolonged detention or refugee migration.

Torture victims and detainees often experience direct effects of their traumatic experiences that interfere with interpersonal functioning following release. Residual trauma effects can interfere with intimacy, empathy, emotional expressiveness, control, sexuality, and regulation of anger and aggression toward family members (see below and Carroll, Rueger, Foy, & Donahoe, 1985; Matsakis, 1988; Roberts et al., 1982; Shay, 1995). In most societies, important roles of a father are to be the economic provider and to protect the family; significant roles of the mother are to be the caretaker of the children and the household. The adequacy of performance of social and family-role expectations by trauma victims may be compromised by their prolonged absence during detention, their level of functioning following release, and their functioning during migration and resettlement. Following release, adult male and female family members may not be able to function adequately socially or occupationally nor be able to adequately perform family responsibilities because of trauma symptoms such as chronic, disabling reexperiencing of the trauma; physical disability; low morale as a result of disillusionment, guilt, or lowered status; or passivity and physical enervation as an aftermath of imprisonment, torture, or resettlement dependence (Chung & Bemak, 1996).

Many families who experience prolonged separation from a family member, for example, if a father is detained, must, after a period of time, adopt new roles to ensure survival. Often these new roles may involve greater social or economic competence and psychological independence by women and children in the family than were displayed before the detention (Hunter, 1986). If the detained family member later rejoins the family, both the returned member and the other family members may have a difficult time adjusting to the changed functioning of family members during the detention. This adjustment could be especially difficult because detainees, being in a situation of severe deprivation, may conserve or accentuate predetention behavioral patterns and attitudes. Resettlement in a foreign country can also create significant stress between husbands and wives and between parents and children. The country of resettlement may provide social role models, particularly of behavior by women and adolescents, that are at variance with traditional norms in the family's culture of origin (see, for example, the discussion by Lipson and Miller, 1994, of conflicts regarding models of women's roles in Afghan refugee women in the United States). During refugee adaptation, children often acculturate much more quickly, learn a new language much more competently, and establish social relations much more quickly than their parents do. This accelerated adaptation can lead to intergenerational conflicts (Rick & Forward, 1992).

Trauma, Anger, and Aggression

Emotional dysregulation is a common difficulty in survivors of combat, detainment, and torture. Undercontrol or overcontrol of anger and hostility can be a risk factor for explosive aggression toward family members. Clinicians treating war veterans have described rage attacks in combat veterans, sometimes triggered by war reminders or interpersonal stress and at times appearing with seemingly no precipitants. Often traumatized war veterans or torture survivors fear turning their rage on loved ones and adopt socially avoidant behavior to prevent uncontrolled outbursts of violence (Hierholzer, Munson, Peabody, & Rosenberg, 1992; Matsakis, 1988; Shay, 1995). A national study of Vietnam war veterans 15 years after the end of the war reported that 16% of the sample had committed an act of severe physical aggression involving kicking or beating or using a weapon in the prior year (Zatzick et al., 1997). Although many trauma victims have difficulty with irritability and anger, a relatively small proportion of trauma survivors have significant problems with repetitive and serious anger and aggression. Thus, among a group of Vietnam veterans with posttraumatic stress disorder (PTSD) who committed on the average about five physically aggressive acts targeted at their partner, a subgroup of 9% of the veterans committed at least 13 partner-directed aggressive acts in the prior year (Jordan et al., 1992). Anger and irritability can result from the consequences of torture, including head injury, exhaustion because of sleep difficulties, and low frustration tolerance because of general hyperarousal.

Additional Considerations

Those survivors of torture or war trauma who migrate to avoid war or political violence often experience additional significant family stress in refugee camps, which are often violent and have few social, educational, or employment opportunities. In addition to family conflict and anger that may potentiate spousal and child-directed violence, torture and trauma survivors and their families may not have access to social resources that buffer the likelihood of stress catalyzing domestic violence, such as emotional and child-care support from friends and extended family members. Thus, one of the legacies of the Pol Pot atrocities in Cambodia is that many battered Cambodian women have no parents left who could provide safe shelter or intervene to protect them (Zimmerman, 1994).

Some effects of torture and related trauma, such as physical disabilities, depression, a general lack of energy, or a greater appreciation of the negative effects of violence and positive regard for the value of a family, could decrease the likelihood of engaging in domestic violence. In addition to the role of trauma symptoms on engagement in domestic violence, the effects of traumatic experiences can play a role in being a victim of domestic violence, especially for women survivors of torture and related trauma. Both research reports (e.g., Jordan et al., 1992) and clinical accounts (Matsakis, 1988) describe relationship violence directed at traumatized male combat veterans by their wives. Such aggression is often related to frustration in coping with the veterans' symptoms or stress associated with increased responsibilities arising from the veterans' dysfunction.

For many war-trauma refugees, domestic violence is a continuation of family violence experienced before trauma exposure. Studies of women refugees from Central America revealed high rates of domestic violence predating and continuing through experiences of war trauma (Farias, 1991; Jenkins, 1991). Many such women fled persecution or danger in their homeland in part to escape ongoing domestic violence. In such cases, factors associated with domestic violence in nontraumatized populations are relevant (e.g., psychopathy in the perpetrator, culturally sanctioned physical aggression for suspected infidelity, or alcohol and drug abuse).

ARE THE CHARACTERISTICS OF DOMESTIC VIOLENCE DIFFERENT IN FAMILIES THAT HAVE EXPERIENCED SEVERE TRAUMA?

Domestic violence in families of survivors of torture and related trauma manifests characteristics that are different from typical manifestations of family violence. In addition to cultural differences, major differences are (a) the influence of the effects of traumatic experiences on the family functioning of traumatized individuals, (b) shared and secondary trauma in the family as a whole, and (c) the role of sexual trauma on intimate relationships.

Individual Trauma

Torture and other trauma experiences can have a profound effect on interpersonal interactions and the capacity for positive marital and other family relationships. Exposure to severe trauma results in very high rates of chronic and incapacitating posttraumatic stress symptoms, depression, and other trauma-related symptoms. Thus, in a study of 160 torture victims, Somasundaram (1993) found that 85% were diagnosed with PTSD; almost 90% suffered from physical tiredness; 80% had memory and concentration difficulties; 65% had severe somatic symptoms, such as headaches and fainting; 50% exhibited extreme distrust and suspiciousness; 40% exhibited irritability and aggressiveness; 40% exhibited social withdrawal; and 25% experienced sexual dysfunction. Crocq, Macher, Barros-Beck, Rosenberg, and Duval (1993) reported that in a sample of approximately 500 former POWs assessed more than 40 years after release, more than 75% still experienced intrusive reexperiencing of captivity-related trauma, 60% to 70% reported active avoidance of thoughts and activities that might remind them of war or captivity trauma, about half reported social isolation or estrangement, and about 40% had frequent anger outbursts. The type and severity of psychological symptoms were related to length of captivity, severity of abuse during captivity, and head injuries.

Effects of torture trauma can directly affect intimate and family relationships. These effects include the posttraumatic symptoms of reexperiencing or preoccupation with trauma reminders; affective and social avoidance or withdrawal; hyperarousal and irritability because of jumpiness, hypervigilance, and sleep deprivation; difficulties with basic cognitive processing of memory, attention, and learning; somatic symptoms, such as pain or disability from injuries, headaches, and stress-exacerbated illnesses; demoralization, distrust, a sense of a foreshortened future, and lack of ambition; and personality changes, especially passivity and detachment (Herbst, 1992; Shay, 1995; Turner & Gorst-Unsworth, 1993).

Torture victims and detainees also may have adopted coping behaviors that, although adaptive during detention, are maladaptive in their family interactions after release from detention. Such coping strategies include emotional numbing, dissociating, perseverative engagement in mental gymnastics, shutting out stimulation, and focusing on the body (Silove, McIntosh, & Becker, 1993). Thus, many torture survivors have difficulty tolerating high levels of stimulation, especially social stimulation, and may withdraw from social interactions or avoid interpersonal conflicts. Trauma survivors may also adopt coping methods to deal with trauma symptoms and dysphoria, such as drug and alcohol use, lengthy work hours, and prolonged absences from home, that have a negative effect on family relationships. A survey of counselors who provided treatment to wives of traumatized Vietnam veterans indicated that their primary problems in their relationship with their husbands were fear of their husbands' explosive rage, feelings of loneliness and social isolation, and coping with their husbands' trauma symptoms, especially social and emotional withdrawal (Matsakis, 1988).

Studies of trauma survivors have, in general, shown that severity of posttraumatic stress symptoms has a much greater effect on functioning than just exposure to traumatic events. Thus, in the study of Vietnam war veterans reported above, twice as many combat veterans with PTSD (one third of the sample) committed acts of severe physical aggression as did combat veterans without PTSD (Zatzick et al., 1997). Combat veterans with PTSD are less likely to be married and had more divorces, more occupational and residential instability (35% homeless or vagrant), and more violent episodes (25% had committed more than 13 acts of aggression in the prior year and 50% had been arrested or jailed more than once as an adult) than veterans without PTSD (Friedman, 1992). Byrne and Riggs (1996) reported that exposure to combat was not related to relationship aggression in veterans who did not have serious trauma symptoms.

The effects of torture on family functioning is exemplified in the following excerpt:

> They told me that I was their pet dog. They made me walk on my hands and knees and bark. They fed me scraps of orange peels which they threw on the floor. They would kick me in the ribs and sometimes hit me with a thorn-like branch. I have no right to complain because I was treated better than the other prisoners. You may find this hard to believe—on the day the police let me go, I couldn't stand up. I walked like a dog back to my house. I was so humiliated.

> Now that I'm free, you would think that I could forget what happened and start living a normal life. When I was picked up by the police, I became a different person. Now I can't work. I can't concentrate. I am afraid that I will be abducted again. I no longer know how to be affectionate to my family. At the worst of times, it's like I'm no longer in the present. I'm back there again. At night I have horrible dreams—when I wake up, I hear myself barking. My wife tries to comfort me, telling me that I am safe, that they can't hurt me anymore. But I don't see her face, I see theirs. I feel this rage and lash out at her. Only after beating her, do I realize what I've done. I'm not hurting the torturers, I'm hurting my own wife. And when night comes, I huddle in the corner.... The other night my little girl came to cover me with a blanket. I was afraid that I was going to hurt her. I know that I frighten her—her eyes tell me so and sometimes I think she tries to stay away from me. My wife, she's a good woman, but she threatened to take the children and leave unless I got my life back together. So now I am talking to a counselor on a weekly basis. My family and I go to a family counselor as well. Together, we are finally beginning to understand how my experience has affected us all. (Testimony given to Sister Dianna Ortiz; used by permission.)

Family Trauma

With few exceptions (e.g., Bentovim, 1992; Figley & Kleber, 1994; Solomon, 1993), trauma has been investigated as an individual event, and little attention or conceptualization has been focused on shared or group trauma. Trauma has direct and indirect effects on the family members of a torture survivor. Families of trauma victims can be affected in several ways.

- Family members may have directly experienced their own traumas of physical or sexual assault; danger; witnessing acts of brutality; significant losses; and traumas associated with interrogation of family members, with house searches, with internal displacement, and with migration and resettlement (Macksoud, Aber, & Cohn, 1996; Pynoos & Nader, 1993). Often, individual or shared traumatic experiences are not discussed or acknowledged in families. This lack of sharing is particularly true of trauma exposure and reactions of children, which are often underestimated and minimized by adults (Almqvist & Brandell-Forsberg, 1997). Pynoos and Nader (1988), for example, described trauma symptoms in children and adolescents who witnessed the rape of their mother. Almost all of the children and adolescents experienced severe traumatic stress symptoms, including frequent upsetting thoughts of the event; fear of future attacks and counterphobic behavior and fantasies; intrusive thoughts and sensory images; subjective distress when exposed to traumatic reminders and avoidance of such reminders; increased experience of and expression of negative emotions, including anger, irritability, aggression, depression, and anxiety; and, with younger children, repetitive traumatic play themes. Children exposed to violence and other types of traumatic experiences often adopt behaviors or exhibit symptoms, such as anxiety, fearfulness, dependency, and clingingness, as well as aggression, anger, and oppositional behavior, that may place them at increased risk of triggering parental frustration, anger, and aggression (Westermeyer & Wahmanholm, 1996).
- Family interactions may provide traumatic reminders to trauma survivors that trigger reexperiencing of the trauma or avoidant behavior (e.g., remaining children may trigger reexperiencing of events leading to the traumatic death of a child).
- Family members may acquire contagious emotional reactions through interacting with or imitating traumatized family members.
- Families may develop interaction patterns in reaction to the symptomatology or dysfunction of the trauma survivor, for example, children assuming a caregiving role, attempting to "rescue" the survivor, denying symptomatology or dysfunction of the survivor, or assuming physical or behavioral symptoms to maintain family cohesion (Jaffa, 1993).
- Family members may experience additional family-focused trauma resulting from the behavior of traumatized individuals (e.g., neglect of emotional or physical needs of children by trauma-preoccupied parents or psychological abuse or physical assaults fueled by trauma-related rage reactions).

The effect of war trauma on a child is expressed in the following excerpt:

> My father came home with a hearing impairment.... His resentment today toward his
> deafness is still eating him up inside, because it has gradually gotten worse over the
> years. He had changed a great deal when he got home. His nightmares and diving into
> the bushes from his fear from the war were a few things I heard and saw. His drinking
> got a lot worse, and so did his anger. Violence entered our house for the first time
> roughly a year later from his return from 'Nam. He physically abused me and the rest of
> the family. Verbal abuse was almost all the time. I never, never knew what to expect.... It
> seemed like he had his own war he was fighting inside himself, and, with the effects of
> alcohol, he couldn't control his unbelievable rage that would explode in front of any-
> body. My resentment toward my mother grew also. I felt she didn't care for us kids or
> else she would protect us from this insane man.... (Matsakis, 1988, p. 185; used with
> permission.)

In addition, families can experience secondary strains resulting from the traumatic experiences of individual family members, including stress from uncertainty
regarding the fate of family members, economic deprivation associated with absence or dysfunction of a family economic provider, and change in family roles in
reaction to symptoms or disability of the traumatized family members (e.g., a child
assuming primary role as an economic provider or parent figure). Numerous studies have found that the strongest protective factor against emotional and behavior
problems in children is the mental health and coping ability of the parents, which
may be seriously compromised in some traumatized families (see, for example,
Almqvist & Brandell-Forsberg, 1997).

Sexual Trauma

Experiencing sexual trauma can have a particularly deleterious effect on intimate relationships of trauma survivors. Women in war zones or political conflicts
experience rape and sexual assault at high rates (Friedman, 1992; Roe, 1992).
Men and children may be forced to watch their wives, daughters, or mothers being
raped. Moreover, many torture survivors, both males and females, have experienced sexual torture designed to permanently destroy their sexuality (Agger &
Jensen, 1993). Sexual trauma is particularly potent in giving rise to chronic PTSD
in both men and women. Additional symptoms associated with sexual trauma include acute and chronic depression, feelings of hopelessness and powerlessness,
feelings of being contaminated or dirty, chronic anxiousness or fearfulness, guilt
feelings, and somatization of symptoms.

Combat veterans with PTSD experience a number of problems related to sexual
intimacy, including lack of interest in sex, flashbacks during sex, sadistic fantasies
arising in reaction to sexual torture, physical pain during sex, and impotence (Matsakis,
1988; Solomon, 1993). These problems are described as follows by one veteran:

> I never thought I'd get so calloused that I wouldn't care how my wife felt. But right now
> all her desires to love and kiss me are just a pain to me. Outright nuisances! I wish she'd
> just go away. I've been thinking about 'Nam lately. The thoughts just interfere with
> everything. My depression takes over and I'm an utter flop in bed.... I had nightmares.

I tried to turn them off ... but I couldn't stop the dream, the horror. At the end of the dream, I was so angry I wanted to kill somebody, something. The last thing on my mind was sex. (Matsakis, 1988, p. 61–62; used with permission.)

In addition to direct effects on sexual functioning of trauma survivors, changed views of sexual status can often play a role in marital conflict and dissatisfaction in intimate relationships. Many societies view a woman's honor to be based on monogamy or sexual purity. In such societies, rape victims may be ostracized, especially in cultures that view victimization experiences as a punishment for past sins or as destiny because of accumulated karma. Rape often leaves a woman viewed as devalued by her husband or creates anger in the woman or guilt in the male for failure to protect the woman. In cultures in which chastity or monogamy is a prerequisite for marriage, the wife may be abandoned by the husband (Somasundaram, 1993). For these reasons, sexual trauma is seriously underreported in torture and refugee populations (Herbst, 1992; McCloskey, Fernandez-Esquer, Southwick, & Locke, 1995).

SHOULD APPROACHES TO TREATMENT AND PREVENTION OF DOMESTIC VIOLENCE BE DIFFERENT FOR FAMILIES THAT HAVE EXPERIENCED TRAUMA?

Interventions for domestic violence in industrialized society include (a) police and court interventions (e.g., arrest, prosecution, protection orders); (b) batterer treatment programs, which are often court mandated, are usually conducted in groups, usually focus on dominance and control issues, and often use confrontation and group pressure to attempt to effect change in individual group members; (c) victims services, which include shelter housing and associated services that are often intended to help victims establish an independent household or take legal action against their perpetrator; and (d) couples treatment, which is usually employed only with moderately abusive couples in which both partners want to maintain the relationship and end the violence. In developing countries, family members, neighbors, or local leaders may be the primary intervenors to stop violent episodes and to provide shelter to victims; legal, religious, or customary separation and divorce may also be recognized as a remedy for chronic domestic violence.

No strong evidence shows that these approaches are particularly effective, especially for more seriously violent couples. Beyond the question of effectiveness, most of these approaches are probably not appropriate for addressing domestic violence in families that have experienced severe trauma. Thus, most refugees from war or political violence have had specific kinds of experiences, such as police-administered torture, unjust legal proceedings, and inhumane treatment during processing of asylum requests, that would make them unlikely to turn to police and governmental authorities for help with personal or family problems. Trauma survivors in a country of resettlement who become perpetrators are likely, if referred for batterer treatment, to experience language and cultural value differences in batterers' groups and risk retraumatization from confrontational or group pressure techniques. Refugee victims of domestic violence are unlikely to report domestic violence or to seek shelter services because of fear of authorities; fear of compromising refugee status or asylum applications; anxiety about the fragile mental state of the survivor; ignorance of domestic violence laws, especially if from a culture that sanctions physical abuse of wives; and lack of awareness of services for domestic violence victims in the host country. Moreover, victimized refugee women often do not have the economic or social resources to establish independent households because of language and work-skill deficits and lack of social support. In many societies, marital dissolution is not socially accepted or is viewed as shameful by victims. Finally, in many societies, discussion of personal or family problems in front of strangers is dissonant with cultural norms (Morris & Silove, 1992).

Domestic violence intervention must specify what must be changed to decrease or eliminate domestic violence. Assessment of the history and context of domestic violence is important in planning adequate interventions because, as discussed above, there are cultural differences in valuation of emotional and family-role functioning as well as a large number of etiological and contextual factors in domestic violence (e.g., jealousy and possessiveness may be a dominant factor in some cases of domestic violence; in other cases, physical abuse may be directly related to the substance abuse of the perpetrator). Traumagenic effects may play a role in the perpetration of domestic violence or the victimization; however, one should not necessarily assume that all types of dysfunction result from trauma exposure. As indicated previously, some instances of domestic violence in families continue the abuse that preceded trauma exposure, and an important part of treatment assessment is to clarify the role of trauma symptoms in episodes of relationship aggression.

The frequency and severity of domestic violence is an overriding consideration in planning intervention, and different types of interventions should be used for different levels of severity of domestic violence. Ethically, the safety of family members is the primary consideration. In domestic violence situations in which family members are in danger of injury or death, legal intervention or support for removal of family members from danger is the only justifiable intervention. Interventions for relatively infrequent and mild to moderate aggression in which there is low risk of injury can focus on controlling anger and aggression (DiGiuseppe, Eckhardt, Tafrate, & Robin, 1994), improving family communication, providing social support to the family, reducing family conflicts, promoting positive interactions, and developing a family plan to defuse escalation of anger during conflicts and to prevent acts of physical aggression. Such intervention efforts are unlikely to be effective unless the physical aggression is distressing to the perpetrator or the perpetrator is threatened with family dissolution. For more severe cases of domestic violence or cases in which physical aggression is not distressing to the perpetrator, interventions to protect victims include safety planning, legal interventions, legal or other outside monitoring of the perpetrator's behavior, and support for termination of the relationship. Explosive rage may be amenable to psychopharmacologic treatment (Kavoussi & Coccaro, 1996; Maiuro & Avery, 1996).

Current treatment for torture and severe trauma victims often focuses on reducing individual trauma symptoms in survivors, usually by guiding and supporting the survivor in telling his or her "trauma story" (e.g., Ochberg, 1993). It is often assumed that individual trauma symptoms drive functional disabilities and that amelioration of trauma symptoms will improve family, social, and work functioning. The efficacy of individual trauma-focused treatment has not been adequately tested. It is possible that, given the complexity of interactions between functioning and symptomatology, improvement in family functioning of the survivors' families might be a potent factor in reduction of symptom severity and in improved functioning in other areas. This possibility should be assessed in future research.

Many torture and trauma rehabilitation programs now include collateral or conjoint family treatment in an array of services provided to survivors and their families (Rehabilitation and Research Centre for Torture Victims, 1996). Family intervention approaches generally aim to support the reintegration of survivors into their families, to allow them to engage in positive family interactions, and to increase family support for the survivor(s). Family intervention approaches can be arrayed on a continuum according to the degree of mutual involvement of family members. At the most individualistic end of the continuum, treatment programs may involve family members in treatment only to the extent that doing so supports the individual treatment of the survivor. In such programs, the individual or shared trauma of other family members may not be assessed. Further along the continuum would be programs that provide individual trauma-focused treatment for some or all family members who have been exposed to traumatic events. Other programs that have individually focused treatment involve family members more by providing supportive services to help families function in the host country (e.g., assistance in applying for social benefits, educational placement for children, job training and placement). At the most family-focused end of the continuum, some treatment programs do provide joint therapy for all members of the family (e.g., Jaffa, 1993). These programs may use traditional family therapy goals and techniques, including identifying and analyzing negative interaction patterns, promoting disclosure and communication between family members, and developing joint family problem-solving processes. Family interventions that are more trauma focused target, in addition, shared family trauma (Bar-On, 1996; Figley, 1989). Such programs might focus not only on telling individual "trauma stories," but also on achieving a family consensus on a "family trauma story." Interventions with families that include significant aggression would also focus on reducing verbal, psychological, and physical aggression and on promoting positive marital interactions and parenting behavior (e.g., O'Leary, 1996).

No research studies have been done of the efficacy of family-focused trauma intervention in contrast to individual-focused trauma intervention (Allen & Bloom, 1994). Levy and Neumann (1987) reported their clinical impression that family treatment of soldiers with combat stress reaction facilitated the soldiers' improvement.

A number of significant clinical issues are apparent in the implementation of family treatment approaches with traumatized families, including secondary traumatization of family members by exposure to disclosure of individual trauma, compounding of secondary traumatization because of trauma to multiple family members, strain on the coping resources of trauma survivors because of participation in intense family interactions during family treatment, and suitability of family approaches in different ethnic groups (Morris & Silove, 1992; Rosenheck & Thomson, 1986).

Much of the research described in this chapter has relevance for the improved treatment and understanding of torture survivors and their loved ones. It is clear that more research is needed that will specifically focus on the unique needs of the family of the survivor so that those who provide services and set policies can better understand how the effects of torture can be long lasting and far reaching, extending well beyond the individual.

REFERENCES

Agger, I., & Jensen, S. B. (1993). The psychosexual trauma of torture. In J. P. Wilson & B. Raphael (Eds.), *International handbook of traumatic stress syndromes* (pp. 685–702). New York: Plenum Press.

Allen, S. N., & Bloom, S. L. (1994). Group and family treatment of post-traumatic stress disorder. *Psychiatric Clinics of North America, 17*(2), 425.

Almqvist, K., & Brandell-Forsberg, M. (1997). Refugee children in Sweden: Post-traumatic stress disorder in Iranian preschool children exposed to organized violence. *Child Abuse and Neglect, 21*(4), 351–366.

Bar-On, D. (1996). Attempting to overcome the intergenerational transmission of trauma: Dialogue between descendants of victims and of perpetrators. In R. J. Apfel & B. Simon (Eds.), *Minefields in their hearts: The mental health of children and communal violence* (pp. 165–188). New Haven, CT: Yale University Press.

Bentovim, A. (1992). *Trauma-organized systems: Physical and sexual abuse in families (Systemic thinking and practice).* New York: Brunner/Mazel.

Byrne, C. A., & Riggs, D. S. (1996). The cycle of trauma: Relationship aggression in male Vietnam veterans with symptoms of posttraumatic stress disorder. *Violence and Victims, 11*, 213–223.

Carroll, E. M., Rueger, D. B., Foy, D. W., & Donahoe, C. P. (1985). Vietnam combat veterans with posttraumatic stress disorder: Analysis of marital and cohabiting adjustment. *Journal of Abnormal Psychology, 94*, 329–337.

Cascardi, M., & Vivian, D. (1995). Context for specific episodes of marital violence: Gender and severity of violence differences. *Journal of Family Violence, 10*, 265–293.

Choi, A., & Edelson, J. (1995). Advocating legal interventions in wife assaults: Results from a national survey of Singapore. *Journal of Interpersonal Violence, 10*, 243–258.

Chung, R. C., & Bemak, F. (1996). The effects of welfare status on psychological distress among Southeast Asian refugees. *Journal of Nervous and Mental Disease, 184*, 346–353.

Counts, D. A., Brown, J. K., and Campbell, J. C. (Eds.). (1992). *Sanctions and sanctuary: Cultural perspectives on the beating of wives.* Boulder, CO: Westview Press.

Crocq, M. A., Macher, J. P., Barros-Beck, J., Rosenberg, S. J., & Duval, F. (1993). Posttraumatic stress disorder in World War II prisoners of war from Alsace-Lorraine who survived captivity in the USSR. In J. P. Wilson & B. Raphael (Eds.), *International handbook of traumatic stress syndromes* (pp. 253–261). New York: Plenum Press.

Crowell, N. A., & Burgess, A. W. (Eds.). (1996). *Understanding violence against women.* Washington, DC: National Academy Press.

Cunningham, M., & Silove, D. (1993). Principles of treatment and service development for torture and trauma survivors. In J. P. Wilson & B. Raphael (Eds.), *International handbook of traumatic stress syndromes* (pp. 751–762). New York: Plenum Press.

DiGiuseppe, R., Eckhardt, C., Tafrate, R., & Robin, M. (1994). The diagnosis and treatment of anger in a cross-cultural context. *Journal of Social Distress and the Homeless, 3,* 229–261.

Eckhardt, C. I., Babour, K. A., & Stuart, G. L. (1997). Anger and hostility in maritally violent men: Conceptual distinctions, measurement issues, and literature review. *Clinical Psychology Review, 17,* 333–358.

Farias, P. J. (1991). Emotional distress and its socio-political correlates in Salvadoran refugees: Analysis of a clinical sample. *Culture, Medicine, and Psychiatry, 15,* 167–192.

Fernandez, M. (1997). Domestic violence by extended family members in India: Interplay of gender and generation. *Journal of Interpersonal Violence, 12,* 433–455.

Figley, C. R. (1989). *Helping traumatized families.* San Francisco: Jossey-Bass.

Figley, C. R., & Kleber, R. J. (1994). Beyond the "victim": Secondary traumatic stress. In R. J. Kleber, C. R. Figley, & B. P. R. Gersons (Eds.), *Beyond trauma: Cultural and societal dynamics* (pp. 75–98). New York: Plenum Press.

Friedman, A. R. (1992). Rape and domestic violence: The experience of refugee women. *Women and Therapy, 13*(2), 65–78.

Herbst, P. (1992). From helpless victim to empowered survivor: Oral history as a treatment for survivors of torture. *Women and Therapy, 13*(2), 141–155.

Hierholzer, R., Munson, J., Peabody, C., & Rosenberg, J. (1992). Clinical presentation of PTSD in World War II combat veterans. *Hospital and Community Psychiatry, 43*(8), 816–820.

Hunter, E. J. (1986). Families of prisoners of war held in Vietnam. *Evaluation and Program Planning, 9,* 243–251.

Hunter, E. J. (1993). The Vietnam prisoner of war experience. In J. P. Wilson & B. Raphael (Eds.), *International handbook of traumatic stress syndromes* (pp. 297–303). New York: Plenum Press.

Jaffa, T. (1993). Therapy with families who have experienced torture. In J. P. Wilson & B. Raphael (Eds.), *International handbook of traumatic stress syndromes* (pp. 715–723). New York: Plenum Press.

Jenkins, J. H. (1991). The state construction of affect: Political ethos and mental health among Salvadoran refugees. *Culture, Medicine, and Psychiatry, 15,* 139–166.

Jordan, B. K., Marmar, C. R., Fairbank, J. A., Schlenger, W. E., Kulka, R. A., Hough, R. L., & Weiss, D. S. (1992). Problems in families of male Vietnam veterans with posttraumatic stress disorder. *Journal of Consulting and Clinical Psychology, 60*(6), 916–926.

Kahana, B., Harel, Z., & Kahana, E. (1988). Predictors of psychological well-being among survivors of the Holocaust. In J. Wilson, Z. Harel, & B. Kahana (Eds.), *Human adaptation to extreme stress: From the Holocaust to Vietnam* (pp. 171–192). New York: Plenum Press.

Kavoussi, R. J., & Coccaro, E. F. (1996). Biology and pharmacological treatment of impulse-control disorders. In J. M. Oldham, E. Hollander, & A. E. Skodol (Eds.), *Impulsivity and compulsivity* (pp. 119–142). Washington, DC: American Psychiatric Press.

Korbin, J. E. (1991). Child maltreatment and the study of child refugees. In F. L. Ahearn & J. L. Athey (Eds.), *Refugee children: Theory, research, and services* (pp. 39–49). Baltimore: Johns Hopkins University Press.

Lavik, N. J., Hauff, E., Skrondal, A., & Solberg, O. (1996). Mental disorders among refugees and the impact of persecution and exile: Some findings from an outpatient population. *British Journal of Psychiatry, 169,* 726–732.

Levinson, D. (1989). *Family violence in cross-cultural perspective.* Newbury Park, CA: Sage.

Levy, A., & Neumann, M. (1987). Involving families in the treatment of combat reactions. *Journal of Family Therapy, 9*(2), 177–188.

Lipson, J. G., & Miller, S. (1994). Changing roles of Afghan refugee women in the United States. *Health Care for Women International, 15*, 171–180.

Macksoud, M. S., Aber, J. L., & Cohn, I. (1996). Assessing the impact of war on children. In R. J. Apfel & B. Simon (Eds.), *Minefields in their hearts: The mental health of children and communal violence* (pp. 218–230). New Haven, CT: Yale University Press.

Maiuro, R. D., & Avery, D. H. (1996). Psychopharmacological treatment of aggressive behavior: Implications for domestically violent men. *Violence and Victims, 11*, 239–261.

Matsakis, A. (1988). *Vietnam wives.* Kensington, MD: Woodbine House.

McCloskey, L. A., Fernandez-Esquer, M. E., Southwick, K., & Locke, C. (1995). The psychological effects of political and domestic violence on Central American and Mexican immigrant mothers and children. *Journal of Community Psychology, 23*, 95–116.

Morris, P., & Silove, D. (1992). Cultural influences in psychotherapy with refugee survivors of torture and trauma. *Hospital and Community Psychiatry, 43*, 820–824.

Ochberg, F. M. (1993). Posttraumatic therapy. In J. P. Wilson & B. Raphael (Eds.), *International handbook of traumatic stress syndromes* (pp. 773–783). New York: Plenum Press.

O'Leary, K. D. (1996). Physical aggression in marriage can be treated within a marital context under certain circumstances. *Journal of Interpersonal Violence, 11*, 450–452.

Pynoos, R. S., & Nader, K. (1988). Children who witness the sexual assault of their mothers. *Journal of the American Academy of Child and Adolescent Psychiatry, 27*(5), 567–572.

Pynoos, R. S., & Nader, K. (1993). The children of Kuwait after the Gulf Crisis. In L. A. Leavitt & N. A. Fox (Eds.), *The psychological effects of war and violence on children* (pp. 181–195). Hillsdale, NJ: Erlbaum.

Rehabilitation and Research Centre for Torture Victims. (1996). *Annual report.* Copenhagen: Author.

Rick, K., & Forward, J. (1992). Acculturation and perceived intergenerational differences among Hmong youth. *Journal of Cross-Cultural Psychology, 23*, 85–94.

Roberts, W. R., Penk, W. E., Gearing, M. L., Robinowitz, R., Dolan, M. P., & Patterson, E. T. (1982). Interpersonal problems of Vietnam combat veterans with symptoms of posttraumatic stress disorder. *Journal of Abnormal Psychology, 91*(6), 444–450.

Rodriguez, C. M., & Green, A. J. (1997). Parenting stress and anger expression as predictors of child abuse potential. *Child Abuse and Neglect, 21*(4), 367–377.

Roe, M. (1992). Displaced women in settings of continuing armed conflict. *Women and Therapy, 13*(2), 89–104.

Rosenheck, R., & Thomson, J. (1986). "Detoxification" of Vietnam war trauma: A combined family-individual approach. *Family Process, 25*, 559–570.

Shay, J. (1995). *Achilles in Vietnam: Combat trauma and the undoing of character.* New York: Atheneum.

Silove, D., McIntosh, P., & Becker, R. (1993). Risk of retraumatization of asylum-seekers in Australia. *Australian and New Zealand Journal of Psychiatry, 27*, 606–612.

Sinnerbrink, I., Silove, D., Field, A., Steel, Z., & Manicavasagar, V. (1997). Compounding of preimmigration trauma and postimmigration stress in asylum-seekers. *Journal of Psychology, 131*, 463–470.

Solomon, Z. (1993). *Combat stress reaction: The enduring toll of war.* New York: Plenum Press.

Somasundaram, D. J. (1993). Psychiatric morbidity due to war in northern Sri Lanka. In J. P. Wilson & B. Raphael (Eds.), *International handbook of traumatic stress syndromes* (pp. 333–348). New York: Plenum Press.

Tseng, W. S., & Hsu, J. (1991). *Culture and family: Problems and therapy.* New York: Haworth Press.

Turner, S. W., & Gorst-Unsworth, C. (1993). Psychological sequelae of torture. In J. P. Wilson & B. Raphael (Eds.), *International handbook of traumatic stress syndromes* (pp. 703–713). New York: Plenum Press.

Westermeyer, J., & Wahmanholm, K. (1996). Refugee children. In R. J. Apfel & B. Simon (Eds.), *Minefields in their hearts: The mental health of children and communal violence* (pp. 75–103). New Haven, CT: Yale University Press.

Wilson, J. P., & Raphael, B. (Eds.). (1993). *International handbook of traumatic stress syndromes*. New York: Plenum Press.

Zatzick, D. F., Marmar, C. R., Weiss, D. S., Browner, W. S., Metzler, T. J., Golding, J. M., Stewart, A., Schlenger, W. E., & Wells, K. B. (1997). Posttraumatic stress disorder and functioning and quality of life outcomes in a nationally representative sample of male Vietnam veterans. *American Journal of Psychiatry, 154*(12), 1690–1695.

Zimmerman, C. (1994). *Plates in a basket will rattle: Domestic violence in Cambodia.* Phnom Penh, Cambodia: Project Against Domestic Violence.

V

Clinical Issues for Survivors
of Torture

16

Assessment, Diagnosis, and Intervention

JAMES M. JARANSON, J. DAVID KINZIE, MERLE FRIEDMAN,
SISTER DIANNA ORTIZ, MATTHEW J. FRIEDMAN, STEVEN
SOUTHWICK, MARIANNE KASTRUP, and RICHARD MOLLICA

The consequences of torture and other extreme interpersonal trauma show many similarities across groups of survivors. Thus, data about assessment and intervention approaches with other traumatized populations are potentially valuable for survivors of torture. However, determining with accuracy the generalizability of findings from one group to another is challenging. The differences in the physical, psychological, sociocultural, and economic variables, both within and between disparate groups, have significant implications for assessment approaches, diagnostic validity, and treatment interventions. Because of the scarcity of empirical data specifically on the assessment and treatment of torture survivors, little consensus exists about which assessment and intervention approaches are best to use.

Even the categorization of other survivors of trauma into discrete groups is not easy. For example, survivors of torture may be refugees, asylum-seekers, or

JAMES M. JARANSON • Department of Psychiatry, University of Minnesota, St. Paul, Minnesota 55108-1300.   J. DAVID KINZIE • Department of Psychiatry, Oregon Health Sciences University, Portland, Oregon 97201.   MERLE FRIEDMAN • Psych-Action, Senderwood, Bedfordview, Gauteng 2007, South Africa.   SISTER DIANNA ORTIZ • Guatemalan Human Rights Commission, Washington, D.C. 20017.   MATTHEW J. FRIEDMAN • Dartmouth University, and the National Center for Post-Traumatic Stress Disorder, White River Junction, Vermont 05009.   STEVEN SOUTHWICK • Department of Psychiatry, Yale University School of Medicine, West Haven, Connecticut 06516.   MARIANNE KASTRUP • Rehabilitation and Research Center for Torture Victims, Borgergade 13/P.O. Box 2107, DK-1014 Copenhagen, Denmark.   RICHARD MOLLICA • Harvard Program in Refugee Trauma, Department of Psychiatry, Harvard University, Cambridge, Massachusetts 02138.
The Mental Health Consequences of Torture, edited by Ellen Gerrity, Terence M. Keane, and Farris Tuma. Kluwer Academic/Plenum Publishers, New York, 2001.

immigrants. If so, they live outside their countries of origin and may differ from exiles returning to their home countries or survivors of long-term oppression in their own countries. They may have been persecuted for strongly held political beliefs or because of their ethnic or socioeconomic backgrounds. They differ in their cultural backgrounds and may cope in different ways (Morris & Silove, 1992). They may be veterans, former prisoners of war, or survivors of holocausts. They may have been physically or sexually assaulted. They may have witnessed homicide and mass violence or suffered through war. They may have family members, including children, who were tortured or traumatized. They are at higher risk for multiple traumas, as are other survivors discussed in this chapter. Despite these high levels of trauma exposure, some evidence suggests that survivors can recover in good health and lead meaningful and productive lives (Basoglu, Paker, Ozmen, Tasdemir, & Sahin, 1994).

A primary characteristic of torture is the deliberate and systematic infliction of physical or mental suffering. Government-sanctioned torture (United Nations, 1989) can occur for any reason, such as extracting a confession, but the actual purpose is to make the survivor serve as an example to his or her community, thereby weakening political opposition, consolidating political power, and deterring others from political activity. Torture that occurs in cults or in domestic situations may be perpetrated for entirely different reasons; but in general, torture is imposed for purposes of control and degradation.

Torture is different from trauma that occurs as a result of natural disasters because of the intensely personal nature of the assault. Rather than being caused by environmental forces, torture and other interpersonal forms of trauma are deliberately inflicted by one or more human beings whose identities may not necessarily be known to the survivor. Child abuse, whether sexual or physical, shares this intensely personal attribute and may be even more psychologically damaging because the perpetrator is often known to the survivor. Rape can cross these categories—it can be child abuse, violence against an adult, or a part of systematic state-sponsored torture (Swiss & Giller, 1993). In all cases of extreme interpersonal trauma, the objective is to demonstrate control of the perpetrators over the survivor.

Determining the most effective methods of assessment and treatment of the survivor of torture is difficult in the absence of fundamental information and data. The perspectives of clinicians, researchers, survivors, and human rights activists are all important. Clinicians have a wealth of experience from practice with treated populations; however, in general, it is not based on a scientific or theoretical foundation. Most knowledge that currently exists on the topics of the assessment and treatment of torture survivors is not validated by scientific methods, such as randomized, placebo-controlled clinical trials or through the use of sound psychometric methods. It is clear that the field of torture treatment is in an early stage, one that resembles the extent of knowledge in the rape treatment field, the posttraumatic stress disorder (PTSD) field, and related areas some 20 years ago.

The development of the torture treatment field is viewed from a variety of perspectives. Seasoned, experienced clinicians who work with torture survivors are concerned that studying their patient populations with standard scientific rigor presents both ethical and logistical problems. Sensitive, capable researchers feel that the scientific method, appropriately applied, can provide answers to questions that are critically important to clinicians, policymakers, and advocates. Survivors of torture feel that researchers and clinicians often do not understand their suffering and may harm them further. Human rights activists have as their primary objective the prevention of the traumatic event entirely.

The complexity of this situation is the basis for a critically necessary dialogue among all concerned but also poses a serious challenge to progress in this field. It is valuable to note that these same issues were salient in other fields and that they have been overcome substantially in the past 20 years. Consequently, the focus of this chapter is a review of the current treatment for torture survivors, a discussion of a scientific framework for reviewing the existing assessment and intervention approaches for a variety of traumatized populations, and a presentation of proposed clinical guidelines with the inclusion of scientific evidence, when available, for particular approaches to assessment and intervention.

ASSESSMENT

Standardized psychological assessment measures are often used with survivors of trauma (a) in research studies; (b) in the screening of high-risk populations, such as refugees, for possible referral by public health, immigration, or education personnel; and (c) in the first part of the intervention strategy at a treatment facility. However, many survivors live in countries where health professionals and specialized services are scarce and where access to health care is limited. Friends, family, teachers, lawyers, community or religious leaders, and traditional healers may be their primary perceived sources of psychological help.

Under ideal circumstances, where health care resources are available and accessible, torture survivors may initially seek help from a general medical clinic, whether in the home country, in the refugee camp, or in countries of resettlement. Often, primary care clinicians may recognize depression in a patient, yet not realize the patient is a survivor of torture. Knowing that the patient is a member of a group at high risk for torture (e.g., refugees, asylum-seekers, or those involved in radical political activity in their own countries) will assist the primary care practitioner in providing optimal care. Having a history of experiencing torture may mean that presumably innocuous situations, such as a visit to the doctor, may precipitate reexperiencing symptoms in a torture survivor. Therefore, survivors may be reluctant to talk about their lives. Many times, torture survivors are fearful of being touched or examined. Merely sitting in a waiting room might remind the torture survivor of periods of enforced waiting. A doctor or nurse wearing a white coat may remind the survivor of other doctors who were responsible for assisting torturers. An electrocardiogram might remind the victim of electrical torture. Dental work may trigger recollections of dental extractions during torture. Referrals or consultations may be needed during treatment, as the situation may require expertise in physical or psychological trauma, crosscultural issues, particular languages, or other social or legal needs of the survivor.

Whereas assessment in more specialized settings starts with the basics of any good evaluation, certain aspects of the evaluation process must be emphasized when assisting survivors of extreme interpersonal trauma. Survivors particularly need support from professionals who are well acquainted with the survivor's world. Lack of such knowledge is likely to lead to significant errors in assessment and evaluation. The establishment of rapport between the specialist and the survivor is crucial because the survivor needs to be an active participant in treatment. The trust of the survivor is needed in the assessment, diagnosis, and any subsequent intervention. No matter how uncommunicative or withdrawn the survivor may be, simply by being in the same room, he or she has offered the specialist the opportunity to build trust. First and foremost, however, the environment must be safe and feel safe to the survivor. If these conditions are not met, the survivor is unlikely to continue with any intervention.

Professionals who are expert in this area recognize that the assessment of torture survivors is extremely complicated. A major difficulty in conducting a diagnostic interview with a survivor of torture is that it can stimulate memory of traumatic events and activate or reactivate PTSD symptoms (Kinzie, 1989). Consequently, a preliminary treatment plan may need to be formulated at the initial interview. Systematic reevaluation of established patients may prove to be the most critical way of obtaining accurate information and data from torture survivors (Kinzie et al., 1990). Even among experts in the most trauma-sensitive programs, the following difficulties have been encountered:

- Patients may have multiple psychiatric disorders, including depression, anxiety reactions, substance abuse, schizophrenia, and PTSD. Accompanying these diagnoses there may be long-term personality changes, including paranoia and suspiciousness that result from exposure to torture and other forms of traumatic life experiences (Bensheim, 1960; Kluznik, Speed, Van Valkenberg, & Magraw, 1986; Ostwald & Bittner, 1968; Venzlaff, 1967).
- The symptoms of PTSD may appear and disappear over time, particularly the intrusive symptoms. These symptoms may not be present at the time of the interview, posing a diagnostic dilemma for any cross-sectional or one-time effort at assessment.
- The symptoms of avoidance, numbing, and amnesia may prevent the patient from reporting information about the trauma and other symptoms.
- The information may be so disturbing that it is difficult for the interviewer to reliably assess the patient or to gather objective data.
- The patient may decompensate, thus precluding and postponing a thorough clinical assessment.

In the interview process, most survivors recommend that the survivor be allowed to tell his or her story at a pace that is comfortable. Interviewers who are too aggressive may produce an exacerbation of reexperiencing symptoms. The interview should be interactive while the interviewer supports, probes, and questions the patient. The interviewer needs to monitor both the patient's nonverbal and verbal communication, noting if questions are too painful or if the patient wants to explain or clarify further. Survivors may be reticent to tell their stories or, if they do, may seem paradoxically less upset than one would expect following horrible torture experiences. This flat effect could well be a function of dissociation from the cognitive aspects of the torture.

Any bond that may develop between the therapist and the patient begins during the initial interview; thus, therapy can begin at that time, often with a discussion of the reason and origin of the survivor's symptoms. Although the often-used statement, "These are normal responses to abnormal circumstances," can be helpful for the patient, it is not always true. Some individuals are more adversely affected and disabled by their experiences.

Ideally, assessment is done as part of treatment and is completed in settings in which psychopharmacological and psychological treatments are available. The assessment should include a thorough mental status examination, physical examination, and laboratory tests, in addition to a comprehensive psychological and neuropsychological examination. In addition, historical data are gathered including information about the patient's level of function in the periods preceding and following the traumatic experience. Preexisting psychiatric and physical conditions, personality maladjustment, and exposure to prior traumatic experiences (as victim or perpetrator) are part of a comprehensive assessment. Particularly important is a history of head trauma, with or without loss of consciousness, at any time in the survivor's past. For refugees and asylum-seekers, postmigration factors need to be explored to include the stressors of displacement, acculturation, and alterations in social support systems (Steel & Silove, in press) as distinct from the effects of torture and related traumatic events.

DIAGNOSES

The physical consequences of politically motivated or government-sanctioned torture have been well documented elsewhere (e.g., Rasmussen, 1990; Skylv, 1992). The neuropsychiatric symptoms are often difficult to diagnose correctly because of the multiplicity of symptoms and the frequency of comorbidity. The fourth edition of the *Diagnostic and Statistical Manual of Mental Disorders* (DSM-IV; American Psychiatric Association, 1994) includes not only those who have experienced torture and other extreme trauma, but also those who have witnessed or been confronted with actual death or serious injury or have been threatened with death or serious injury, either to themselves or to someone else. As noted earlier in this chapter, PTSD is not the sole psychiatric diagnosis among survivors; in some samples, it may not even be the most common. Major depression is extremely common, often found concurrently with PTSD (Turner & Goest-Unsworth, 1990), but comorbidity with substance abuse and other anxiety disorders is also seen. In studies by Basoglu et al. (1994), the most common diagnosis among torture survivors was PTSD, whereas depression, anxiety, and substance abuse were less frequent diagnoses.

Whether the PTSD diagnosis is valid for torture survivors is a topic that has generated considerable controversy. Although survivors have suffered from a life-threatening event, they are often concerned about being labeled with diagnoses such as PTSD. Allodi (1991) defined two categories of torture treatment settings with a geographic designation: the "North" and the "South." Countries of final resettlement, such as the industrialized nations in the continents of Europe, North America, and Australia, fall into the "North" category, whereas totalitarian "Third World" countries where torture is practiced, as well as countries of initial refuge, are part of the "South" category of treatment settings. So-called "Northern" countries have developed diagnostic systems, for example, DSM-IV (American Psychiatric Association, 1994) and *International Classification of Diseases* (World Health Organization, 1992), based on the medical model (or syndrome approach) to diagnosis. Clinicians in the "Southern" countries argue against this approach, particularly the applicability of the PTSD diagnosis to survivors of torture and extreme trauma, claiming that it is a western ethnocentric concept (Chakraborty, 1991) or that PTSD-related symptoms are in fact normal responses following torture and do not warrant a psychiatric diagnosis.

One argument in favor of the universality of the PTSD approach is based on existing biologically based research indicating that many symptoms of posttraumatic stress have biological correlates. For example, neurobiological changes that can occur in survivors of posttraumatic stress are (a) hyperarousal and hyperreactivity of the sympathetic nervous system; (b) increased sensitivity and augmentation of the acoustic–startle eyeblink reflex; (c) a reducer pattern of auditory cortical event-related potentials; (d) abnormal noradrenergic, hypothalamic–pituitary–adrenocortical, and endogenous opioid systems; (e) possible differences in the volume of the hippocampus between PTSD and non-PTSD patients; and (f) abnormal sleep patterns (Friedman & Jaranson, 1994). Neurobiologically, the evidence in favor of a crosscultural posttraumatic stress syndrome is greatest for the hyperarousal cluster of symptoms, especially the startle response. Jablensky et al. (1994) asserted that because posttraumatic stress symptoms appear in many nonwestern survivors, the claim that the PTSD diagnosis is ethnocentric is unfounded.

The second argument that claims that because PTSD symptoms are commonly observed, they are therefore normal, can also be refuted with a public health analogy. The fact that posttraumatic stress may be statistically frequent in traumatic situations does not exclude it as a disorder or illness. Posttraumatic stress can be considered a pathogen not unlike, for example, the cholera bacterium, which causes illness in most members exposed to a contaminated water supply. Although most exposed become ill, this does not make cholera normal or, for that matter, untreatable. Likewise, PTSD is observed in many of those individuals exposed to torture or extreme trauma, yet it is a treatable disorder (Jaranson, 1998).

PTSD was never conceptualized as a diagnosis that would encompass the entire range of responses following torture (Friedman & Jaranson, 1994). Genefke and Vesti (1998) have proposed a broader construct, a "torture syndrome," that includes most of the PTSD symptoms but extends beyond this one diagnosis. The torture syndrome has not yet been validated but is one promising direction for future research that will shed more light on the North–South discussions. In the meantime, much of the research on torture survivors that has been conducted with control or comparison groups has identified outcomes of PTSD and other psychiatric sequelae but has not provided support for a separate torture syndrome (Basoglu et al., 1994). For example, in Basoglu's controlled studies of nonrefugee survivors studying the effects of torture per se, 33% had lifetime PTSD. Furthermore, 18% had current PTSD after a mean of 5 years, suggesting a chronic course of illness (Westermeyer & Williams, 1998). These figures suggest that PTSD is extremely common after torture, although neither a universal nor "normal" response.

Other concepts have focused on the long-term effects on personality and worldview, including complex PTSD (Herman, 1993) and continuous traumatic stress response (Dowdall, 1992). Especially when torture is prolonged over many years or when the survivor is young when tortured, many fundamental personality changes can occur. Long-term sequelae often include somatization, comorbidity, dissociation, lability of affect, difficulty with relationships, inability to trust, changes in the way one looks at oneself or the world, and inappropriate risk taking.

On the basis of case reports from clinical experience, torture appears to be such an extreme stressor that it reduces many differences across cultures; the symptoms of PTSD appear in individuals from many different countries (Jaranson, 1993). However, this does not mean that cultural factors are insignificant. In fact, cultural differences have been identified as important factors in the diagnosis of PTSD (Marsella, Friedman, & Spain, 1993; Westermeyer, 1989). Cultural differences occur, but these differences are found predominantly in the way that the symptoms are expressed and in the ways in which the individual interprets what has happened or looks at the world (Friedman & Jaranson, 1994).

INTERVENTION ISSUES

Overview of Treatment

The study of the treatment of trauma has a long history. In 1919, Mott described both the hysterical symptoms and neurasthenic symptoms (which are very similar to the modern diagnosis of PTSD) experienced by trauma patients and concluded that the hysterical symptoms could be removed by suggestion or hypnosis. However, the neurasthenic symptoms, particularly nightmares, were extremely resistant to treatment. A great deal of psychoanalytic treatment, particularly between the World Wars and after the Holocaust, was devoted to treating victims of trauma, but the results were mixed and generally poor (De Wind, 1971). As PTSD emerged in the 1980s as a diagnostic category, it became increasingly clear that the symptoms of the disorder might respond differentially to treatment. One of the first studies of severely traumatized individuals with the third edition of the *Diagnostic and Statistical Manual of Mental Disorders* (DSM-III; American Psychiatric Association, 1980) criteria for PTSD showed that 6 of the 12 Cambodian refugees treated no longer had PTSD 1 year later, in large part because specific intrusive symptoms—nightmares and reexperiencing—had been reduced (Boehnlein, Kinzie, Rath, & Fleck, 1985).

Clinicians working with torture survivors often find themselves responding to many needs of survivors of torture, and they find that treatment is complicated, time consuming, and fraught with difficulties for a number of reasons.

- Severely traumatized individuals may have disorders that are persistent. Treatment protocols need to take this into account, with regularly scheduled reevaluation. Because symptoms appear and disappear over time, treatment plans should adjust to a changing pattern. For example, if hyperarousal symptoms should reemerge, then pharmacological or focused behavioral treatment may be needed.
- Symptoms such as chronic avoidance, numbing, personality changes, suspiciousness, paranoia, and substance abuse frequently complicate the clinical picture.
- Some patients are extremely sensitive to any new life stresses, and their symptoms may be exacerbated. However, some torture survivors show increased resiliency following treatment, even to subsequent realistic threats of arrest and torture (Basoglu & Aker, 1996).
- Few double-blind, well-controlled studies on treatment of PTSD in torture survivors have been conducted; those that have been completed are inconclusive and provide little data on which to base treatment. However, such randomized controlled trials of behavioral treatment of war veterans, rape survivors, and other groups have been done and provide excellent data from which treatment of torture survivors can be cautiously generalized. Recently, a randomized controlled trial of cognitive and behavioral treatment of PTSD showed that both treatments were effective in treating PTSD (Marks, Lovell, Noshirvani, Livanou, & Thrasher, 1998).
- The bond between therapist and patient develops over time. All treatment programs need to recognize and address the burden on the therapist that accompanies the sharing of traumatic experiences.

Many survivors feel that they bear the ultimate responsibility for their own recovery. Health professionals offer emotional support, therapeutic advice, pharmacological treatment, and other assistance. However, it must be clear to the survivor that the working relationship is collaborative and that the survivor is more than simply a passive participant in the treatment process. The survivor's role may vary based on psychotherapeutic approach. The role of the therapist is quite different when using psychodynamic, client-centered, or cognitive–behavioral approaches, but all therapies depend on the efforts of the patient to change. Insofar as virtually all treatments work through a focus on the traumatic experiences, it is important that survivors be informed of this early in treatment. A focus on the trauma may result in exacerbation of symptoms in the short term. If uninformed, the survivor may feel betrayed or controlled again, as if repeating the experience of torture, and the trust in the treating professional may be compromised. By simply asking the patient for input, the therapist sends a message that the survivor's opinion is valued, that honesty exists in the therapeutic relationship, and that the therapist is not trying to control the survivor. Education about the psychology of torture and its effects must be discussed during assessment or early in the intervention. This information may alleviate the guilt of the survivor for having been tortured, or forced to torture others, and help the survivor understand that it was not his or her fault. Education may also include the larger effect of politically motivated torture as a crime against the individual, the family, the society, and all of humanity.

General Principles in Therapy with Traumatized Patients

Although no standard set of rules applies to all interventions, the following general principles are based on specific theoretical approaches that underlie the treatment of severely traumatized patients:

- Do no harm. Aggressive and insensitive treatments and evaluations can exacerbate patients' symptoms and contribute to severe complications (Solomon, Gerrity, & Muff, 1992).
- Conduct a functional analysis of the patient's primary problems and focus treatment on the individual patient's treatment needs, which may mean to reduce symptoms, limit disability, increase an understanding of PTSD, increase personal freedom, or some other need.
- Show respect to patients by allowing them to express their stories at their own rate. Do not encourage or press for catharsis and ventilation.
- Have a single person (primary care physician, therapist, or psychiatrist) take responsibility for coordinating the integration of the variety of treatments and services that may be needed.
- Use pharmacotherapy to help in the treatment of intrusive symptoms and impaired sleep, nightmares, hyperarousal, startle reaction, and irritability as needed. Antidepressants in combination with clonidine (Kinzie & Leung, 1989) have been shown to be helpful.
- Provide supportive therapy by maintaining regular and predictable meetings in which there is continuity, warmth, and modeling of positive and negative emotions (Kinzie et al., 1988; Kinzie, Sack, & Riley, 1994).
- Support the physical, social, and medical needs of patients, particularly the patients who are refugees. These needs may include medical, food, housing, and financial requirements.
- Recognize that cultural differences may exist in patients' needs to focus on the traumatic events. For example, Morris and Silove (1992) found that refugees from South America were more receptive to providing recollection of trauma, whereas this approach was not helpful for Indo-Chinese refugees. Similarly, patient involvement in political or public activities will vary based on individual choice, cultural factors, and stage of recovery.

- Explore the value of group therapy for socializing and supportive activities (Kinzie et al., 1988). For some patients, this experience can help reestablish a sense of family and preserve cultural values for refugees.
- Support the traditional religious beliefs of patients. These beliefs may provide an explanation or an acceptance of life or may be part of a search for existential meaning as part of a therapeutic goal.
- Understand that many patients need to maintain the therapeutic relationship with the clinician over an extended period and may require long-term rehabilitation and support.

The context in which survivors of torture seek help partially determines both their perceptions of the experience and the treatment intervention. Treatment of torture survivors can occur in their countries of origin, as well as in countries of initial or final resettlement. Allodi (1991) stated that torture in the "North" is viewed as resulting in the medical and psychological consequences of traumatic stress. In the "South," torture is viewed as part of the sociopolitical process, requiring preventive action and social change. The chosen philosophical stance can dictate the approach to treatment, and a survivor's perspective about these issues may be important in the development of a treatment goal.

One commonality of the two approaches is the goal of empowerment, or regaining a sense of control lost during torture. A medical–psychological treatment approach empowers the individual by validating his or her experiences, facilitating effective reprocessing of the experience, and encouraging active engagement in living. Empowerment within the larger society or community has the more explicit goals of reintegrating the individual into the political process as evidence of healing. An equally important goal is the documentation of the torture and extreme trauma to record the truth, provide the survivors with validation of their own experiences, and expose the perpetrators. Because the survivor and his or her own community have been affected, the survivor may be encouraged to participate in social action groups in the larger community. In some instances, this participation has been seen as part of treatment, although there have been no systematic evaluations of such approaches.

In the early stages of treatment, torture survivors need safety. Immediate needs are establishing trust, stabilizing physical illness, and reducing symptoms. Medications in the early stages may help psychotherapy to progress. Often, survivors initially find it easier to talk about their physical symptoms and their social needs than about their psychological symptoms. This may be particularly so in countries in transition, such as South Africa, where, despite disappearance of the initial threat of violence and trauma, high rates of crime and community violence may inhibit the restoration of a sense of safety.

In the later stages, as survivors begin new lives, they may have a different set of social needs. Physical limitations may have occurred as a result of the torture, and torture survivors may need to adjust to these changes, as well as psychologically deal with the torture experience so that they can shape their future. They may engage in tasks of adjustment such as learning about the sequelae of torture, mourning their losses, and engaging with their families once again.

Individual responses to different types of traumatic events vary, but certain standard treatment elements may be helpful to trauma survivors. Treatment for torture survivors ideally benefits from a multidisciplinary approach (Bøjholm & Vesti, 1992; Garcia-Peltoniemi & Jaranson, 1989; Ortmann, Genefke, Jakobsen, & Lunde, 1987) because the sequelae of torture are both acute and chronic and may include physical, psychological, cognitive, and sociopolitical problems. There is no consensus about the best treatment method, however, and treatment effectiveness studies are formed on a specific method or population and are therefore less generalizable across trauma groups.

The potential risk of secondary gain must be recognized when both documentation of evidence and treatment are combined as part of treatment services. With relatively few skilled professionals available to work with trauma survivors, these roles are often difficult to separate. A conflict may exist between providing treatment and providing evidence of need for social security disability, asylum, or workers' compensation applications.

In countries where torture is still practiced, treatment resources are usually limited. Concepts such as mental health may not be well understood or accepted, and there may be few available psychologists or psychiatrists. Ordinarily, primary care physicians or community health workers provide most of the local mental health services for victims. Treatment emphasizes a more community-based intervention approach and can be affected by safety and political issues (Parong, 1998; Parong, Protacio-Marcelino, Estrado-Claudio, Pagaduan-Lopez, & Cabildo, 1992).

The cost–benefit ratio in rehabilitation programs has also not been assessed. Because resources are scarce and the need is great, especially in developing countries, short-term treatments with demonstrated efficacy are more useful. Practical training programs are needed in the delivery of the best and most feasible psychological treatment methods for on-site health and mental health care workers.

SPECIFIC INTERVENTION STRATEGIES

Specific intervention strategies for veterans and prisoners of war; holocaust survivors; survivors of rape, sexual assault, physical assault, homicide, and mass violence; civilians in war; and children and families may be found in other chapters of this book. The rest of this chapter focuses on intervention strategies that have been used to help survivors of torture, existing evidence for the effectiveness of these strategies, and the techniques found to be most effective in survivors of other traumatic events.

Psychotherapy

The psychotherapy literature for survivors of torture was reviewed by Chester and Jaranson (1994). They noted that the primary treatment, at least in countries of final resettlement, has been psychotherapy, but that no controlled treatment–outcome studies of psychotherapy have been completed. Many authors have described treatments that appear to be helpful for torture survivors. For example, Somnier and Genefke (1986) and Vesti and Kastrup (1992) provided an excellent overview of the "insight" therapy used by the Rehabilitation and Research Centre for Torture Victims (RCT) in Copenhagen. Varvin and Hauff (1998) described relational psychotherapy, while Drees (1989) presented basic guidelines for short-term treatment of depression in torture survivors. Cognitive–behavioral (Basoglu, 1992a, 1998) and insight-oriented approaches, such as psychodynamic therapy (Allodi, 1998; Bustos, 1992), are frequently used treatment methods with torture survivors. Other approaches described in the literature include supportive therapy, desensitization, family therapy, group therapy (Fischman & Ross, 1990), play therapy, psychosocial therapy, and giving testimony (Vesti & Kastrup, 1992).

A metaanalysis of controlled clinical trials of behavioral, cognitive, and psychodynamic treatment of combat veterans, crime victims, and the severely bereaved has shown that psychotherapeutic intervention reduces PTSD symptoms and that these effects persist after treatment is terminated (Sherman, 1998). The most compelling evidence for effective psychotherapeutic treatment of PTSD is in the area of cognitive–behavior therapy (Keane, Albano, & Blake, 1992). One caveat is that severely traumatized individuals may require longer-term treatment than the relatively short-term approach of behavior therapy. Some case studies suggest that behavioral treatment may be effective with torture survivors, but controlled treatment studies are needed to confirm its effectiveness with this population.

Certain common elements can be found among the various modalities of treatment that have been tried, but controlled studies are needed to identify the specific elements that are effective in these treatment approaches. Most treatments involve telling the trauma story, which might involve imaginal exposure and habituation to trauma memories with consequent cognitive change (Basoglu, 1992a). Common elements in various forms of psychotherapy, such as "insight therapy" (and concurrent physiotherapy used at the RCT), giving testimony, and cognitive–behavioral treatment have been discussed by Basoglu (1992a). Although retelling the trauma story for reframing and reworking is a central tenet in treatment (Mollica, 1988), treating torture survivors must be done in a safe setting, with the appropriate timing, and with acknowledgment of cultural variations in the expression and interpretation of these memories.

Many clinicians fear that the retelling of traumatic memories can be risky if catharsis and abreaction are part of this task, but this risk has not been confirmed by controlled studies. However, if there is no follow-up intervention, most clinicians believe that the retelling alone will likely cause more problems than it solves. Often a need exists for continuing care once the trauma is revealed.

Most psychotherapy approaches are typically not based on one consistent theory. Treatment outcome studies are necessary to determine the efficacy of an approach. Multidisciplinary rehabilitation approaches contain many interventions on different levels, and no analytical outcome evaluation has been carried out to identify the effective components of these rehabilitation programs. For example, the RCT rehabilitation model involves strong behavioral elements, such as exposure elements in a lengthy physiotherapy process and detailed medical investigation. In addition, this model includes a focus on the trauma story during insight psychotherapy, which involves imaginal exposure.

PTSD is a chronic condition, and psychotherapy is a crucial component of a rehabilitation program. Medications may also be effective, but the literature has shown that relapse is common on discontinuation of medication for treatment of most anxiety disorders, including PTSD. Some case studies have shown that this situation may be true for PTSD in torture survivors (Basoglu, Marks, & Sengun, 1992). More recent research (Basoglu et al., 1994) has shown that severity of torture predicts PTSD but not depression, whereas lack of social support relates to depression but not to PTSD. This finding implies that treatment that mobilizes support may help with depression but may not have an effect on PTSD. Specific psychotherapy interventions with proven efficacy may be required to deal specifically with PTSD symptoms. It is important to deal with PTSD symptoms because survivors with severe PTSD may not be able to access and utilize social support (Keane et al., 1992). In a current review of PTSD treatment, Keane et al. (1992) reported that the psychological treatments also tend to have the greatest effect on the intrusive or positive symptoms, whereas the numbing and restricted affect remain relatively unchanged.

Pharmacotherapy

Smith, Cartaya, Mendoza, Lesser, and Lin (1998) reviewed the conceptual basis for pharmacotherapy and the literature supporting treatment with psychotherapeutic agents. In comprehensive reviews, Lin, Poland, and Nagasaki (1993), and Lin, Poland, and Anderson (1995) discussed the biological basis for ethnicity and its implications for pharmacotherapy. Given the high prevalence of torture-related disorders in refugees, an understanding of pharmacokinetics across ethnic and racial groupings is invaluable for the clinician.

Indications for drug treatment (Blank, 1995) are to (a) decrease overwhelming symptoms that require rapid reduction for the patient to function; (b) provide help if no psychotherapy is available or if psychotherapy is proceeding slowly; (c) facilitate psychotherapy by reducing hyperarousal, intrusions, numbing, and avoidance; (d) reduce comorbid symptoms, particularly panic and depression; and (e) improve impulse control, reducing rage and violence.

Jaranson (1991), in a review of pharmacotherapy for refugees, also stressed the importance of starting medication for highly symptomatic patients even if the initial evaluation and assessment are still in process. However, the clinician should assess concurrent use of traditional or folk medications, over-the-counter medications, or substances with abuse potential that may alter the effect of prescribed medications. Alternatives or supplements to medication, such as acupuncture, hypnosis, relaxation, massage, or medicinal teas, have also been used, although there is little scientific support for the efficacy of these treatments (Hiegel, 1994).

Psychotropic agents from virtually all the major psychopharmacologic categories have been used to treat survivors of extreme trauma. Some crosscultural research and clinical experience indicate that prescribing smaller doses of psychotropic medications than recommended for Whites can effectively treat survivors who belong to non-White groups (Jaranson, 1991; Lin et al., 1995; Lin, Poland, & Nagasaki, 1993). Both pharmacokinetic (metabolic) and pharmacodynamic (brain receptor) differences have been demonstrated (Lin et al., 1993).

Aside from biological response differences, cultural factors and attitudes also affect medication compliance (Jaranson, 1991). For example, refugees and torture survivors may take medication only until symptoms begin to remit, rather than continuing for the full course of treatment. Consequently, they may take antidepressant medication for less time than required for maximum therapeutic effect. If psychotropic medications do work, survivors may tend to share them with family members or friends who suffer from similar symptoms (Jaranson, 1991), creating further complications for these people. In one study, medication compliance among Southeast Asian refugees was shown to be poor, based on antidepressant blood levels, even when the patients reported they were taking the medication as prescribed (Kroll et al., 1989). Kinzie (1985) demonstrated that poor compliance can be improved with patient education that includes information on how medication works, how long it will need to be taken, what can be expected, and what side effects are possible.

The results from randomized, controlled medication effectiveness trials show a moderate, but clinically meaningful, effect at posttreatment. A series of randomized trials was published between 1987 and 1991. These early investigations focused primarily on tricyclic antidepressants (TCAs) and monoamine oxidase inhibitors (MAOIs). Despite some very promising leads from these early trials, results were too inconsistent and modest to stimulate further research until selective serotonin reuptake inhibitors (SSRIs) became available in recent years.

TCAs, SSRIs, and clonidine have all been found useful for some symptoms of PTSD (Kinzie & Leung, 1989). TCAs are the most studied psychopharmacologic agents, but, because of their relative lack of potency, side effects, and failure to reduce avoidance or numbing symptoms, they have been replaced by SSRIs as first-line drugs in PTSD treatment. There have been three randomized clinical trials with TCAs involving 124 patients, as well as numerous case reports and open trials (Braun, Greenberg, Dasberg, & Lerer, 1990). Results have been mixed and generally modest in magnitude. In their analysis of 15 randomized trials, open trials, and case reports involving TCA treatment for PTSD, Southwick et al. (1994) found that 45% of patients showed moderate to good global improvement following treatment, whereas MAOIs produced global improvement in 82% of patients who received them. As with MAOIs, most improvement was due to reductions in reexperiencing rather than avoidance or numbing or arousal symptoms. A minimum of 8 weeks of treatment with either TCAs or MAOIs was necessary to achieve positive results.

MAOIs, such as phenelzine, produced excellent reduction of PTSD symptoms during an 8-week randomized clinical trial, in two open trials, and in several case reports. In other studies, it was reported to be less effective (VerEllen & van Kammen, 1990). Southwick et al. (1994) reviewed all published findings (randomized trials, open trials, and case reports) concerning MAOI (phenelzine) treatment for PTSD. They found that MAOIs produced moderate to good global improvement in 82% of all patients, primarily because of reduction in reexperiencing symptoms such as intrusive recollections, traumatic nightmares, and PTSD flashbacks. Insomnia also improved. No improvement was found, however, in PTSD avoidance, numbing, hyperarousal, depression, anxiety, or panic symptoms. In summary, most published reports have shown that MAOIs effectively reduce some PTSD symptoms. In practice, however, most clinicians appear reluctant to prescribe these agents because of concerns about the risk of administering these drugs to patients who may ingest alcohol or certain illicit drugs or who may not adhere to necessary dietary restrictions.

SSRIs have revolutionized pharmacotherapy and are beginning to emerge as the first choice of clinicians treating PTSD patients. The SSRIs generally have fewer side effects and are less lethal if the suicidal patient takes an overdose. In the only published randomized clinical trial of an SSRI in PTSD, fluoxetine produced a marked reduction in overall PTSD symptoms, especially with respect to numbing and arousal symptoms (van der Kolk et al., 1994). In addition, a number of open trials and case reports have appeared concerning fluoxetine, sertraline, and fluvoxamine (Friedman, 1996). In general, investigators have been impressed by the capacity of SSRIs to reduce the numbing symptoms of PTSD, as other drugs tested thus far do not seem to have this property. However, most studies of SSRIs are inconclusive and have not been conducted specifically with torture survivors.

Trazodone and nefazodone are serotonergic antidepressants with both SSRI and serotonin blockade properties. They also exert alpha-adrenergic blockade and strong sedative effects. Recently, trazodone has received renewed attention because of its capacity to reverse the insomnia caused by SSRI agents, such as fluoxetine and sertraline. Nefazodone is closely related to trazodone with respect to mechanism of action, but it appears to have greater potency. Multisite trials with nefazodone and PTSD are currently in progress.

Although it is well established that adrenergic dysregulation is associated with chronic PTSD (Friedman & Southwick, 1995; Yehuda & McFarlane, 1997), no randomized clinical trials with either the beta-adrenergic antagonist, propranolol, or the alpha-2 agonist, clonidine, have been conducted, despite the fact that positive findings with both drugs were reported as early as 1984 (Kolb, Burris, & Griffiths, 1984). It should be noted that positive reports of open trials with both drugs continue to be published. In addition, preliminary success has been achieved with the adrenergic alpha-2 agonist, guanfacine, which has a longer half-life (18 to 22 hours) than clonidine.

Because of their proven anxiolytic potency, benzodiazepines have been prescribed widely for PTSD patients in some clinical settings. However, only four studies of benzodiazepine treatment for PTSD have been published. In a randomized clinical trial (Post, Weiss, & Smith, 1995) and two open label studies, alprazolam and clonazepam were no better than placebo in reducing core PTSD symptoms, although modest reductions in generalized anxiety were observed. Because the use of benzodiazepines in PTSD has questionable efficacy and poses problems of addiction, these drugs are generally prescribed with caution.

One theory has proposed that, following exposure to traumatic events, limbic nuclei become kindled or sensitized so that, henceforth, they exhibit excessive responsivity to less intense trauma-related stimuli (Friedman & Southwick, 1995). Based on this theoretical perspective, several open trials of anticonvulsant or antikindling agents have been conducted. In five studies, carbamazepine produced reductions in reexperiencing and arousal symptoms, whereas in three studies, valproate produced reductions in avoidance or numbing and arousal symptoms but not in reexperiencing symptoms (Glover, 1993).

Spurred by the hypothesis that emotional numbing in PTSD might result from excessive endogenous opioid activity, an open trial of the narcotic antagonist, nalmefene, was conducted (Friedman, 1991). Some Vietnam veterans with PTSD exhibited reduced numbing, whereas the other participants showed either no improvement or a worsening of anxiety, panic, and hyperarousal symptoms.

Before the empirical and conceptual advances of the past 15 years, PTSD patients were often considered by treating physicians to have psychotic disorders. Indeed, the intense agitation, hypervigilance (that sometimes appeared to be paranoid delusions), impulsivity, and dissociative states seemed to call for neuroleptic treatment. It now appears that most of these symptoms will respond to antiadrenergic or antidepressant drugs and that antipsychotic medications are usually prescribed for the rare PTSD patient who exhibits frank paranoid behavior, overwhelming anger, aggressivity, psychotic symptoms, fragmented ego boundaries, self-destructive behavior, and frequent flashback experiences marked by auditory or visual hallucinations of traumatic episodes (Friedman & Yehuda, 1995).

Most drugs tested in PTSD studies were developed as antidepressants and later shown to have efficacy against panic and other anxiety disorders. Given high comorbidity rates of PTSD and the symptomatic overlap of PTSD, major depression, panic disorder, and generalized anxiety disorder (Stout, Kilts, & Nemeroff, 1995), it is reasonable to have tested such drugs with PTSD. Yet PTSD appears to be distinctive in a number of ways. First, its symptoms seem to be more complex than affective or other anxiety disorders, and, second, its underlying pathophysiology appears to be qualitatively different. For example, abnormalities in the hypothalamic–pituitary–adrenocortical system are markedly different from those present in major depressive disorders despite similarities in clinical phenomenology. We have just begun to explore a variety of pharmacotherapeutic approaches for PTSD.

However, because long-term follow-up studies have not been conducted, no conclusions about medications having a lasting effect on PTSD can be drawn. In a review of 255 English-language reports, it was found that there were only 11 clinical trials that employed a randomized design (Solomon et al., 1992). From this review, the authors concluded that medications showed a modest, but clinically meaningful effect, and that more research was needed.

Other Medical Services

Primary care medicine (Chester & Holtan, 1992), nursing, and physiotherapy are important components in the care of torture survivors. Holtan (1998) described the importance of the primary care physician and the psychiatrist working in close collaboration to more effectively coordinate care. However, in countries where torture is still practiced, mental health resources are usually limited.

Some of the most critical ways in which primary care physicians can help torture survivors include (a) detecting physical evidence of the torture, which is useful both for treatment and for support of asylum claims (Randall & Lutz, 1991); (b) reassuring the survivor that, when physical sequelae are not detected, he or she has been spared permanent physical damage from the torture; (c) preparing the survivor, through education and reassurance, that psychotropic medication and psychotherapy may be useful treatments; and (d) ruling out infectious and metabolic diseases that may masquerade as psychiatric disorders.

Nursing also has a role in the care of torture victims. Jacobsen and Vesti (1989) articulated the nurse's role to include (a) providing support for the survivor in difficult circumstances; (b) supporting victims in their attempts to recover and maintain their emotional and physical health; (c) educating and guiding survivors to acquire better lifestyles by improving their diet, exercising, and engaging in other health prevention activities; and (d) educating the survivor about the effects and side effects of prescribed medications.

Physiotherapy (Prip, Amris, & Marcussen, 1994; Prip, Tivold, & Holten, 1995) has been used in some centers for many years as an integral part of an interdisciplinary treatment team. An important benefit of physiotherapy includes, of course, modulation of acute and chronic pain. Physiotherapy sessions also provide numerous opportunities for exposure and habituation to reminders of the trauma, which may decrease the fear, anxiety, or distress associated with trauma cues (Basoglu, 1992b). Psychotherapeutic treatment appears to proceed more effectively when combined with physiotherapy, but the reasons for this perceived effect have not been established.

Social Services

Social service needs for most survivors are of primary importance. Social support and social validation are important aspects of general recovery from trauma (Janoff-Bulman, 1992). In resettlement countries, the refugee and asylum-seeker adjusting to a new society and culture often encounter additional stressful experiences with housing, finances, or asylum applications. Many clinicians believe the healing cannot proceed effectively unless the survivor has these social service needs met. In countries that still practice torture, social work is often not recognized as a discipline. Nonetheless, social service needs are usually great, and local health workers, primary medical care practitioners, and others will need to meet the social needs of the patient.

COMMUNITY APPROACHES

Government-sponsored torture affects the larger community and society, as well as the individual, and often community interventions are needed. In some parts of the world, family, community, and societal resources no longer exist.

Linking the individual to the new community by the use of language and employment training, art, music, and other programs has been a focus of this effort. The use of scientific methods to evaluate community interventions is difficult and complex, and few scientific studies of community intervention have been attempted. In one review article, Scott and Dixon (1995) evaluated studies of the effects of a comprehensive treatment approach (assertive community treatment, or ACT) and a more narrowly focused case management approach on the use and costs of mental health services, as well as clinical and social outcomes for individuals with chronic mental illness. They concluded that ACT programs reduced hospital recidivism rates and that case management did so less consistently. The ACT programs also reduced psychiatric symptoms, improved social function, and promoted independent living.

Dixon and Lehman (1995) also reviewed the evidence for the efficacy and effectiveness of psychoeducational family interventions as part of the treatment of schizophrenics and found reduced rates of patient relapse and improved patient functioning and family well-being. In addition, multifamily groups for selected subgroups of patients were of superior benefit (McFarlane et al., 1995). In addition to psychoeducation, behavioral problem solving, family support, and crisis management were the most frequently used approaches. Dixon and Lehman (1995) recommend developing interventions for members of patients' broader support systems.

A Community Approach in South Africa

In South Africa, a Truth and Reconciliation Commission was established to promote healing in a country traumatized by years of oppression. Many survivors of torture and extreme trauma identified themselves and gave testimony, but others chose not to do so, usually because of a lack of trust in the system. For all survivors, the question for the community is how to support recovery both individually and collectively and, from a broader perspective, what kind of interventions would enhance the future functioning of the entire South African society.

Whereas individual recovery is the fundamental goal of the clinician, South Africa's circumstances also demanded social or national reconciliation. Reconciliation, a substantive healing process reflecting restoration rather than retribution, implies that all involved parties ultimately move toward friendship. Such an approach must accommodate both individual and group processes, should be context and culture sensitive, and should deal not only with victims but also with perpetrators and bystanders. This approach seeks improvement not only in the functioning of the individual but also in the functioning of the society, community, and nation.

The Three-Part Reconciliation Model

A clinically based intervention rooted in an understanding of traumatic stress may provide some support for the ongoing approach to reconciliation; a model for reconciliation is proposed, based on related traumatic stress research. The three parts of the model are (a) acknowledgment, (b) apology, and (c) reparation.

Acknowledgment

Bearing witness, giving testimony, and creating memorials (e.g., in the form of literature, poetry, art, and sculpture) acknowledge that the traumatic event happened. The issue of memory is central for both victims and perpetrators of oppression. The entire debate over the veracity of recovered memories underscores the need for discovery of the "truth" and the importance of the acknowledgment of such truth to validate the experience of the survivor and his or her suffering. Agger and Jensen (1996) emphasized the significance of testimony as a part of therapy for survivors of state terrorism in Chile. It is the combination of both the telling of the story, in this case in a public forum, and the manner in which it is heard and understood that is part of the healing. Herman (1992) described how, in individual work, "this work of reconstruction actually transforms the traumatic memory so that it can be integrated into the survivor's life" (p. 174). Therefore, in the public forum, the survivors telling their stories and the nation acknowledging their veracity transform the private traumatic memory into public memory. This public memory can then be integrated into the historical memory of the nation.

Apology

Apology is an important step in the healing process. A sincere apology on the part of the specific perpetrator to the victim implies in-depth reflection on the violation, some understanding of the suffering, and a genuine sense of remorse. It not only serves to verify the traumatic experience and suffering of the victim, but it also directly addresses the relationship of the victim to the perpetrator. Acts of acknowledgment and apology by the perpetrator "rehumanize" the victim, allowing him or her to reestablish and confirm a cognitive schema regarding self and others. It is also the ultimate way that the survivor's suffering may be recognized. The act of apology, following acknowledgment, justifies the internal world of the victim and assists in the establishment of a sense of meaning (Blackwell, 1993; Casella & Motta, 1990). The victim then becomes empowered to accept or reject the apology. The power balance shifts, which is a significant step in emergence from the victim posture. In a sincere apology, perpetrators are remorseful for their acts and seek pardon for them; it is not possible to legislate an apology. When an apology is not made, when it is perceived to be inadequate, or when the victim is not yet ready to accept it, the seeking of justice has no psychological advantage (Lagos, 1988, 1994).

Reparation

Reparation, or repair of the damage, attempts to provide resources to those who have lost them. Reparations allow a survivor to feel that the oppression is over and that they have an equal chance of living a reasonable life. It is different for each person and for each family. Each must determine what form the reparation will take. Reparation may involve efforts to rehabilitate.

Implications

This three-tiered model attempts to assertively move victims of oppression and violence to a new role of being survivors. Herman (1992) described how it is the compensation fantasy, fueled by "the desire for victory over the perpetrator that erases the humiliation of the trauma. When the compensation fantasy is explored in detail, it usually includes psychological components that mean more to the patient than any material gain. The compensation may represent an acknowledgment of harm, an apology, or a public humiliation of the perpetrator" (p. 190).

Herman suggests that this fantasy paradoxically keeps the survivor's fate and recovery tied to the whims of the perpetrator. These aspects of the compensation fantasy may also operate at the public level. Forgiveness is a complicated and individual process that may be arrived at in due course. For example, Eckhart (1988) warned that forgiving too easily may perpetuate the evil.

For the individual, questions exist as to whether offering testimony will have positive effects. Giving testimony on a single occasion may open up the therapeutic process, but it may require additional support from the community and perhaps even ongoing interventions. Interventions should be culturally appropriate, but they may include mass ceremonies, emphasizing rituals of importance for the entire nation (Agger & Jensen, 1996). Bystanders, who form an integral part of the past, present, and future of the country, may need to be involved. Attitudinal changes necessary for true reconciliation must be predicated on acknowledgment of all past roles in the society broadly. Forgiveness of the perpetrators by the survivors should be an outcome that is hoped for, but not expected at such an early stage in the process of reconciliation.

Assessment of the Truth Commission Model

Although there are no systematic studies of the effects of acknowledgment, apology, and reparation on the psychological functioning of individual torture survivors, the literature on issues potentially relevant to this model is extensive. For example, the psychology literature touches on related issues, including the effects of aggression on individuals, of helplessness in the face of aggression, of a sense of injustice and vengeance, and of issues related to retribution or monetary or symbolic compensation.

Some outcome studies of U.S. reconciliation programs for victims of other traumatized populations have been completed. Umbreit (1994) found that victims participating in a victim–offender reconciliation program were very satisfied, with more than 90% stating they were fairly treated and that the mediator and the restitution agreement were fair. In a large-scale evaluation of four victim–offender mediation programs, 79% of the victims and 87% of the offenders were satisfied with the mediation. Fear of revictimization by the same offender lessened and offenders were more likely to pay the restitution agreed on. Victim impact panels require convicted alcohol-impaired offenders to listen to a panel of bereaved or injured victims describe the effect on their lives. In a survey on the effect of participation (Mercer, Lorden, & Lord, 1994), 82% of the victims claimed that the process aided their healing; they also reported a better sense of well-being and purpose in their lives, less anxiety, and less anger at the perpetrators. In addition, victims used less anxiolytic medication.

This model uses psychoanalytic concepts (Herman, 1992) as well as cognitive–behavioral techniques (Janoff-Bulman, 1992) and extrapolates them to the society. It is possible that interventions on the individual level may improve symptoms of depression, anxiety, and posttraumatic stress even if problems on the larger sociopolitical level are not adequately addressed. For example, good treatment results have been demonstrated in settings in which perpetrators of torture have virtually complete immunity from legal prosecution for their crimes (Basoglu et al., 1994). However, for long-term gains at the societal level, an approach such as that taken by the Truth and Reconciliation Commission may well bolster the effectiveness of treatments aimed at the individual.

RESEARCH RECOMMENDATIONS

Based on the current state of the field, the needs for future research include the following areas.

- A prospectively designed study of the symptoms of torture patients with PTSD is needed. Such a study would include the persistence of PTSD symptoms, of concentration and learning problems, of ability to work, and of health problems. Many studies have shown survivors to have increased vulnerability to stress. This vulnerability needs to be documented further. If such vulnerability is confirmed, it would have implications on treatment philosophy and disability evaluations.
- The effects of pharmacotherapy need to be studied.
  - General issues: Research designs need to consider and include psychological and social variables. Chronic symptoms may be slow to change, although one might expect that subjective distress would be the first to change, then symptoms, then functioning. A great deal of evidence suggests that psychopharmacology helps certain symptoms, particularly intrusive symptoms of sleep disturbance in PTSD, and research is needed to see if this is universally true among refugees in various cultures. Studies, especially among groups with chronic PTSD, should be carried out over a longer time period. Currently, 6 to 12 weeks is a typical time frame, while 6 to 12 months may be more appropriate. The effects to measure include not only PTSD symptoms but also demoralization, distress, functioning (work, education, family life, participation in psychological treatment),

interactions with psychotherapy, ability to gain control over violent impulses, reduction of hyperarousal, and changes in drug or alcohol use (Blank, 1995).

— Specific pharmacologic agents: Further research on adrenergic alpha-2 agonists (such as clonidine and guanfacine), on SSRIs and other serotonergic agents, and on anticonvulsants with antikindling or sensitization properties is needed. Efforts to develop psychopharmacologic agents specifically for PTSD should be a high priority. From this perspective, promising future directions might be to test drugs that antagonize the actions of corticotropin releasing factor, the substance that appears to play such a central role in the stress response (Krystal, Bennett, Bremner, Southwick, & Charney, 1995). Another promising direction for future research might be to design drugs that can reverse the dissociative symptoms associated with PTSD (Krystal et al., 1995).

• Comorbidity needs to be studied. Much of the American experience with veterans has concentrated on substance abuse problems, but there is great variability in the abuse of substances across traumatized populations. Research is needed to document the extent to which substance abuse is a problem among PTSD patients from different cultures.

• The value of insight therapy for torture survivors needs to be carefully studied. Many groups have emphasized psychodynamic insight, understanding, and reintegration for people of various cultures, whereas others have found this approach to treatment to be uniquely western and therefore unacceptable. The differential effects of different types of psychotherapy should be studied with particular emphasis on long-term follow-up studies, the value of groups, and the advantages of indigenous treatments. Most of the latter have also never been subjected to any systematic evaluation.

• Treatment programs should be carefully evaluated. Many treatment programs espouse an avoidance of discussing the traumatic events associated with torture. They take a more palliative approach to treating survivors. Others advocate a more directive, trauma-focused approach. The relative effectiveness of each should be studied, and the benefits and problems for refugees and trauma survivors of various cultures examined.

• Combination studies that address the relative contributions of psychological and psychopharmacologic treatments would address the needs of many clinicians actively treating torture survivors with PTSD and related disorders such as depression. Combination studies would make a valuable contribution to the clinical literature.

REFERENCES

Agger, I., & Jensen, S. B. (1996). *Trauma and healing under state terrorism.* London: Zed Books.
Allodi, F. (1991). Assessment and treatment of torture victims: A critical review. *Journal of Nervous and Mental Disease, 179*, 4–11.

Allodi, F. (1998). The physician's role in assessing and treating torture and the PTSD syndrome. In J. Jaranson & M. Popkin (Eds.), *Caring for victims of torture* (pp. 89–106). Washington, DC: American Psychiatric Press.

American Psychiatric Association. (1980). *Diagnostic and statistical manual of mental disorders* (3rd ed.). Washington, DC: Author.

American Psychiatric Association. (1994). *Diagnostic and statistical manual of mental disorders* (4th ed., pp. 427–428). Washington, DC: Author.

Basoglu, M. (1992a). Behavioural and cognitive approach in the treatment of torture-related psychological problems. In M. Basoglu (Ed.), *Torture and its consequences: Current treatment approaches* (pp. 402–429). Cambridge: Cambridge University Press.

Basoglu, M. (Ed.). (1992b). *Torture and its consequences: Current treatment approaches.* Cambridge: Cambridge University Press.

Basoglu, M. (1998). Behavioral and cognitive treatment of survivors of torture. In J. Jaranson & M. Popkin (Eds.), *Caring for victims of torture* (pp. 131–148). Washington, DC: American Psychiatric Press.

Basoglu, M., & Aker, T. (1996). Cognitive–behavioural treatment of torture survivors: A case study. *Torture, 6*(3), 61–65.

Basoglu, M., Marks, I. M., & Sengun, S. (1992). Amitriptyline for PTSD in a torture survivor: A case study. *Journal of Traumatic Stress, 5*(1), 77–83.

Basoglu, M., Paker, M., Ozmen, E., Tasdemir, O., & Sahin, D. (1994). Factors related to long-term traumatic stress responses in survivors of torture in Turkey. *Journal of the American Medical Association, 272,* 357–363.

Bensheim, H. (1960). Die K. Z. Neurose den rassischen verfolgtern: Ein beitrag zur psychopathologie der neurosen [The concentration camp neurosis of the racially persecuted: A contribution on the psychopathology of neuroses]. *Der Nervenarzt, 31,* 462–469.

Blackwell, R. D. (1993). Disruption and reconstitution of family, network, and community systems following torture, organized violence, and exile. In J. P. Wilson & B. Raphael (Eds.), *International handbook of traumatic stress syndromes* (pp. 733–741). New York: Plenum Press.

Blank, A. S., Jr. (1995). *A biopsychosocial review of the pharmacotherapy of PTSD.* Presented at the Fourth European Conference on Traumatic Stress, Paris, France.

Boehnlein, J. K., Kinzie, J. D., Rath, B., & Fleck, J. (1985). One year follow-up study of posttraumatic stress disorder among survivors of Cambodian concentration camps. *American Journal of Psychiatry, 142,* 956–959.

Bøjholm, S., & Vesti, P. (1992). Multidisciplinary approach in the treatment of torture survivors. In M. Basoglu (Ed.), *Torture and its consequences: Current treatment approaches* (pp. 299–309). Cambridge: Cambridge University Press.

Braun, P., Greenberg, D., Dasberg, H., & Lerer, B. (1990). Core symptoms of posttraumatic stress disorder unimproved by alprazolam treatment. *Journal of Clinical Psychiatry, 51,* 236–238.

Bustos, E. (1992). Psychodynamic approaches in the treatment of torture survivors. In M. Basoglu (Ed.), *Torture and its consequences: Current treatment approaches* (pp. 333–347). Cambridge: Cambridge University Press.

Casella, L., & Motta, R. W. (1990). Comparison of characteristics of Vietnam veterans with and without posttraumatic stress disorder. *Psychological Reports, 67,* 595–605.

Chakraborty, A. (1991). Culture, colonialism, and psychiatry. *Lancet, 337,* 1204–1207.

Chester, B., & Holtan, N. (1992). Working with refugee survivors of torture. *Western Journal of Medicine, 157,* 301–304.

Chester, B., & Jaranson, J. (1994). The context of survival and destruction: Conducting psychotherapy with survivors of torture. *National Center for Post Traumatic Stress Disorder Clinical Newsletter, 4*(1), 17–20.

De Wind, E. (1971). Psychotherapy after traumatization caused by persecution. *International Psychiatric Clinics, 8,* 93–114.

Dixon, L. B., & Lehman, A. F. (1995). Family interventions for schizophrenia. *Schizophrenia Bulletin, 21*, 631–643.

Dowdall, T. (1992). Torture and the helping profession in South Africa. In M. Basoglu (Ed.), *Torture and its consequences: Current treatment approaches* (pp. 452–471). Cambridge: Cambridge University Press.

Drees, A. (1989). Guidelines for a short-term therapy of a torture depression. *Journal of Traumatic Stress, 2*, 549–554.

Eckhart, A. L. (1988). Forgiveness and repentance: Some contemporary considerations and questions. In Bauer, Y., Eckhart, A., Littell, F., Franklin, H., Maxwell, E., Maxwell, R., & Patterson, D. (Eds.). *Remembering for the future: Working papers and addenda* (pp. 571–583). New York: Elsevier Science.

Fischman, Y., & Ross, J. (1990). Group treatment of exiled survivors of torture. *American Journal of Orthopsychiatry, 60*(1), 135–142.

Friedman, M. J. (1991). Biological approaches to the diagnosis and treatment of post traumatic stress disorder. *Journal of Traumatic Stress, 4*, 67–91.

Friedman, M. J. (1996). Biological alterations in PTSD: Implications for pharmacotherapy. In E. Giller & L. Weisaeth (Eds.), *Bailliere's clinical psychiatry: International practice and research: Posttraumatic stress disorder* (Vol. 2, Part 2, pp.245–262). London: Bailliere Tindall.

Friedman, M. J., & Jaranson, J. (1994). The applicability of the posttraumatic concept to refugees. In T. Marsella, T. Bornemann, S. Ekblad, & J. Orley (Eds.), *Amidst peril and pain: The mental health and well-being of the world's refugees* (pp. 207–227). Washington, DC: American Psychological Association.

Friedman, M. J., & Southwick, S. M. (1995). Towards pharmacotherapy for PTSD. In M. J. Friedman, D. S. Charney, & A. Y. Deutch (Eds.), *Neurobiological and clinical consequences of stress: From normal adaptation to PTSD* (pp. 465–481). Philadelphia: Lippincott–Raven.

Friedman, M. J., & Yehuda, R. (1995). PTSD and co-morbidity: Psychobiological approaches to differential diagnosis. In M. J. Friedman, D. S. Charney, & A. Y. Deutsch (Eds.), *Neurobiological and clinical consequences of stress: From normal adaptation to PTSD* (pp. 429–446). Philadelphia: Lippincott–Raven.

Garcia-Peltoniemi, R., & Jaranson, J. (1989). *A multidisciplinary approach to the treatment of torture victims*. Abstract and presentation at the Second International Conference of Centres, Institutions and Individuals Concerned with the Care of Victims of Organized Violence, San Jose, Costa Rica.

Genefke, I., & Vesti, P. (1998). The diagnosis of governmental torture. In J. Jaranson & M. Popkin (Eds.), *Caring for victims of torture* (pp. 43–59). Washington, DC: American Psychiatric Press.

Glover, H. (1993). A preliminary trial of nalmefane for the treatment of emotional numbing in combat veterans with post-traumatic stress disorder. *Israel Journal of Psychiatry and Related Science 30*, 255–263.

Herman, J. (1992). *Trauma and recovery*. New York: Basic Books.

Herman, J. (1993). Sequelae of prolonged and repeated trauma: Evidence for a complex posttraumatic syndrome (DESNOS). In J. Davidson & E. Foa (Eds.), *Posttraumatic stress disorder: DSM-IV and beyond* (pp. 213–228). Washington, DC: American Psychiatric Press.

Hiegel, J. P. (1994). Use of indigenous concepts and healers in the care of refugees: Some experiences from the Thai border camps. In T. Marsella, T. Bornemann, S. Ekblad, & J. Orley (Eds.), *Amidst peril and pain: The mental health and well-being of the world's refugees* (pp. 293–309). Washington, DC: American Psychological Association.

Holtan, N. (1998). How medical assessment of victims of torture relates to psychiatric care. In J. Jaranson & M. Popkin (Eds.), *Caring for victims of torture* (pp. 107–113). Washington, DC: American Psychiatric Press.

Jablensky, A., Marsella, A., Ekblad, S., Janason, B., Levi, L., & Bornemann, T. (1994). Refugee mental health and well-being: Conclusions and recommendations. In T. Marsella, T.

Bornemann, S. Ekblad, & J. Orley (Eds.), *Amidst peril and pain: The mental health and well-being of the world's refugees* (pp. 327–339). Washington, DC: American Psychological Association.

Jacobsen, L., & Vesti, P. (1989). Treatment of torture survivors and their families: The nurse's function. *International Nursing Review, 36,* 75–80.

Janoff-Bulman, R. (1992). *Shattered assumptions.* New York: Free Press.

Jaranson, J. (1991). Psychotherapeutic medication. In J. Westermeyer, C. L. Williams, & A. N. Nguyen (Eds.), *Mental health services for refugees* (pp. 132–145). Washington, DC: U.S. Government Printing Office.

Jaranson, J. (1993, June–July). *Torture, PTSD, and culture.* Presented at the Scientific Institute on Ethnocultural Aspects of Post-Traumatic Stress and Related Stress Disorders: Issues, Research, and Directions, Honolulu, HI.

Jaranson, J. (1998). The science and politics of rehabilitating torture survivors: An overview. In J. Jaranson & M. Popkin (Eds.), *Caring for victims of torture* (pp. 15–40). Washington, DC: American Psychiatric Press.

Keane, T. M., Albano, A. M., & Blake, D. D. (1992). Current trends in the treatment of post-traumatic stress symptoms. In M. Basoglu (Ed.), *Torture and its consequences: Current treatment approaches* (pp. 363–401). Cambridge: Cambridge University Press.

Kinzie, J. D. (1985). Overview of clinical issues in the treatment of Southeast Asian refugees. In T. Owan (Ed.), *Southeast Asian mental health: Treatment, prevention, services, training, and research* (pp. 113–135). Rockville, MD: U.S. Department of Health and Human Services.

Kinzie, J. D. (1989). Therapeutic approaches to traumatized Cambodian refugees. *Journal of Traumatic Stress, 2,* 75–79.

Kinzie, J., Boehnlein, J., Leung, P., Moore, L., Riley, C., & Smith, D. (1990). The prevalence of posttraumatic stress disorder and its clinical significance among Southeast Asian refugees. *American Journal of Psychiatry, 147,* 913–917.

Kinzie, J., & Leung, P. (1989). Clonidine in Cambodian patients with posttraumatic stress disorder. *Journal of Nervous and Mental Disease, 177,* 546–550.

Kinzie, J. D., Leung, P. K., Bui, A., Keopraseuth, K. O., Rath, B., Riley, C., Fleck, J., & Ades, M. (1988). Group therapy with Southeast Asian refugees. *Community Mental Health Journal, 24,* 157–166.

Kinzie, J. D., Sack, R. L., & Riley, C. M. (1994). The polysomnographic effects of clonidine on sleep disorders in posttraumatic stress disorder: A pilot study with Cambodian patients. *Journal of Nervous and Mental Disease, 182,* 585–587.

Kluznik, J. C., Speed, N., VanValkenberg, C., & Magraw, R. (1986). Forty-year follow-up of United States prisoners of war. *American Journal of Psychiatry, 143,* 1443–1446.

Kolb, L. C., Burris, B. C., & Griffiths, S. (1984). Propranolol and clonidine in the treatment of the chronic post-traumatic stress disorders of war. In B. A. van der Kolk (Ed.), *Post-traumatic stress disorder: Psychological and biological sequelae* (pp. 97–107). Washington, DC: American Psychiatric Press.

Kroll, J., Habenicht, M., Mackenzie, T., Yang, M., Chan, S., Vang, T., Nguyen, T., Ly, M., Phommesouvanh, B., Nguyen, H., Vang, Y., Souvannasoth, L., & Cabugao, R. (1989). Depression and posttraumatic stress disorder in Southeast Asian refugees. *American Journal of Psychiatry, 146*(12), 1592–1597.

Krystal, J., Bennett, A., Bremner, J., Southwick, S., & Charney, D. (1995). Toward a cognitive neuroscience of dissociation and altered memory functions in post-traumatic stress disorder. In M. J. Friedman, D. S. Charney, & A. Y. Deutch (Eds.), *Neurobiological and clinical consequences of stress: From normal adaptation to post-traumatic stress disorder* (pp. 239–269). Philadelphia: Lippincott–Raven.

Lagos, D. (1988). Professional ethics–social ethics–mental health and impunity. In Psychological Assistance to Mothers of "Plaza de Mayo" Group (Ed.), *Psychological effects of political repression* (pp.157–162). Buenos Aires, Brazil: Sudamericana/Planeta.

Lagos, D. (1994). Argentina: Psychosocial and clinical consequences of political repression and impunity in the medium term. *Torture*, *4*(1), 13–15.

Lin, K., Poland, R., & Anderson, D. (1995). Psychopharmacology, ethnicity, and culture. *Transcultural Psychiatric Research Review*, *32*, 3–40.

Lin, K., Poland, R., & Nagasaki, G. (Eds.). (1993). *Psychopharmacology and psychobiology of ethnicity*. Washington, DC: American Psychiatric Press.

Marks, I. M., Lovell, K., Noshirvani, H., Livanou, M., & Thrasher, S. (1998). Treatment of posttraumatic stress disorder by exposure and/or cognitive restructuring: A controlled study. *Archives of General Psychiatry*, *55*(4), 317–325.

Marsella, A. J., Friedman, M. J., & Spain, E. H. (1993). Ethnocultural aspects of posttraumatic stress disorder. In J. M. Oldham, M. B. Riba, & A. Tasman (Eds.), *Review of psychiatry 12* (pp. 157–181). Washington, DC: American Psychiatric Press.

McFarlane, W. R., Lukens, E., Link, B., Dushay, R., Deakins, S. A., Newmark, M., Dunne, E. J., Horen, B., & Toran, J. (1995). Multiple family group and psychoeducation in the treatment of schizophrenia. *Archives of General Psychiatry*, *52*, 679–687.

Mercer, D., Lorden, R., & Lord, J. (1994). *Drunken driving victim impact panels: Victim outcomes*. Report funded by the Department of Health and Human Services, National Institute of Mental Health, Grant #1-R01-MH48987.

Mollica, R. (1988). The trauma story: The psychiatric care of refugee survivors of violence and torture. In F. M. Ochberg (Ed.), *Post-traumatic therapy and victims of violence* (pp. 295–314). New York: Brunner/Mazel.

Morris, P., & Silove, D. (1992). Cultural influence in psychotherapy with refugee survivors of torture and trauma. *Hospital and Community Psychiatry*, *43*, 820–824.

Mott, F. W. (1919). *War neurosis and shell shock*. London: Oxford University Press.

Ortmann, J., Genefke, I., Jakobsen, L., & Lunde, I. (1987). Rehabilitation of torture victims: An interdisciplinary treatment model. *American Journal of Social Psychiatry*, *7*(3), 161–167.

Ostwald, P., & Bittner, E. (1968). Life adjustment after severe persecution. *American Journal of Psychiatry*, *124*(10), 1393–1400.

Parong, A. (1998). Caring for survivors of torture: Beyond the clinics. In J. Jaranson & M. Popkin (Eds.), *Caring for victims of torture* (pp. 229–242). Washington, DC: American Psychiatric Press.

Parong, A., Protacio-Marcelino, E., Estrado-Claudio, S., Pagaduan-Lopez, J., & Cabildo, M. (1992). Rehabilitation of survivors of torture and political violence under a continuing stress situation: The Philippine experience. In M. Basoglu (Ed.), *Torture and its consequences: Current treatment approaches* (pp. 483–510). Cambridge: Cambridge University Press.

Post, R. M., Weiss, S. R. B., & Smith, M. A. (1995). Sensitization and kindling: Implications for the evolving neural substrates of posttraumatic stress disorder. In M. J. Friedman, D. S. Charney, & A. Y. Deutch (Eds.), *Neurobiological and clinical consequences of stress: From normal adaptation to posttraumatic stress disorder* (pp. 203–224). Philadelphia: Lippincott-Raven.

Prip, K., Amris, K., & Marcussen, H. (Eds.). (1994). Physiotherapy to torture survivors. *Torture Quarterly, Supplementum No. 1*. Copenhagen, Denmark: International Rehabilitation Council for Torture Victims.

Prip, K., Tivold, L., & Holten, N. (Eds.). (1995). *Physiotherapy for torture survivors: A basic introduction*. Copenhagen: International Rehabilitation Council for Torture Victims.

Randall, G., & Lutz, E. (1991). *Serving survivors of torture*. Washington, DC: American Association for the Advancement of Science.

Rasmussen, O. V. (1990). Medical aspects of torture. *Danish Medical Bulletin*, *37*, 1–88.

Scott, J. E., & Dixon, L. B. (1995). Assertive community treatment and case management for schizophrenia. *Schizophrenia Bulletin*, *21*, 657–668.

Sherman, J. J. (1998). Effects of psychotherapeutic treatments for PTSD: A metaanalysis of controlled clinical trials. *Journal of Traumatic Stress*, *11*(3), 413–435.

Skylv, G. (1992). The physical sequelae of torture. In M. Basoglu (Ed.), *Torture and its consequences: Current treatment approaches* (pp. 38–55). Cambridge: Cambridge University Press.

Smith, M., Cartaya, O., Mendoza, R., Lesser, I., & Lin, K. (1998). Conceptual models and psycho-pharmacologic treatment of torture victims. In J. Jaranson & M. Popkin (Eds.), *Caring for victims of torture* (pp. 149–169). Washington, DC: American Psychiatric Press.

Solomon, S., Gerrity, E., & Muff, A. (1992). Efficacy of treatments for posttraumatic stress disorder. *Journal of the American Medical Association, 268,* 633–638.

Somnier, F., & Genefke, I. (1986). Psychotherapy for victims of torture. *British Journal of Psychiatry, 149,* 323–329.

Southwick, S. M., Yehuda, R., Giller, E. L., & Charney, D. S. (1994). Use of tricyclics and mono-amine oxidase inhibitors in the treatment of PTSD: A quantitative review. In M. M. Murburg (Ed.), *Catecholamine function in post-traumatic stress disorder: Emerging concepts* (pp. 293–305). Washington, DC: American Psychiatric Press.

Steel, Z., & Silove, D. (in press). The psychosocial cost of seeking asylum. In A. Y. Shalev, R. Yehuda, A. C. McFarlane (Eds.), *International handbook of human response to trauma.* New York: Plenum Press.

Stout, S. C., Kilts, C. D., & Nemeroft, C. B. (1995). Neuropeptides and stress: Preclinical findings and implications for pathophysiology. In M. J. Friedman, D. S. Charney, & A. Y. Deutch (Eds.), *Neurobiological and clinical consequences of stress: From normal adaptation to PTSD* (pp. 103–123). Philadelphia: Lippincott–Raven.

Swiss, S., & Giller, J. E. (1993). Rape as a crime of war: A medical perspective. *Journal of the American Medical Association, 270,* 612–615.

Turner, S., & Goest-Unsworth, C. (1990). Psychological sequelae of torture: A descriptive model. *British Journal of Psychiatry, 157,* 475–480.

Umbreit, M. S. (1994). *Victim meets offender: The impact of restorative justice and mediation.* Monesy, NY: Criminal Justice Press.

United Nations. (1989). Convention against torture and other cruel, inhuman, and degrading treatment or punishment. In United Nations (Ed.), *Methods of combating torture* (p. 17). Geneva, Switzerland: United Nations Centre for Human Rights.

van der Kolk, B. A., Dreyfuss, D., Michaels, M., Shera, D., Berkowitz, R., Fisler, R. & Saxe, G. (1994). Fluoxetine in posttraumatic stress disorder. *Journal of Clinical Psychiatry, 55,* 517–522.

Varvin, S., & Hauff, E. (1998). Psychotherapy with patients who have been tortured. In J. Jaranson & M. Popkin (Eds.), *Caring for victims of torture* (pp. 117–129). Washington, DC: American Psychiatric Press.

Venzlaff, U. (1967). *Die psychoreaktiven störungen nach entschädigungspflichtigen ereignissen: Die sogenannten unfallneurosen* [Psychoreactive disturbances following compensable events: The so-called accident neuroses]. Berlin: Springer-Verlag.

VerEllen, P., & van Kammen, D. P. (1990). The biological findings in post-traumatic stress disorder: A review. *Journal of Applied Social Psychology, 20,* 1789–1821.

Vesti, P., & Kastrup, K. (1992). Psychotherapy for torture survivors. In M. Basoglu (Ed.), *Torture and its consequences: Current treatment approaches* (pp. 348–362). Cambridge: Cambridge University Press.

Westermeyer, J. (1989). Cross-cultural care for PTSD: Research, training and service needs for the future. *Journal of Traumatic Stress, 2*(4), 515–536.

Westermeyer, J., & Williams, M. (1998). Three categories of victimization among refugees in a psychiatric clinic. In J. Jaranson & M. Popkin (Eds.), *Caring for victims of torture* (pp. 61–86). Washington, DC: American Psychiatric Press.

World Health Organization. (1992). *The ICD-10 classification of mental and behavioral disorders: Clinical descriptions and diagnostic guidelines.* Geneva, Switzerland: Author.

Yehuda, R., & McFarlane, A. C. (Eds.). (1997). Psychobiology of posttraumatic stress disorder. *Annals of the New York Academy of Sciences, 821.*

17

Measurement Issues

ANTHONY J. MARSELLA

This chapter discusses the general principles and procedures of measurement in understanding the mental health consequences of torture and related violence and trauma experiences for adults. (Measurement issues related to children are discussed in chapter 14 in this volume.) Measurement issues related to the mental health consequences of torture have only recently received attention, although there is a vast amount of literature on related areas (Carlson, 1997; Goldberger & Breznitz, 1993; Wilson & Keane, 1997). In the interest of brevity, however, this chapter will limit its discussion to three important areas: principles of measurement, procedures, and measurement instruments.

The consequences of torture and related violence and trauma create challenges for mental health researchers and clinicians to address these problems with professional expertise (Basoglu, 1992; Marsella, Friedman, Gerrity, & Scurfield, 1996; McFarlane, van der Kolk, & Weisaeth, 1998; Ochberg, 1988; van der Kolk, McFarlane, & Weisaeth, 1996; Wilson & Raphael, 1993). Because measurement is the foundation for scientific and clinical knowledge, the quality of the measurement process is a determining factor in improving our understanding of the needs of survivors and in developing appropriate treatment methods for their mental health problems (Carlson, 1997; Sutker, Uddo-Crane, & Allain, 1991; Wilson & Keane, 1997).

In this context, "measurement" refers to the systematic process used by clinicians and researchers to document, assess, and verify the individual's experiences of torture, violence, and trauma and their mental health consequences. Measurement also provides the foundation for subsequent knowledge development, policy formation, and clinical practice. Accurate measurement is based on

ANTHONY J. MARSELLA • Department of Psychology, University of Hawaii, Honolulu, Hawaii 96821.

The Mental Health Consequences of Torture, edited by Ellen Gerrity, Terence M. Keane, and Farris Tuma. Kluwer Academic/Plenum Publishers, New York, 2001.

precise psychometric standards regarding the validity and reliability of measurement materials and processes (Denzin & Lincoln, 1994; Herman, Morris, & Fitz-Gibbon, 1987; Isaac & Michael, 1995; Pedhazur & Schmelken, 1991).

Meeting rigorous psychometric standards in the measurement process is a formidable task under normal life circumstances. This task becomes substantially more difficult in the case of torture survivors because of unique validity and reliability challenges. Nonetheless, research on the measurement of torture and trauma has progressed considerably within the last decade (Jaranson & Popkin, 1998; Kahana, Harel, & Kahana, 1989; Kantemir, 1994; Keane, Kaloupek, & Weathers, 1996; Keane, Wolfe, & Taylor, 1987; Mollica et al., 1992; Sutker et al., 1991; Wilson & Keane, 1997).

BASIC PRINCIPLES OF MEASUREMENT

Validity and Reliability

The foundation of all measurement is validity (i.e., the extent to which an instrument measures what it purports to measure) and reliability (i.e., reproducibility) (Isaac & Michael, 1995; Pedhazur & Schmelken, 1991). To be of value, all instruments and other methods used in the assessment of survivors of torture and extreme trauma must meet criteria for these two psychometric standards. Table 1 provides a brief review of relevant validity and reliability issues associated with the measurement and evaluation of survivors of torture and extreme trauma.

In research and clinical practice with torture and trauma survivors, validity and reliability are critical concerns, especially regarding psychiatric diagnoses such as posttraumatic stress disorder (PTSD) and depression, experiences with violence and substance abuse, problems in functioning and disability, and sources of support for recovery. Concern for reliability and validity issues has led to the development of a number of related psychometric concepts, such as utility analysis, sensitivity

Table 1. Challenges to Measurement Validity and Reliability

- Sources of the data (e.g., survivor, family member, records)
- Accurate recall of the experience
- Errors related to use of interpreters
- Distortion and interference from associated emotions (e.g., fear, anxiety, guilt, depression, anger)
- Survivor willingness and motivation to discuss or share the experience
- Lack of valid and reliable instruments
- Negative consequences accompanying recall and sharing (e.g., onset of symptomatology)
- Lack of skilled and experienced measurement professionals to conduct assessments
- Ethnic, racial, and gender differences between survivors and assessors
- Cultural equivalence and sensitivity of materials (i.e., language, concepts, norms, scales)
- Presence of multiple problems and comorbidity (these may exist in different domains of functioning, including medical, psychiatric, familial, and occupational functioning)
- Sampling errors

(i.e., the extent to which a measure can identify "true" cases of the disorder), specificity (i.e., the extent to which a measure can identify "true" noncases of a disorder), positive and negative predictive value, and referent value.

Approaches to Measurement

Under the best of circumstances, measurement should proceed from a conceptual framework that organizes the process and the meaning of the activities. Several theories have been proposed for organizing the process of measurement with trauma survivors. For example, Keane, Wolfe, and Taylor (1987) proposed a method for measuring the psychological effects of trauma exposure that incorporates (a) assessment of the stressor variable (rape, disaster, combat), (b) symptom measurement, and (c) the use of multiple indices of PTSD. They also noted the importance of integrating statistical and clinical decision-making procedures. However, this effort focuses on only a limited portion of the range of variables that influence the immediate and long-term mental health consequences of torture and trauma. Van der Kolk (1987) suggested a more complex measurement approach that considers (a) biological factors, (b) the developmental level at the time of trauma, (c) the severity of the trauma, (d) the social context of the individual both before and after the trauma, and (e) life events that occur prior and subsequent to the trauma.

Marsella (1984, 1987) took a more comprehensive approach in describing the context of psychopathology and suggested the use of ecological or interactional conceptual models for understanding psychopathology. While this conceptual approach has not been used with torture survivors, it does offer a useful approach for fully capturing the specifics of torture, violence, and trauma experience. Table 2 lists useful categories for developing clinical treatment and healing plans.

Biological and genetic measures are sometimes part of assessment, although very little is known about the genetic potential for vulnerability or resilience (Carlson, 1997; R. Davidson, 1992). In addition, research has shown that extreme traumatic events can alter important neurological substrates (e.g., neurotransmitters, hippocampus, hormones), creating secondary biopsychological problems (see chapter 5 in this volume).

The following are equivalences to consider in evaluating the process of measurement and in selecting instruments:

1. Cultural Equivalence. Measurement instruments and approaches are usually based on western assumptions and concepts. As such, they are "ethnocentric" to western society and may have little validity when applied to nonwestern people. Ethnocentrism refers to the tendency to view reality from one's own cultural experience and perspective. By doing so, the traditions, behaviors, and practices of people from other cultures may be considered inferior, deviant, or even pathological, and generalizations are inappropriately made (e.g., "a healthy person is always autonomous and independent") (Dana, 1993; Marsella & Kameoka, 1989). Ethnocentric bias can be prevented by adopting procedures that ensure

**Table 2. Different Categories of Measurement Topics for
Torture and Mass Violence Survivors**

I. **Examples of torture experience variables**
  1. Parameters of events that occurred (e.g., frequency, severity, duration,
     controllability, predictability)
  2. Situation of events (e.g., location, people present, gender, age, profession
     of perpetrators)
  3. Emotions experienced
  4. Historical and political background

II. **Examples of demographic variables**
  1. Age
  2. Gender
  3. Education
  4. Social class
  5. Religion
  6. Ethnicity/race
  7. Height, weight, body type
  8. Marital status and family parameters

III. **Examples of person variables**
  1. Current emotions elicited (e.g., fear, horror, anxiety, guilt, disgust)
  2. Trauma history (e.g., accidents, crime, poverty, abuse, disasters, war)
  3. Premorbid personality (e.g., hardiness, sense of coherence)
  4. Social resources (social networks and support system)
  5. Life change and stress history
  6. Prior health state and medical conditions
  7. Genetic history

IV. **Examples of disorders**
  1. Depression
  2. Anxiety
  3. Psychosis
  4. PTSD
  5. Substance abuse
  6. Dissociation
  7. Somatic problems
  8. Idiomatic and indigenous complaints

---

cultural equivalence, that is, by ensuring that the instruments used are applicable or relevant to the client's ethnocultural characteristics. For measurement to
transcend ethnic and cultural boundaries, and thus to be both valid and reliable,
linguistic, conceptual, scale, and normative equivalence are needed (Dana, 1993;
Marsella & Kameoka, 1989).

  2. **Linguistic Equivalence.** This term refers specifically to the language of the
instrument and is concerned mainly with translation. Thus, many western tests
(e.g., Minnesota Multiphasic Personality Inventory, Beck Depression Inventory)
have been translated into other languages so that they can be used with different
ethnocultural groups. Accurate translation is best achieved when back translation
methods are used. As a single technique, the simple translation of materials from

one language into another is no guarantee that the instrument is valid or appropriate for use in another culture. Other kinds of psychometric equivalences that ensure cultural validity are also needed.

3. **Conceptual Equivalence.** This term refers to the similarity in the nature and meaning of a concept, which can run deeper than mere translation. For example, in the United States, the word "dependency" is associated with immaturity, childishness, helplessness, and many other negative terms because American society places a positive value on individual "independence." Conversely, Asian cultures place a positive value on "interdependence," and this value is reflected in the child-rearing practices and family relationships of those cultures.

To determine conceptual equivalence, we recommend that ethnosemantic procedures be used to identify similarity in meanings and behavior patterns (Marsella, 1987). These procedures provide a foundation for testing, establishing cultural equivalence, or both. In essence, ethnosemantic procedures involve (a) eliciting the universe of terms in a particular domain (e.g., the emotions), (b) ordering the terms according to various dimensions (e.g., good–bad, strong–weak), (c) assessing their meaning through word association and antecedent–consequence methods, and (d) mapping their behavioral or action components through observation or behavior intention scales.

4. **Scale Equivalence.** This term refers to the cultural comparability of the scales that are used in the assessment instrument. For example, the Minnesota Multiphasic Personality Inventory uses a true–false scale format. In many nonwestern cultures, however, answering questions as simply "true" or "false" is extremely difficult because situational factors rather than overriding principles determine the appropriate action or behavior. Many nonwestern cultural groups are also unfamiliar with Likert and Thurstone scales, since such linear or graduated rating scales are not part of how a concept or life situation is evaluated.

5. **Normative Equivalence.** Normative equivalence requires that norms be available for the specific group being studied. For example, if the norms for a particular personality test are based on western college students but the test is being used with Vietnamese immigrants, questions may be raised about the validity of such information. This kind of equivalence is frequently part of the discussion about intelligence tests, but the same degree of care is needed with any psychological test.

Quantitative and Qualitative Approaches

Quantitative measurement approaches, including standardized tests, structured diagnostic interviews, questionnaires, and tasks, have great value and have proven their worth within the mental health field. However, combining qualitative (e.g., narrative history) and quantitative (e.g., self-report depression scale) measurement approaches provides more opportunities to gain insights into a survivor's problems and resources. Table 3 lists some of the strengths of both approaches. Self-report scales are often used for measuring symptomatology, disabilities, and various aspects of the traumatic experience. Attention to issues such as compliance motivation, social desirability, overreporting, intellectual capacity, and complexity of

Table 3. Strengths of Quantitative and Qualitative
Measurement Instruments and Methods

Quantitative instruments and methods
- Are useful for nomenthetic approaches and generalizations to populations
- Generate numerical data capable of being combined, scored, and analyzed mathematically; are concerned with amount
- Generate "objective" data because of numerical status
- Reduce errors associated with "interpretation" because of variations in perceptions among scorers
- Permit the development of large databases with common scoring procedures and methods
- Generate norms for comparison purposes
- Limit costs of test administration, scoring, and interpretation
- Standardize administration, scoring, and interpretation
- Emphasize internal validity and external validity indices and reliability (i.e., consistency) of measures

Qualitative instruments and methods
- Are useful for idiographic approaches and individual cases
- Preserve real-life context of events being studied; are concerned with the essence of the nature of things, not the amount
- Preserve the naturalistic context rather than controlling or manipulating variables
- Seek meanings, interpretations, and symbols
- Acknowledge social construction of reality for both researcher and subject; emphasize multiple realities
- Emphasize credibility, transferability, dependability, and confirmability of data
- Can adjust research methods and approaches to specific topics under study; promote strong concern for ethnocentrism, sexism, and ageism
- Value opinions, interpretations, and perceptions of researcher

questions is important. A posttest interview about patient perceptions of the measurement materials and process can assist in reducing problems (Simon, 1995).

Qualitative measures refer to methods that incorporate concepts central to human perception (phenomenology) and an acknowledgment of multiple realities (Denzin & Lincoln, 1994; Isaac & Michael, 1995; Marsella, in press). Qualitative approaches represent a particularly valuable approach for the measurement of torture and trauma survivors because they provide an opportunity to use the survivor's own words, experiences, and reality. Through techniques such as narration, oral history, ethnographic interviews, and other approaches, a rich and detailed account of the survivor's experience can emerge. Further, this can occur within the context of the survivor's reality and terms. As such, qualitative research has emerged as a resource for indexing variation and possibility rather than constraining it. Qualitative approaches have introduced a new vocabulary to measurement activities, including such terms as "hermeneutics," "constructivism," "deconstruction," "ethnomethodology," "discourse analysis," and "psychobiography." With these concepts have come new methods that emphasize "qualitative" approaches to understanding and validating experience and knowledge.

Holistic Approach

A medical examination must be part of a comprehensive assessment, and the results need to be considered in determining the presence or absence of mental health and related psychosocial problems. Frequently, depression, anxiety, and psychosis may be a function of neurological or anatomical diseases such as hypothyroidism, hypoglycemia, cardiovascular impairment, and brain injuries, including substance abuse. In most instances, survivors will present with multiple physical problems. This situation requires a broad-based multidisciplinary and multifocus measurement effort. A full understanding of the survivors' problems and resources demands a holistic orientation that considers biological, psychological, social, and spiritual domains of functioning. These different domains are typically interactive in their effects and consequences, indicating that simplistic approaches to measurement can result in serious errors. Thus, any measurement activities must proceed from a firm foundation in which any medical illnesses, impairments, or both, have been identified and evaluated as potential contributors to mental health problems.

MEASUREMENT PROCEDURES

Many procedural issues are important in the measurement of the mental health consequences of torture. Some of these are discussed briefly in the following sections.

Establishing the Purposes of Measurement

The purposes of measurement may differ for the torture survivor, the helping agencies, and researchers. Thus, it is essential that the primary reason for conducting the measurement be identified and communicated clearly before proceeding. For survivors, the purposes of measurement typically include diagnosis, placement, referral, treatment and service planning, and resource and ability appraisal. But for helping agencies, the purposes of measurement are often primarily administrative, including record keeping, reimbursement for services, research and evaluation, legal disposition, service planning policies, advocacy, and political lobbying. The primary goal of researchers may be to complete a scientific study that will enhance clinical or research knowledge.

These differences may place survivors and others in conflicting positions, which can create tension and result in noncompliance. Although administrative needs are important, the clinical welfare and well-being of survivors are more important (Silove, 1996; Silove, Tarn, Bowles, & Reid, 1991). Not placing the well-being of survivors first can result in distrust and suspicion, and the survivor may ultimately terminate treatment and other assessment procedures.

Among the most important decisions for the measurement researcher and professional to make is to specify the substantive areas to be addressed. The following areas related to psychopathology and psychosocial adjustment are often measured for research, clinical, and administrative purposes:

- Symptomatology
- Diagnosis
- Neuropsychological functioning
- Current stressors
- Trauma history
- Culture shock and acculturation problems
- Coping and resources, including defense mechanisms, personal predispositions, social networks and supports, and spiritual strengths and resources
- Quality-of-life levels

Many survivors have suggested that any measurement activities should begin by providing survivors with the opportunity to tell their story in their own words. As one survivor said, "It is easier for me to tell you my story in my words." Formal measurement techniques may then follow more easily. Measurement is accompanied by many moral, ethical, professional, and technical issues and complexities. Measurement and evaluation, when it is required, must be conducted with primary concern for the survivor's welfare and well-being. Mollica (1996) has outlined the critically important ethical and moral obligations of professionals who work with survivors of torture and related violence and trauma.

Establishing Trust

Establishing a trusting relationship between survivors and researchers and other professionals (including interpreters, when they are part of the process) is essential. Every effort must be made to develop trust through the communication of concern, empathy, and compassion for survivors. The establishment of trust may be challenged by ethnic and gender differences between survivors and researchers and other professionals. The survivors may have a justifiable fear and distrust of authorities because of past abuses. To the extent that researchers and other professionals can communicate a genuine understanding and appreciation of the survivor's past and present circumstances, the validity and reliability of assessment efforts can be improved. No amount of technical skill can overcome the problems associated with insensitivity and disrespect. For measurement activities to be valid, reliable, and useful, it is essential that researchers and other professionals learn to establish a supportive and trusting relationship with survivors.

Informed Consent

The obligation to obtain informed consent is an ethical standard of all research and clinical practice, and survivors must be told the purposes and consequences of the measurement activities, including the potential risks associated with the tasks. Survivors must be informed that they do not have to answer any questions, especially questions that may potentially harm their health, legal situation, or other aspects of their lives. Every effort must be made to ensure that survivors understand all aspects of the measurement activities—especially confidentiality risks—since many survivors may be seeking political asylum and their responses may affect the processing of their applications.

The Role of Interviewers

Because of the serious difficulties that the torture and trauma experience poses for establishing positive relationships with researchers and professionals, the question of who should conduct mental health measurements should be considered. There are times when the researcher and other professionals should yield the task to other survivors or to friends and family members, with appropriate training as needed. For many survivors, even well-meaning researchers and professionals are often symbolically associated with larger institutional or governmental systems that perpetrated the abuses and brutalities. Thus, researchers and other professionals may wish to consider conducting measurement activities either in cooperation or in consultation with survivor peers, friends, and family members.

Location and Timing Issues

The location and timing of measurement activities are also important to successful measurement. It may be difficult for survivors to come to clinics and offices, especially if frequent visits are needed; thus, outreach activities may be required. Further, the formality of the clinic or office may make the survivors less willing to cooperate and share their experiences. Consideration should be given to the use of the survivors' homes (or another environment viewed as safe) as the site of any measurement activities. This option also provides an opportunity to observe the home life and housing circumstances of survivors and may offer additional information regarding life contexts.

Because of the difficulties associated with recalling and sharing torture and trauma experiences, care must be taken regarding the frequency of the measurement activities. While the reliability (consistency) of the survivors' reports is a critical concern, reiteration can lead to retraumatization and to distortion of the experiences. In addition, because survivors are often compelled to retell their story to numerous officials, they may be less motivated to comply with further measurement activities, especially if their previous encounters have been aversive, inconsequential, or both.

MEASUREMENT INSTRUMENTS

Specific measures have been developed for use with survivors of traumatic events. Because of space limitations, this section lists only three of the most important types of measurement instruments: PTSD symptom and diagnostic measures, other diagnostic measures, and trauma history measures. As noted previously, when possible, efforts should also be made to measure personality predispositions, cognitive and intellectual functioning, family and social resources, and current stressors (e.g., life changes).

PTSD Symptom and Diagnostic Measures

PTSD Interviews

- Clinician-Administered PTSD Scale (CAPS) (Blake et al., 1995)
- Structured Interview for PTSD (SI-PTSD) (J. Davidson, Smith, & Kudler, 1989)
- PTSD Symptom Scale Interview (PSS-I) (Foa, Riggs, Dancu, & Rothbaum, 1993)

PTSD Questionnaires and Scales

- Mississippi Combat-Related PTSD Scale (Keane, Caddell, & Taylor, 1988)
- Indo-Chinese PTSD Screening Schedule (Mollica, Wyshak, & Lavelle, 1987)
- Harvard Trauma Questionnaire (HTQ) (Mollica et al., 1992)
- Clinician Administered PTSD Scale (Blake et al., 1995)
- Trauma Symptom Inventory (Briere, 1995)
- PTSD Symptom Scale (PSS) (Foa, et al. 1993)
- Post-Traumatic Diagnostic Scale (PDS) (Foa, Cashman, Jaycox, & Perry, 1997)
- Davidson Trauma Scale (DTS) (J. Davidson et al., 1997)

Other Diagnostic Measures

The assessment of trauma-related disorders such as depression, anxiety, dissociation, and psychosis involves the use of a number of well-known instruments that employ either self-report (e.g., Beck Depression Inventory, SCL-90) or interview (e.g., Present State Examination, Structured Clinical Interview for the fourth edition of the *Diagnostic and Statistical Manual of Mental Disorders*) formats. These instruments are reviewed in any current psychiatry or clinical psychology textbook.

Trauma History Measures

Taking trauma history is a necessary part of any full measurement protocol with torture and extreme trauma survivors because it indexes the cumulative trauma burden imposed on survivors throughout their lives. In recent years, numerous trauma history questionnaires have been developed. These measures were recently reviewed by Norris and Riad (1997). Clinicians and researchers generally use several different measures simultaneously to provide convergent validation. Among the most popular are the following:

- Trauma History Questionnaire (THQ) (Green, 1995)
- Traumatic Events Questionnaire (TEQ) (Vrana & Lauterbach, 1994)
- Potential Stressful Events Interview (Kilpatrick, Resnick, & Freedy, 1991)
- Trauma Assessment for Adults (TAA)–Self Report (Resnick, Falsetti, Kilpatrick, & Freedy, 1996)
- Evaluation of Lifetime Stressors (ELS) (Krinsley, 1996)
- Trauma Stress Schedule (TSS) (Norris, 1990)
- Impact of Event Scale–Revised (IES-R) (Weiss & Marmar, 1997)

SUMMARY OF MEASUREMENT ISSUES

The following list summarizes the points discussed in this chapter.

- The purposes and procedures of measurement should be clarified for all participants at the outset.
- The primary concern for any measurement activity with torture survivors is the immediate and long-term welfare of survivors.
- Complete informed consent should be obtained from participating survivors, in keeping with moral, ethical, legal, and scientific principles.
- Whenever possible, measurement should use multiple data sources (i.e., self-report, family, interviewer's observations, life records, objective tasks, and interpreter debriefings).
- The validity and reliability of measurement materials should be determined within the full context of the survivor's situation.
- The scope and complexity of problems in the context of the survivors' lives require that careful attention be given to the full range of biological, psychological, social, and spiritual domains of functioning.
- The time available for measurement activities may be limited because of personal and other circumstantial factors. Thus, priorities in measurement should be determined at the outset.
- Qualitative measurement approaches are a valuable complement to quantitative approaches. The combined use of these approaches often enhances the breadth and depth of the information provided by the survivor.
- Ethnocultural factors are among the many factors that must be considered in measurement with torture survivors—linguistic, conceptual, scale, and normative equivalences of the measures should be well established.
- The multiple purposes of measurement may conflict with one another. Care is needed to support cooperative collaboration whenever possible. Measurement may serve multiple purposes simultaneously, including diagnosis, placement referral, treatment, reimbursement for services, research, and legal disposition.

- The focus of measurement should be on the positive and negative aspects of functioning, including psychopathology and psychosocial adjustment. Narrative reports by survivors are often a valuable part of assessment procedures.
- Researchers and other professionals need to explore the relevance and possible application of new developments in measurement theory and practice for survivors, including item-response theory, signal detection theory, latent-construct identification, micro-response analysis, structural-equation modeling, ethnosemantic procedures, and qualitative methods.
- Efforts should be made to improve the training of researchers and other professionals working with survivors of torture, to improve testing and measurement skills.
- More research is needed on the development of specific measures that focus directly on the consequences of the torture experience.

REFERENCES

Basoglu, M. (Ed.). (1992). *Torture and its consequences: Current treatment approaches.* Cambridge: Cambridge University Press.

Blake, D., Weathers, F., Nagy, L., Kaloupek, D., Gusman, F., Charney, D., & Keane, T. (1995). The development of the clinician-administered PTSD Scale. *Journal of Traumatic Stress, 8,* 75–90.

Briere, J. (1995). *Trauma Symptom Inventory: Professional manual.* Odessa, FL: Psychological Assessment Resources.

Carlson, E. (1997). *Trauma assessments: A clinician's guide.* New York: Guilford Press.

Dana, R. (1993). *Multicultural assessment perspectives for professional psychology.* Boston: Allyn & Bacon.

Davidson, J., Book, S., Colbert, J., Tupler, L. A., Roth, S., David, D., Hertzberg, M., Mellman, T., Beckham, J. C., Smith, R. D., Davidson, R. M., Kate, R., & Feldman, M. E. (1997). Assessment of a new self-rating scale for post-traumatic stress disorder. *Psychological Medicine, 27*(1), 153–160.

Davidson, J., Smith, R., & Kudler, H. (1989). Validity and reliability of the DSM-III-R criteria for post-traumatic stress disorder: Experience with a structured interview. *Journal of Nervous and Mental Disease, 177,* 336–341.

Davidson, R. (1992). Emotion and affective style: Hemispheric substrates. *Psychological Science, 3,* 39–43.

Denzin, N., & Lincoln, Y. (Eds.). (1994). *Handbook of qualitative research.* Thousand Oaks, CA: Sage.

Foa, E. B., Cashman, L., Jaycox, L., & Perry, K. (1997). The validation of a self-report measure of PTSD: The Post-Traumatic Diagnostic Scale (PDS). *Psychological Assessment, 9*(4), 445–451.

Foa, E. B., Riggs, D., Dancu, C., & Rothbaum, B. (1993). Reliability and validity of a brief instrument for assessing PTSD. *Journal of Traumatic Stress, 6,* 459–474.

Goldberger, L., & Breznitz, S. (Eds.). (1993). *Handbook of stress.* New York: Free Press.

Green, B. (1995). *Trauma history questionnaire.* Unpublished instrument [Available from the author, Department of Psychiatry, Georgetown University, Washington, DC].

Herman, J., Morris, L., & Fitz-Gibbon, C. (Eds.). (1987). *Program evaluation kit.* Thousand Oaks, CA: Sage.

Isaac, S., & Michael, W. (1995). *Handbook of research and evaluation.* San Diego, CA: EDITS.

Jaranson, J., & Popkin, M. (Eds.). (1998). *Caring for victims of torture.* Washington, DC: American Psychiatric Press.

Kahana, B., Harel, Z., & Kahana, E. (1989). Clinical and gerontological issues facing survivors of the Nazi Holocaust. In P. Marcus & A. Rosenberg (Eds.), *Healing their wounds: Psychotherapy with Holocaust survivors and their families.* New York: Praeger.

Kantemir, E. (1994). Studying torture survivors: An emerging field in mental health. *Journal of the American Medical Association, 272,* 400–401.

Keane, T., Caddell, J., & Taylor, K. (1988). Mississippi Scale for combat-related PTSD. *Journal of Consulting and Clinical Psychology, 56,* 85–90.

Keane, T., Kaloupek, D., & Weathers, F. (1996). Ethnocultural considerations in the assessment of PTSD. In A. Marsella, M. Friedman, E. Gerrity, & R. Scurfield (Eds.), *Ethnocultural aspects of PTSD* (pp. 183–205). Washington, DC: American Psychological Association Press.

Keane, T., Wolfe, J., & Taylor, K. (1987). Post-traumatic stress disorder: Evidence for diagnostic validity and methods of psychological assessment. *Journal of Clinical Psychology, 43,* 32–43.

Kilpatrick, D., Resnick, H., & Freedy, J. (1991). *The potential stressful events interview.* Unpublished instrument [Available from the authors, Department of Psychology, Medical University of South Carolina, Charleston, SC].

Krinsley, K. (1996). Psychometric review of the evaluation of lifetime stressors questionnaire and interview. In B. Stamm (Ed.), *Measurement of stress, trauma, and adaptation* (pp. 160–162). Lutherville, MD: Sidran Press.

Marsella, A. J. (1984). An interactional model of psychopathology. In W. O'Connor & B. Lubin (Eds.), *Ecological approaches to clinical and community psychology* (pp. 232–250). New York: Wiley.

Marsella, A. J. (1987). The measurement of depression: Cross-cultural perspectives. In A. J. Marsella, R. Hirschfeld, & M. Katz (Eds.), *The measurement of depression* (pp. 376–395). New York: Guilford Press.

Marsella, A. J. (in press). Qualitative research in psychology: Issues and directions. *South Pacific Journal of Psychology.*

Marsella, A. J., Friedman, M., Gerrity, E., & Scurfield, R. (Eds.). (1996). *Ethnocultural aspects of PTSD.* Washington, DC: American Psychological Association Press.

Marsella, A. J., & Kameoka, V. (1989). Ethnocultural issues in the assessment of psychopathology. In S. Wetzler (Ed.), *Measuring mental illness: Psychometric assessment for clinicians* (pp. 229–256). Washington, DC: American Psychiatric Press.

McFarlane, A., van der Kolk, B., & Weisaeth, L. (Eds.). (1998). *Comprehensive text on post-traumatic stress.* Cambridge: Cambridge University Press.

Mollica, R. (1996). Human rights reflections in daily medical practice. *Medical Journal of America, 165,* 594–595.

Mollica, R., Caspi-Yavin, Y., Bollini, P., Truong, T., Tor, S., & Lavelle, J. (1992). The Harvard Trauma Questionnaire: Validating a cross-cultural instrument for measuring torture, trauma, and PTSD in Indo-Chinese refugees. *Journal of Nervous and Mental Disease, 180,* 111–116.

Mollica, R., Wyshak, G., & Lavelle, J. (1987). The psychosocial impact of war trauma and torture on Southeast Asian refugees. *American Journal of Psychiatry, 144,* 1567–1572.

Norris, F. (1990). Traumatic stress schedule. *Journal of Applied Social Psychology, 20,* 1704–1718.

Norris, F., & Riad, J. (1997). Standardized self-report measures of civilian trauma and posttraumatic stress disorder. In J. Wilson & T. Keane (Eds.). *Assessing psychological trauma and PTSD* (pp. 7–42). New York: Guilford Press.

Ochberg, F. (Ed.). (1988). *Post-traumatic therapy and victims of violence.* New York: Brunner/Mazel.

Pedhazur, E., & Schmelken, L. (1991). *Measurement, design, and analysis: An integrated approach.* Hillsdale, NJ: Erlbaum.

Resnick, H. S., Falsetti, S., Kilpatrick, D. G., & Freedy, J. R. (1996). Assessment of rape and other civilian trauma-related PTSD: Emphasis on assessment of potentially traumatic events. In T. W. Miller (Ed.), *Theory and assessment of stress life events.* Madison, CT: International Universities Press.

Silove, D. (1996). Torture and refugee trauma: Implications for nosology and treatment of PTSD syndromes. In F. Mak & C. Nadelson (Eds.), *International review of psychiatry* (pp. 211–232). Washington, DC: American Psychiatric Press.

Silove, D., Tarn, R., Bowles, R., & Reid, J. (1991). Psychosocial needs of torture survivors. *Australian and New Zealand Journal of Psychiatry, 25,* 481–490.

Simon, R. (1995). *Post-traumatic stress disorder in litigation.* Washington, DC: American Psychiatric Press.

Sutker, P., Uddo-Crane, M., & Allain, A. (1991). Clinical and research assessment of post-traumatic stress disorder: A conceptual overview. *Journal of Consulting and Clinical Psychology, 3,* 520–530.

van der Kolk, B. (Ed.). (1987). *Psychological trauma.* Washington, DC: American Psychiatric Press.

van der Kolk, B., McFarlane, A., & Weisaeth, L. (Eds.). (1996). *Traumatic stress: The effects of overwhelming experience on mind, body, and society.* New York: Guilford Press.

Vrana, S., & Lauterbach, D. (1994). Prevalence of traumatic events and post-traumatic psychological symptoms in a non-clinical sample of college students. *Journal of Traumatic Stress, 7,* 289–302.

Weiss, D., & Marmar, C. (1997). The impact of event scale—revised. In J. Wilson & T. Keane (Eds.), *Assessing psychological trauma and PTSD* (pp. 399–411). New York: Guilford Press.

Wilson, J., & Keane, T. (Eds.). (1997). *Assessing psychological trauma and PTSD.* New York: Guilford Press.

Wilson, J., & Raphael, B. (Eds.). (1993). *International handbook of traumatic stress syndromes.* New York: Plenum Press.

18

Mental Health Services Research
Implications for Survivors of Torture

KATHRYN M. MAGRUDER, RICHARD MOLLICA, and MERLE FRIEDMAN

This chapter describes mental health services delivery models that are potentially useful for the development of treatment programs for survivors of torture. Delivering appropriate and effective mental health care to those who have survived the absolute worst experiences of their lives is a complicated issue for many reasons. There are relatively few formal programs for survivors of torture, and in many countries where the need is greatest, resources and other support to establish new programs are severely limited. Furthermore, personal circumstances vary widely for survivors of torture and related violence and trauma; that is, some are refugees in countries of resettlement, some are in refugee camps, others stay in their home countries, and yet others have been tortured in a foreign country and have returned to their home country. Health care delivery systems also differ, varying from country to country, within countries, and even depending on the socioeconomic status of specific groups. The challenge for health services administrators, then, is to develop systems that are responsive to these diverse circumstances, as well as practical. For this reason, this chapter emphasizes ways in which existing systems can be made more responsive and effective in the provision of mental health care for survivors of torture.

KATHRYN M. MAGRUDER • Department of Psychiatry and Behavioral Sciences, Medical University of South Carolina, Charleston, South Carolina 29425.   RICHARD MOLLICA • Harvard Program in Refugee Trauma, Department of Psychiatry, Harvard University, Cambridge, Massachusetts 02138.   MERLE FRIEDMAN • Psych-Action, Senderwood, Bedfordview, Gauteng 2007, South Africa.
The Mental Health Consequences of Torture, edited by Ellen Gerrity, Terence M. Keane, and Farris Tuma. Kluwer Academic/Plenum Publishers, New York, 2001.

Descriptions of health systems typically center around four components: (a) the structure and organization of the system, (b) the process of care, (c) the intended outcomes of care, and (d) access to care. This chapter will address these components, drawing on examples and studies that bear on mental health care delivery in general and that may have special applicability to caring for survivors of torture.

STRUCTURE AND ORGANIZATION OF THE HEALTH CARE SYSTEM

The Health Care System

The structural characteristics of health care systems vary so widely from country to country that it is difficult to describe a single system. However, most health care systems generally have the basic components discussed below to varying degrees. Primary or general medical care is the backbone of the formal health system. Primary care providers include physicians, nurses, physician assistants, and others (including traditional healers) who deliver primary medical services. Although the type of provider may differ depending on the country, a recent study by the World Health Organization (WHO) shows that mental health problems are common in primary care systems throughout the world and have significant associated disability (Ustun & Sartorius, 1995). This report confirmed internationally the finding by Regier et al. (1993) that in the United States, the primary care system serves as the de facto mental health system as well. Specialty mental health care usually exists in most systems of care, though in limited amounts in developing countries and often only in inpatient settings. Informal care systems—while variable in the type of care provided—are particularly important when dealing with mental health problems and have tremendous potential to expand the capacity to provide services to survivors of torture. Informal care providers are increasingly recognized as important contributors to the health care system.

Primary Care

Many people with mental health problems first interact with the health care system in the primary care clinic. Although primary care providers are not mental health specialists, they have typically received some training in the recognition and treatment of mental health problems and may be the first (and often only) source of care for such problems. As well-meaning as these clinicians may be, however, the structure of primary care can make it very difficult for them to provide optimally effective care for persons with mental health problems.

The amount of time that a primary care practitioner has to devote to a given patient makes it difficult to recognize and treat mental disorders. In many health care systems, the general environment of primary care clinics emphasizes high volume, brief encounters, and low fees. With the average amount of time spent per patient (including paper work) at 15 minutes or less (and this is a luxury in many clinics), it is extremely difficult to attend to the patient's presenting complaints (new and historical), conduct a physical examination, order laboratory and other tests, prescribe medications and other treatment, provide appropriate educational information to the patient, sort out the somatic and psychological complaints that could constitute a mental disorder, and explain the diagnosis and treatment to the patient. Mental health problems, by their very nature, take time to diagnose, time to explain, and time to treat. The logistics of the primary care setting mitigate against dealing effectively with mental disorders. Conditions are often even more difficult in developing countries, where primary clinicians may see up to 200 patients in a single day, and patients do not necessarily see the same nurse or physician from visit to visit.

In one study (Wells et al., 1989), patients in prepaid care were less likely to have their depression recognized than those in fee-for-service care. Whether this is a function of the amount of time the physician spent with each patient or other disincentives under the prepaid structure, a relationship exists between likelihood of recognizing depression and the formal structure of primary care.

Several promising innovative approaches can be used to modify the structure of the primary care system to facilitate recognition and treatment of mental health problems. Katon et al. (1995) have tried a collaborative model to improve treatment. In this model, patients whose depression is recognized and who have agreed to antidepressant treatment are seen by their primary care physician at one visit and then a mental health specialist (in the primary care clinic) at the next visit. These alternating visits continue for about four sessions (about 1 week apart). The primary care physician and the mental health specialist have shared responsibility for the patient, collaborating on the mental health care. Results have shown that for patients with major depression, those under the collaborative care model are about twice as likely to improve as those in the usual care condition. On the other hand, there was no difference between the two models for those with minor (or subsyndromal) depression.

A number of clinical trials are under way or proposed to examine the potential benefit of adding a nonphysician team member in primary care to take on some of the time-consuming functions involved in the recognition, treatment, and monitoring of mental health problems. Pharmacists, social workers, nurses, and other "facilitators" have been suggested. There is increased acknowledgment that in the United States the primary care structure is often the key barrier to improving mental health care in many systems. Physicians cannot be expected to do all that is needed within the time constraints of such primary care structures; therefore, the addition of facilitators is likely to improve care and may also prove cost-effective in the long run.

In many countries, traditional healers are the first line in providing primary care services. For example, in South Africa, about 80% of the black population still consult one of the 300,000 traditional healers at some stage of their life, sometimes while simultaneously consulting a western health worker. The very important role played by traditional healers in dealing with mental health problems in developing countries was strongly emphasized in a recent report (Desjarlais, Eisenberg, Good, & Kleinman, 1995). One of the chief values of consulting a traditional healer for help with a mental health problem is the reduced level of stigma associated with traditional healers compared with the western medical approach. Problems of language and culture are likely to be minimized, and the herbal and other remedies are believed to be effective without the not-inconsiderable side effects sometimes found with psychotropic medications. In addition, traditional healers are part of the local community, and the community containment value in healing mental health problems can be profound. Many of the ancient traditional methods of healing are similar to those employed by western creative arts therapists or psychotherapists. The use of music, dance, art forms, storytelling, and the interpretation of dreams may provide a powerful bridge between traditional forms of healing and western therapies (for more information, see O'Brien, 1995).

The problems associated with recognition and treatment of mental health problems in primary care are highly applicable to the recognition and treatment of survivors of torture and related violence and trauma. It takes a great deal of time to work with survivors of torture in a sensitive, constructive, and effective way. Furthermore, mental health problems of survivors of torture are often compounded by the problems associated with migration and separation from their own culture. The concept of collaborative care is thus a highly relevant concept in the treatment of survivors of torture and related violence and trauma within the primary care context. In addition to training primary care providers in the recognition, treatment, and referral of survivors of torture, other nonphysician facilitators can be trained to deal with mental health problems, including the sequelae of torture. Ideally, these facilitators should be available immediately, onsite, and should be able to work with patients and their families without the time pressures imposed on many primary care providers. By coordinating treatment with the primary care provider, mental health care should be integrated into total health care.

Training programs for local primary care physicians caring for a high number of torture survivors in countries such as Guatemala and Cambodia have successfully used the model of collaborative care in simultaneously preparing primary care physicians, nonphysician health care promoters, and family–child mental health workers. In the United States and other countries of resettlement, the bicultural model that links paraprofessionals from newly arrived immigrant communities to mainstream medical and psychiatric physicians is a promising approach, especially in caring for nonwestern patients (Larson, 1997).

The relevance of providing mental health care to survivors of torture is even more acute in the context of refugee camps, where a high proportion of the population is likely to have been tortured or exposed to torture and related violence and trauma. In refugee camps, primary care providers should expect to see and deal with the mental health sequelae of trauma in most clients. For example, Mollica et al. (1993) found that among Cambodians living in a Thailand–Cambodia border camp (Site 2), 67.9% had symptom scores that indicated depression, with 37.2% having symptoms of posttraumatic stress disorder. Almost all of the adult residents of this border camp had experienced extensive physical and emotional trauma. During the Pol Pot period, 35.8% reported that they had been tortured;

other traumatic events reported by more than half of the respondents were murder of a family member or friend, forced evacuation, being close to death, isolation from others, being forced from family, lack of shelter, brainwashing, ill health and no medical care, forced labor, and lack of food and water. Unfortunately, in this particular border camp, there was no organized system for mental health care. What did exist was a de facto system consisting largely of an unorganized and informal referral system that was difficult to characterize, with few referrals even to the traditional medicine center. As the authors of this report point out, unless the mental health problems of these survivors are addressed, their chances of resuming a productive life on leaving the border camps are in many cases doubtful.

A similar situation exists in Rwanda, where almost an entire population has been traumatized and is now reported to be experiencing profound emotional difficulties (Henderson, van de Velde, Mollica, & Lavelle, 1996). Reports indicate that massive numbers of people are coming to the only psychiatric hospital in the country. In the past, this hospital was essentially the mental health system for the country, as mental health care was noticeably absent from the primary care system. In this and many other situations, responses to mental health crises may be strengthened by enabling primary care systems, including traditional healers, to provide culturally appropriate mental health services.

One approach to accomplishing this goal is the recommendation that a National Trauma Center be established by the Rwandan Ministry of Health (Henderson et al., 1996). As proposed, the center would promote academic excellence, research, and training. Initially with international consultants, but in collaboration with local medical providers (to ensure cultural relevance and sensitivity), such a National Trauma Center might expand the country's capacity to deal with the mental health issues that permeate this population.

Clearly, a key issue relates to training for primary care providers and the facilitators who may be part of the primary care team. Such training should provide them with the expertise to recognize and treat survivors of torture and related violence and trauma and should include collaboration between medical providers and traditional healers. A recent curriculum was established for training Khmer providers in the Thai border camps on the principles and practices of mental health care (Lavelle, Tor, Stedman, Mollica, & Sath, 1993). Though western interventions were part of the training, the curriculum incorporated elements of traditional folk healing, Khmer grassroots counseling, and Buddhist meditation.

In South Africa, traditional healers employ a creative arts approach that may be appropriate in a group context (e.g., to survivors of torture) and thus highly relevant in situations where mental health professionals are lacking. The art medium employed (e.g., music, dance) actually "contains" the person, who can proceed at his or her own pace, reportedly allowing for a safe healing effect to take place through the containing art form (O'Brien, 1995). Initial studies supporting the use of behavioral treatment are encouraging, and more research is needed on such therapeutic interventions for the treatment of torture survivors and their psychosocial problems.

Specialty Mental Health Care

Although primary care remains the most critical component of the mental health care system universally, some countries have specialty mental health care that should be part of the care that is available for survivors of torture and related violence and trauma. Furthermore, without some capacity to care for persons with severe mental illness, the ability of the mental health system to deal with survivors of torture is questionable. The structure of specialty care has undergone rapid transformation in many countries. A description of this evolving structure will highlight possibilities for providing specialized mental health services for survivors of torture and related violence and trauma.

In many countries, access to specialty care is dependent on the referral by the primary care provider, and often there is pressure to limit this access to the most challenging cases. Whether the survivor of torture ever gets to see a specialist may depend entirely on the primary care provider.

Once in specialty care, the patient often finds that there are financial disincentives to continue. For example, in the United States, specialty mental health care is typically reimbursed at a lower rate than other specialty medical care. Furthermore, arbitrary limits are often placed on the annual number of visits or days of care, without evaluating patient need. For the survivor of torture, this limitation may be particularly restrictive, as it often takes time (and repeated visits) for the survivor to develop trust in the therapist, and even more time to make therapeutic progress. It is not surprising that most persons with severe mental illness who seek care eventually find themselves in the public mental health system because their resources are quickly exhausted in getting adequate treatment.

Inpatient mental health care is becoming rarer and rarer in the United States and is used almost exclusively for stabilizing a patient to the point where he or she can be discharged. There is some evidence that community programs are slowly expanding so that the services a patient needs can be provided in the community, with hospitalization reserved for stabilizing persons in acute episodes. While these developments are seen in a positive light by most, it means that almost all public mental health resources are allocated to persons with severe mental illness. These public mental health systems are not necessarily suited for treating the types of mental health sequelae that survivors of torture and related violence and trauma experience. Options for such survivors are often limited and include going back to the primary care system (where there may be problems in the quality and amount of care that can be delivered) and the private mental health system (where there may be financial limitations for many would-be users).

In countries where psychiatrists and other mental health specialists are in short supply, the best use of their talents may be to staff model treatment units and sponsor training programs for primary care providers. Training and collaborative work with primary care providers could be an efficient way of expanding the capacity of such countries to deal with the mental health problems associated with torture and related violence and trauma. Additionally, treatment approaches that combine hospital or clinic and community components (involving both patient and family) may be an efficient method of delivering care to those with severe mental illnesses. For example, McFarlane et al. (1995) have developed a community treatment model that involves working with the patient and his or her family in the hospital and then with a group of families on a biweekly basis in the community for 2 or more years. Such approaches are focused on establishing a social network that can address the problems related to mental illness in the community and family and that involves minimal monitoring of medications and functioning by a mental health professional. These approaches thus may be an efficient way of utilizing mental health specialists.

Larson (1997) proposed that there are two very different treatment approaches for survivors of torture in North America and South America. The "North American" model is based on the premise that torture is a traumatic experience with both medical and psychological consequences. The "South American" model is based on the notion that torture is a tool of the sociopolitical process; therefore, treatment and societal change are intertwined. In further exploring 28 North American (Canadian and U.S.) programs identified as providing care to survivors of torture and organized violence, Larson found that the programs fit into five basic service delivery types: integrated full-service models, full-service referral models, decentralized networks of providers, small group of core staff with no network, and other. The 11 integrated full-service model programs provided or coordinated the full range of services, including psychological, medical, and other services. The six full-service referral models essentially provided a full initial assessment and then made referrals within a referral network. The five decentralized networks consisted of separate providers who occasionally would meet to share ideas. The three "small group of core staff" programs functioned as treatment programs with internal service coordination and external referrals when deemed appropriate. Three "other" programs could not be characterized.

While it has been critically important that at least some specialized programs exist for the treatment of survivors of torture, it is very likely that more will be required, especially in countries where there is great need. Studies of the effectiveness of various treatment models and approaches are also needed to improve and modify treatment approaches.

The Informal System of Care

Increasingly, mental health policymakers recognize that traditional healing and alternative forms of treatment are widely used in all societies (Eisenberg et al., 1993). Nonwestern medical patients, in fact, are identified as concurrently using spiritual and religious institutional-based healing, herbal medicines, and animal-derived potions in addition to many culture-specific treatments such as steaming, cupping, acupuncture, massage, and other physical therapies. Equivalents of mental health counseling are provided by family elders, respected relatives and neighbors, fortune-tellers, and religious clergy from all religious denominations. However, because higher rates of torture and violence are often linked to political and social turmoil and unrest, much of the traditional healing system has been compromised in many societies. Mental health policy for torture survivors is likely to benefit from acknowledging the diversity and powerful effects of traditional healing and developing avenues of mutual cooperation and respect among all elements of the de facto mental health system.

Although rarely studied, the informal system of care has the potential to make major improvements in the lives of persons who have been exposed to torture and related violence and trauma. In such a system, workers can be trained to work exclusively with such survivors. Furthermore, workers may be volunteers or themselves survivors of torture, thereby giving them greater sensitivity in this area. They are also likely to understand the culture of the survivors, which may be extremely important to the effective provision of services.

For example, in South Africa, informal or first-line trauma debriefers have provided the majority of western-based mental health care for crime victims. The services have been provided primarily through volunteers (selected, trained, and supervised) working within organizations such as banks, through clinics serviced by trained volunteers, or through various religious ministries (Friedman, 1997). These informal workers provide a body of service as well as an understanding of issues of trauma throughout the country, which begins the flow of education to the broader community both about the effects of traumatic exposure and the possibilities for care. The informal debriefers also provide screening and referral services for those who need professional care.

The potential for national public policy and educational campaigns to promote healing among survivors of torture and related violence and trauma is discussed in some detail elsewhere in this volume (see chapter 20 in this volume). As an example, in South Africa, there is a state-supported victim empowerment initiative to provide education and training for victim support services in schools and clinics and to develop and provide "best practice" guidelines and training for professionals and volunteers. There is a distinct need to explore alternative approaches to assisting survivors of torture and related violence and trauma; making use of community resources for education and self-help programs appears to be a viable approach.

PROCESS OF CARE

Despite the structural problems noted above, there are a number of recent developments about which to be cautiously optimistic. Here we briefly review several assessment and treatment approaches that may be particularly relevant in discussing the provision of mental health services in various settings. A more thorough, yet focused, discussion of assessment and treatment issues is provided in chapter 16.

First, several screening tools for mental disorders have been developed specifically for use in primary care settings. The PRIME-MD (Spitzer et al., 1994) and the SDDS-PC (Broadhead et al., 1995) are two examples of tools that screen patients for a number of disorders and then go on to formulate a provisional diagnosis. They are designed to cover the common conditions found in primary care and to take as little clinician or physician time as possible. There are now computerized telephone versions of both instruments, which minimize office time and maximize patient convenience. The tools are still so new that we do not have data about their ultimate utility in practice. Use of these instruments may help in improving both the rate and the accuracy of mental health diagnoses. Additional attention to cultural relevance and sensitivity is paramount and will figure importantly in the evaluation and widespread use of such tools.

In addition to the screening instruments, several diagnostic manuals and systems have been developed specifically for primary care. There are now primary care editions of the *Diagnostic and Statistical Manual of Mental Disorders* (4th ed., Primary Care edition) (DSM-IV-PC; American Psychiatric Association, 1996) and the *International Classification of Diseases* (10th edition, Primary Care edition) (ICD-10-PC; World Health Organization, 1996). The DSM-IV-PC retains all of the rigorous diagnostic features of the parent DSM-IV but gives more emphasis to and provides algorithms for the conditions most commonly found in primary care. The ICD-10-PC covers only 20 conditions and provides key diagnostic features, treatment guidance, and advice for patient and family. The *International Classification for Primary Care* (Lamberts & Wood, 1987) covers all medical (including mental health) conditions and includes codes for patient complaints, physician assessment (at the symptom and diagnostic level), tests, and treatment provided. It is compatible with both the DSM-IV and the ICD-10.

An even more recent development, sponsored by WHO, is the publication of mental health educational packets for primary care providers. Designed for physicians and nonphysician providers, these packets cover the basics of diagnosis, treatment, and patient and family counseling. Individual country modifications would allow for the development of a posttraumatic stress disorder packet.

Over the past 20 years, health care providers caring for survivors of torture and related violence and trauma have developed several screening instruments that focus on the traumatic experiences of survivors. These instruments measure DSM-IV symptoms and culture-specific symptoms associated with violence and have established psychometric properties (Mollica et al., 1996). Until 15 years ago, simple screening instruments for interviewing patients who were victims of violence were almost nonexistent. Extensive clinical experience tells us that survivors of trauma did not readily share their experiences with their doctors, nor did the clinical interaction make it easy for them to reveal their symptoms. There are many possible reasons for this phenomenon. In some instances, the survivors may be ashamed of what happened, or they may not feel their trauma is of interest or value to the doctor or nurse. In other cases, health workers have been reluctant to ask survivors about their traumatic experiences, fearing that detailed questions might trigger emotional distress and possibly retraumatize them. In the early 1980s, the Harvard Program in Refugee Trauma (HPRT) discovered that patients from Indo-China who had suffered horrific brutality, including torture, were unable to describe their experiences or symptoms in a standard open-ended psychiatric examination conducted in their own language. Surprisingly, the Hopkins Symptom Checklist-25 (HSCL-25; Derogatis, Lipman, Rickels, Uhlenhuth, & Covi, 1973), a simple screening tool, proved useful in facilitating a psychiatric interview with refugee patients. The HSCL-25 and the Harvard Trauma Questionnaire have been translated into many languages and are being used with traumatized patients throughout the world, including Africa, Asia, and Latin America.

Not surprisingly, the checklists can also help the trauma victim and medical worker build a positive and trusting rapport. We have learned from clinicians that it is not uncommon for the survivor to thank the health provider for the interview, stating that it has been the first time anyone has acknowledged his or her trauma and the suffering associated with it. For example, HPRT's staff working onsite with Japanese earthquake survivors in Kobe found them to be very open and honest in their responses, as well as appreciative of the opportunity to describe their traumatic experiences and problems.

Three major lessons have been learned from the use of simple checklists with trauma survivors:

1. The checklist acknowledges the traumatic life experiences of the survivors and can provide, under appropriate circumstances, permission to elaborate on the details of the trauma.
2. The checklist, as a simple medical test, can help survivors communicate about events and symptoms that might otherwise be emotionally overwhelming in an open-ended interview.
3. The compiled results of screening tests can help to determine the prevalence of symptoms, disorders, and experiences, which can be a powerful piece of information to use when convincing administrators of the need for services and funding for treatment.

There have also been some important improvements in treatments in primary care. The development and widespread use of selective serotonin reuptake inhibitors has made prescribing medications easier for physicians and has improved patient compliance. The publicity surrounding these medications in some parts of the world has caused them to become household words, and, it could be argued, has increased the public's awareness of the availability and effectiveness of mental health treatments. Unfortunately, the cost of these agents is still much higher than the older classes of medications, thereby decreasing their availability to some segments of the population. In some countries, they are not on the national formulary.

In addition to medications, there is some evidence that brief training in problem-solving techniques delivered in the primary care setting can work in addressing depression and perhaps other mental health concerns. An English trial of this brief treatment (compared to amitriptyline and placebo) showed that problem solving was no different from amitriptyline but that both were significantly better than placebo for primary care patients with depression (Mynors-Wallis, Gath, Lloyd-Thomas, & Tomlinson, 1995). A similar trial is currently under way in the United States. Relevant to the mental health treatment of those who have survived torture and related violence and trauma is the fact that these treatments are nonpharmacological and can be learned and administered by nonmental health specialists. It is likely that more targeted treatments can be learned in areas where there are large numbers of persons who have been tortured. As noted earlier, initial studies on the use of brief behavioral and cognitive–behavioral interventions are promising. However, more work is needed regarding the development and use of such approaches for survivors of torture and related violence and trauma.

Also relevant is the development of treatment guidelines for various psychiatric disorders. In particular, the U.S. Agency for Health Care Policy and Research (U.S. Department of Health and Human Services, 1993) has developed guidelines for the treatment of depression by primary care physicians. A test of the effectiveness of the guidelines, when implemented, is currently under way. Positive results would be evidence that guidelines can be incorporated into routine primary care to improve the effectiveness of treatments. As with other approaches to improving mental health treatment, attention will need to be focused on the cultural sensitivity and relevance of these approaches.

What is clear is that primary care physicians need additional training to deal with mental health problems in general, and especially for the mental health problems of torture survivors. Particularly with torture survivors, there is a risk of retraumatization if the issues are not dealt with in a sensitive manner. Though it may take time and training, there are examples of success in countries such as Cambodia, where mental health training programs have been developed and implemented for primary care physicians.

INTENDED OUTCOMES OF CARE

Ideally, the structure and process of care should relate to improving outcomes for patients. Assessing outcomes, however, is sometimes the most complicated part of health services research.

Most outcome assessments at a minimum include levels of symptom change; however, it is clear that there are other important domains as well and that these might figure prominently in the overall goals of treatment. For example, do patients go back to work? Do family relationships improve? Do medical expenses decrease? Is overall quality of life improved? These and other domains of functioning and well-being may be particularly relevant to survivors of torture and related violence and trauma. Additional work is needed regarding the existing instruments that have been developed around these domains and others.

There is a growing sense that recovery from any illness (not just mental illness) is incomplete if the disability (as opposed to the symptoms) associated with that condition is not also improved. It is the disability that creates a burden (economic as well as social) on society (see chapter 6 in this volume). This is reflected in a recent publication by WHO and the World Bank that introduces the concept of disability adjusted life years and looks comparatively at the burden of disability associated with various diseases and conditions (Murray & Lopez, 1996). Because of the prevalence, duration, and high percentage of people who do not seek treatment, depression is the fourth leading cause of disability worldwide, and it is likely to move into second place by 2020.

Traumatic stress outcomes for survivors of torture and related violence and trauma appear on a vast continuum from changes in attitudes (e.g., lack of trust) to physical handicaps (e.g., land mine injuries) that directly affect economic and psychosocial productivity. Similarly, opportunities for employment, skill training, and rehabilitation can vary considerably for traumatized persons and communities in countries of resettlement, refugee camps, and societies where torture is still occurring. Realistic thinking about outcomes of care requires that the physical and mental health professional take into account the standards of functioning that can reasonably be expected of the patient within his or her current situation, considering the cultural expectations and gender-based social roles for participating fully and effectively in the home, neighborhood, and local community (Ingstad & Whyte, 1995).

A model of analysis in planning mental health services that complements the assessment of functioning in individual patients is one that focuses on the level of institutional support necessary to successfully maintain the patient in the community. While the horrific reality of the asylum would seem to be fading throughout the world, the needs of persons with severe mental health conditions who must live in either half-way houses or community asylums (i.e., protected living environments) because of limited mental health resources are important (Watts & Bennett, 1983). In many societies that have experienced mass violence, the patient's family remains the primary structure of protection and social support for even the most disabled individuals. In many societies, the critical role of the family in caring for those individuals with serious and profound mental health conditions in the community is a major policy issue that can influence the overall effectiveness of the system of care. The need to provide assistance to families to relieve the burden of illness placed on family members by the mentally ill is an important policy consideration. The latter is especially important in societies where violence has killed many family members and seriously limited traditional family support roles through ongoing poverty, violence, and displacement (Keane, 1995).

Increasingly, there is acknowledgment that reducing symptomatology alone may be appropriate but not wholly adequate as the goal of treatment. Health care systems that treat survivors of torture are recognizing that the ability to address outcomes in multiple domains of functioning is likely to be very important. Treatment will be incomplete if patients are still unable to return to work or relate to their families. Other domains that may be unique to treating survivors of torture should be documented and included in outcome assessments.

ACCESS TO CARE

General Mental Health Issues

There are many reasons why those who need mental health care do not get appropriate care—even when effective care exists. In many parts of the world, persons in need of mental health care come from ethnic minorities and disadvantaged populations. In addition to the problems they face from their own positions, those in need of care are also confronted by a number of other barriers that create a real access issue.

Having service providers available is one component of access. All too often, appropriate services are unevenly distributed in a country. For example, most mental health specialty services are located in urban areas, and even general medical services are more sparse in rural areas. In developing countries, the maldistribution of services is likely to be even more pronounced. In many countries, psychiatrists are almost exclusively found in the cities, and even psychologists and social workers are scarce in rural areas, with the bulk of health care, including mental health care, being delivered by nurses. Furthermore, the distance one must travel and other transportation issues are key determinants of access. The longer it takes to get to a service provider, the greater the personal cost and the lower the likelihood of accessing that service with the regularity that it takes for effective treatment to take place. Even in urban areas there can be transportation problems, including inconvenient bus schedules and routes with difficult transfer arrangements.

Cost is yet another barrier to accessing mental health treatment. Treatment may be too expensive for many, and health insurance, where it exists, may inadequately cover mental health problems.

Lack of knowledge about mental health problems and about where and how to seek help is an important part of access. Many people do not understand what mental illness is, how it can develop, and how it can be treated. They may fail to understand their own symptoms, particularly in disorders where there are prominent somatic components. They may also fail to understand the connection between past events and current symptomatology—again, especially when the symptoms are predominantly somatic. Even when they recognize that a mental health problem exists, people often do not know where to go for treatment. They think of primary care providers when the care needed is for "medical" (i.e., not mental) problems; therefore, it may be seen as inappropriate to discuss psychological issues.

In countries of resettlement and countries with high rates of torture and related violence and trauma, the medical and mental health systems may not be considered a politically and culturally appropriate and safe domain in which to share the torture experience and its perceived health effects. This is especially the case in nonwestern societies that rely exclusively on primary care physicians for mental health care. In addition, in some societies, primary care physicians are often aware of the health and mental health consequences of violence but do not feel their society has acknowledged their legitimacy in caring for the mental health sequelae of such experiences. In some countries, primary care physicians may have been victims or, in other situations, perpetrators of violence themselves, thus making it difficult for them to address the emotional distress of survivors. This problem is compounded by the lack of traditional healers who might otherwise care for such survivors. All of these issues add to the complexity and challenges of facilitating the motivation and effectiveness of primary care physicians and mental health specialists caring for survivors of torture and related violence and trauma.

Finally, one of the most difficult barriers to overcome is stigma. Individuals feel it and are often reluctant to acknowledge a problem and seek help because of it. Societies express it, causing families and even some health professionals to avoid dealing with stigmatized conditions. Although community and professional education programs are helpful, it is still too often the case that persons with mental health conditions are seen as weak, sinful, or lazy. Thus, even when correctly diagnosed with a mental illness, many individuals will not accept the diagnosis, refusing effective treatment to avoid the stigma of mental illness.

In a recent event that offered voluntary screening for depression, participants who had screened positive for depression were asked why they had not sought treatment. Among those who were severely depressed, the top five reasons for not seeking treatment were as follows (more than one reason could be checked): (a) were not sure where to go (47.5%), (b) thought treatment was too expensive (42.0%), (c) had no insurance (31.2%), (d) did not want others to know (28.4%), and (e) did not recognize depression (28.3%) (Magruder, 1998). Clearly, there are some major issues concerning access that could improve the benefits of treatment for depression to a sizable number of untreated persons in the general population.

Issues Related to Torture

How does all this relate to persons who have survived torture and related violent and traumatic experiences? Often, persons who have been tortured are members of an ethnic or a cultural minority group. Even if they emigrate, they are likely to be in a minority group in their new country—culturally, racially, ethnically, and linguistically. Thus, whatever access issues exist in a given country or area may be amplified by minority status.

In many countries where torture has taken place, mental health resources are slim or nonexistent. The likelihood that appropriate care is available and accessible to someone in need is extremely low. In many countries, it may be difficult to know whether the provider can be trusted. In developing countries, the cost of care may be prohibitive, and thus only life-threatening and the most serious illnesses are brought to medical attention.

Lack of knowledge of where to go for help is likely to be a key issue for survivors of torture. Even in their home country, it may be difficult for them to know that treatment could be available (if, in fact, that is the case). For those who emigrate, the situation may be worse in the new country, where it may be difficult even for native-born persons to successfully navigate the mental health system. Furthermore, for many who would prefer to bury the worst experiences of their lives, it may be difficult to seek help in a new country. Some may not connect their torture experience and their current mental health state, including the relationship of their current symptoms to mental health, making it difficult to articulate the need for treatment. For children and adolescents who have been tortured or have witnessed torture, it may be even more difficult to know how to initiate the help-seeking process. Family members or caretakers may not understand the depths of what these children have been through and the ways in which these experiences may be powerful risk factors for mental health problems and the need for mental health services in the present and in the future.

Clearly, there are many reasons why survivors of torture and related violence and trauma may have a more difficult time in accessing needed mental health care than do others who have untreated mental health problems. Ideally, the structure and organization of the health care system should help to ameliorate some of these access barriers.

CONCLUSION

There is much to be done if our health systems are to be responsive to the needs of those who have survived the experiences of torture and trauma. One important research issue is whether to organize primary care systems in such a way that primary care providers themselves have access to dedicated staff who can do some of the time-consuming parts of the assessment and treatment of torture survivors. Such integrated systems that embody both the medical and the psychosocial needs of survivors are promising, particularly in environments with a lack of mental health resources. Affording primary care providers access to some of the screening and diagnosis instruments, diagnostic manuals, and treatment guidelines that have been developed may make their difficult job easier and, possibly, their treatments more effective.

Mental health specialty systems, where they exist, play a vital role in receiving referrals from primary care. Economic barriers to accessing these systems for those in need are a priority, and more flexible, responsive services for survivors of torture, including community- and residential-based care, might be considered.

Finally, the informal system of care, including the voluntary sector, community, institutions, and families, appears to have great potential in helping survivors of torture to recover to the point where they can participate fully and effectively in the home, neighborhood, and local community. No system of care can be considered successful unless there is improvement in the productivity and quality of life of those who receive care. This should be the ultimate goal of the health care system.

REFERENCES

American Psychiatric Association. (1996). *Diagnostic and statistical manual of mental disorders* (4th ed., Primary Care edition). Washington, DC: Author.

Broadhead, W. E., Leon, A. C., Weissman, M. M., Barrett, J. E., Blacklow, R. S., Gilbert, T. T., Keller, M. B., Olfson, M., & Higgins, E. S. (1995). Development and validation of the SDDS-PC screen for multiple mental disorders in primary care. *Archives of Family Medicine, 4*, 211–219.

Derogatis, L. R., Lipman, R. S., Rickels, K., Uhlenhuth, E. H., & Covi, L. (1973). The Hopkins Symptom Checklist (HSCL): A measure of primary symptom dimensions. In P. Pichot (Ed.), *Psychological measurement: Modern problems in pharmacotherapy*. Basel: S. Karger.

Desjarlais, R., Eisenberg, L., Good, B., & Kleinman, A. (1995). *World mental health: Problems and priorities in low-income countries.* New York: Oxford University Press.

Eisenberg, D. M., Kessler, R. C., Foster, C., Norlock, F. E., Calkins, D. R., & Delbanco, T. L. (1993). Unconventional medicine in the United States: Prevalence, costs, and patterns of use. *New England Journal of Medicine, 328,* 246–252.

Friedman, M. (1997, November). *Trauma in the workplace: Peer service provision in organizations.* Paper presented at the Conference of the International Society of Traumatic Stress Studies, Montreal, Canada.

Henderson, D. C., van de Velde, P., Mollica, R. F., & Lavelle, J. (1996). *The crisis in Rwanda: Mental health in the service of justice and healing.* Cambridge, MA: Harvard Program in Refugee Trauma.

Ingstad, B., & Whyte, S. R. (Eds.). (1995). *Disability and culture.* Berkeley, CA: University of California Press.

Katon, W., Von Korff, M., Lin, E., Walker, E., Simon, G., Bush, T., Robinson, P., & Russo, J. (1995). Collaborative management to achieve treatment guidelines: Impact on depression in primary care. *Journal of the American Medical Association, 273,* 1026–1031.

Keane, F. (1995). *Season of blood.* London: Viking.

Lamberts, H., & Wood, M. (Eds.). (1987). *International Classification of Primary Care.* Oxford, England: Oxford University Press.

Larson, M. A. (1997). *Journeys in healing: Care with survivors of torture and organized violence in the U.S. and Canada: An exploratory study of U.S. and Canadian treatment programs.* Unpublished master's thesis, The University of North Carolina at Chapel Hill, Department of Health Behavior and Health Education, Chapel Hill.

Lavelle, J., Tor, S., Stedman, W., Mollica, R. F., & Sath, S. (1993). *Khmer Mental Health Training and Certification Program on the Thai–Cambodian border: Curriculum.* Cambridge, MA: Harvard School of Public Health.

Magruder, K. M. (1998). Community education and screening programs. In R. Jenkins & T. B. Ustun (Eds.), *Preventing mental illness: Mental health promotion in primary care.* Chichester, England: Wiley.

McFarlane, W. R., Lukens, E., Link, B., Dushay, R., Deakins, S., Newmark, M., Dunne, E., Horen, B., & Toran, J. (1995). Multiple family groups and psychoeducation in the treatment of schizophrenia. *Archives of General Psychiatry, 52,* 679–687.

Mollica, R. F., Caspi-Yavin, Y., Lavelle, J., Tor, S., Yang, T., Chan, S., Pham, T., Ryan, A., & deMarneffe, D. (1996). The Harvard Trauma Questionnaire (HTQ) Manual: Cambodian, Laotian, and Vietnamese versions. *Torture Quarterly Journal on the Rehabilitation of Torture Victims and Prevention of Torture* (Suppl. 1), 19–42.

Mollica, R. F., Donelan, K., Tor, S., Lavelle, J., Elias, C., Frankel, M., & Blendon, R. J. (1993). The effect of trauma and confinement on functional health and mental health status of Cambodians living in Thailand–Cambodia border camps. *Journal of the American Medical Association, 270,* 581–586.

Murray, C. J. L., & Lopez, A. D. (Eds.). (1996). *The global burden of disease.* Cambridge, MA: Harvard University Press.

Mynors-Wallis, L. M., Gath, D. H., Lloyd-Thomas, A. R., & Tomlinson, D. (1995). Randomised controlled trial comparing problem solving treatment with amitriptyline and placebo for major depression in primary care. *British Medical Journal, 310*(6977), 441–445.

O'Brien, M. (1995). *White Paper Western Cape Health Plan.* Unpublished manuscript.

Regier, D. A., Narrow, W. E., Rae, D. S., Manderscheid, R. W., Locke, B. Z., & Goodwin, F. K. (1993). The de facto U.S. mental and addictive disorders service system: Epidemiologic Catchment Area prospective 1-year prevalence rates of disorders and services. *Archives of General Psychiatry, 50,* 85–94.

Spitzer, R. L., Williams, J. B. W., Kroenke, K., Linzer, M., Degruy, F. V., Hahn, S. R., Brody, D., & Johnson, J. G. (1994). Utility of a new procedure for diagnosing mental disorders in primary care: The PRIME 1000 study. *Journal of the American Medical Association, 272*(22), 1749–1756.

U.S. Department of Health and Human Services. (1993). *Depression in primary care: Clinical practice guideline* (AHCPR Publication No. 93-0552). Rockville, MD: Author.

Ustun, T. B., & Sartorius, N. (Eds.). (1995). *Mental illness in general health care: An international study*. Chichester, England: Wiley.

Watts, F. N., & Bennett, D. H. (Eds). (1983). *Theory and practice of psychiatric rehabilitation*. New York: Wiley.

Wells, K. B., Hays, R. D., Burnam, M. A., Rogers, W. H. H., Greenfield, S., & Ware, J. E., Jr. (1989). Detection of depressive disorder in prepaid and fee-for-service practices: Results from the Medical Outcomes Study. *Journal of the American Medical Association, 262*(23), 3298–3302.

World Health Organization. (1996). Diagnostic and management guidelines for mental disorders in primary care. In *International Classification of Diseases* (10th ed., Primary Care edition, chapter 5). Göttingen, Germany: Hogreve and Huber.

19

Professional Caregiver and Observer Issues

J. DAVID KINZIE and BRIAN ENGDAHL

Lok first came to the Indo-Chinese clinic 9 years ago. I cannot forget the initial inter-view nor her story. She was a small Cambodian woman (the nurse's note listed her weight as 113 pounds) who appeared older than her 58 years. Her face reflected fatigue and sadness, yet grace. Ben, the Cambodian mental health worker, had told me a little about her before she came. She was referred from a private physician and had multiple complaints of nausea, headache, arm pain, shoulder pain, and also symp-toms of poor sleep and depression. The private physician was treating her for diabe-tes, and she was on an oral hypoglycemic agent. Ben noted that she had had a very traumatic life in Cambodia. She had suffered many losses with which we now have become familiar from any Pol Pot patient.

After greetings and discussion of physical symptoms, I told her that I understood she had nightmares. She said that they occurred almost nightly and consisted of disturbing thoughts about the death of her children. The nightmares started about 1 year ago and increased to occurring nightly in the last several months. These thoughts also occurred in the daytime and intruded into her consciousness. She could not get any rest from them. When she sat alone, she was constantly flooded with the thoughts, and she would have pain in her chest. At one time, she said she passed out while thinking about the past. She has tried to push the memories out of her mind; it is a tremendous fight to get them out, but they keep coming back. She startles very easily at any sounds or noises. She feels very much on guard all the time. She feels that she will die in the near future. I asked if the nightmares were thoughts of events that really happened. She looked up and said simply, "They really happened."

J. DAVID KINZIE • Department of Psychiatry, Oregon Health Sciences University, Portland, Oregon 97201. BRIAN ENGDAHL • Veterans Administration Medical Center, Minneapo-lis, Minnesota 55417.

The Mental Health Consequences of Torture, edited by Ellen Gerrity, Terence M. Keane, and Farris Tuma. Kluwer Academic/Plenum Publishers, New York, 2001.

She met all the diagnostic criteria for posttraumatic stress disorder. She obviously was quite impaired by the symptoms. I wondered why now she came for treatment. After all, the Pol Pot time in Cambodia was over 6 years ago. She spontaneously mentioned that she had just received a letter from Cambodia that a brother who survived Pol Pot recently was killed as a result of thieves breaking into his house. She began to cry when she said, "and he survived Pol Pot only to have this happen to him." It seems likely that this was a triggering event, a final loss that she felt she could no longer endure, and a reminder of past events and memories.

"What did you do when Pol Pot came to power?" I asked. This was a loaded question. Tears welled up in her eyes almost silently, and they fell down her cheeks. Her respirations increased, she tensed. "They came and dragged my husband away. They took the oldest children, a boy 17, a boy 16, and a girl 14. They were hit over the head until they were almost unconscious, tied up, and dragged around the town. It was 3 days before they died. I could not stop them, and they cried out for me. Before my husband died, they cut him open and took out his liver." There was a long period of silence while she cried, dried her tears, and stopped.

The images of that event filled my own mind, racing from topic to topic. Fantasies of striking back and rescuing them came on, as well as dying in place of them. Thoughts were probably too intense: a brief rage about Pol Pot and his cadres who could destroy life so wantonly. What right did they have to take people and kill them in a brutal fashion? There was even a brief thought of confronting Pol Pot with his evilness; he was still alive somewhere in Cambodia or in Thailand. I remember being angry and then sad, but saying nothing, only a nod to Lok that I understood. I looked at Ben and said, "That's bad." He said, "Yes, that's bad." (Used with permission.)

What is a therapist to think and do when confronted with such stories of horror? How can one be therapeutic and yet handle his or her own reactions? The countertransference issues are intense, complicated, and personal and can be used constructively or destructively. This is why they are a critical part of the therapeutic process.

The goal of this chapter is to discuss issues specific to professional caregivers and observers who are involved with victims and survivors of trauma. Special consideration will be devoted to countertransference reactions and ethical issues.

THERAPIST REACTIONS

When psychoanalysts began therapeutic work with the Jewish survivors of the Holocaust, it soon became clear that the therapists experienced profound reactions to their patients' reports of massive human aggression. It was no longer possible (or perhaps even desirable) to maintain a neutral therapeutic stance. The reactions of these psychoanalysts are described by De Wind (1971) and Chodoff (1975). These intense reactions continued and began to be increasingly reported. Wilson and Lindy's (1994) book, *Countertransference in the Treatment of PTSD*, attests to the importance of this issue. However, because our current understanding of these reactions is supported by so few systematic studies, the foundation of our knowledge is based on personal reports that have been thoughtfully recounted and on widespread observations of common behaviors.

The term *countertransference* in this context is used broadly to encompass all emotional reactions a therapist has toward a patient (Atshul & Sledge, 1989). A similar concept is *empathetic strain*, developed by Wilson and Lindy (1994). The authors maintained that the critical element for therapeutic recovery of traumatic reactions is a "safe" environment—one that includes, even requires, substantial empathy. The rupture of empathy can result in loss of the therapeutic relationship. The intensity of the therapeutic process and the arousal in both the patient and the therapist in response to the traumatic reports can produce unique countertransference (or empathetic strain) reactions.

Wilson and Lindy (1994) divide empathetic strain into two broad categories: (a) overidentification, including enmeshment, overinvolvement, and a loss of boundaries, or disequilibrium, including uncertainty and unmodulated affect; and (b) avoidance, including withdrawal or blank-screen facade and intellectualization, or repression, including denial and distancing. This model has now been supported through experimental validation with the Clinicians' Trauma Reaction Survey (Wilson, 1997). These reactions are complex and interactive within the therapist–patient relationship and depend partially on the nature of the trauma; personal qualities of the therapist, such as training, experience, and personality; and institutional factors, such as political context and adequacy of resources. The theoretical framework provides a basis for further systematic study and research. The effects of countertransference reactions can be quite severe within trauma centers in which caregivers can regularly experience disruptive and painful psychological effects, including suffering some of the symptoms of the patients or responding with disbelief and cynicism (Jaranson, 1995). These reactions, also termed *vicarious traumatizations* (McCann & Pearlman, 1990), may explain some of the internal strife that historically has challenged torture rehabilitation centers.

Some research has explored the details of the countertransference phenomenon. A study by Kinzie (1994) examined the efforts of long-term work with traumatized Indo-Chinese patients and found marked differences between the reactions of the ethnic mental health counselors and the staff psychiatrists. In response to a questionnaire, the counselors almost universally reported very little subjective reaction or symptoms to working with traumatized patients, although there had been observations of avoidance behavior and sometimes even outright rejection by some. However, the psychiatrists described a wider range of reactions, including sadness, horror and disgust, sleep disturbances, aggressiveness and hostility, and loss of impartiality. Despite these subjective symptoms, the psychiatrists showed very few objective signs of actual countertherapeutic reactions. More surprising were the broader effects of the empathetic strain on the psychiatrists outside the therapeutic setting, including an intolerance of other patients with minor problems, a general intolerance of violence, a personal sense of vulnerability, and a strong sense that western medicine and society have failed. They had a sense that their medical education had not prepared them to deal with the evidence of such extreme inhumanity.

A special form of countertransference occurs when the torture survivor and the therapist are working in the dangerous environment where the oppression occurred, for example, in regions of political repression. Chilean therapists working with survivors during the oppression regime in 1985 reported that they were very concerned about their own personal safety, were ambivalent about their role, sometime overidentified with their patients, and feared failure in addition to feeling intense helplessness (Comas-Diaz & Padilla, 1990). Researchers working with Chilean therapists also found themselves drawn into the therapist's world with a temporary loss of boundaries; feelings of denial and avoidance, guilt, and anger; and concern about complicity. They were also concerned about retraumatizing the therapists through their interviews (Agger & Jensen, 1994). These two reports describe many of the countertransference reactions as being similar to the concept of the "wounded healer," in which an assumption exists that suffering facilitates the development of empathy (Halifax, 1981). This is a plausible hypothesis that needs to be tested further.

OTHER CAREGIVER RESPONSES

Rescue and emergency personnel can also have severe reactions to the horrific conditions in which they sometimes work. Police officers, firefighters, paramedics, National Guard members, and other disaster workers often work closely with the remains of maimed bodies, disfigured body parts, and the severe and horrifying human misery of disasters. The effects of working in a disaster situation were found to be comparable to combat stress (Figley, 1981). Even emergency workers not onsite may experience stress in support of those personnel who are directly involved (Beaton, Murphy, Johnson, Pike, & Corneil, 1998; Raphael, 1986). Mitchell and Dyregrov (1993) have described a variety of cognitive, physical, and emotional symptoms among disaster workers; some may not present themselves for months or years.

In a study of secondary disaster victims, Jones (1985) described the effects on Air Force personnel of recovering and identifying human remains from the Jonestown mass suicide. Short-term dysphoria was found in those younger than 25 years, enlisted soldiers, African-Americans, and those with exposure to bodies. In a study of Swedish rescue workers involved in the Armenian earthquake in 1988, professionals (as compared to nonprofessional workers) seemed to express themselves better and had fewer unpleasant experiences over time (Lundin & Bodegard, 1993). Nine percent of the rescue workers responding to the 1989 freeway collapse in San Francisco were found to have symptom levels typical of psychiatric outpatients (Marmar, Weiss, Metzler, Ronfeldt, & Foreman, 1996). Compared with those of lower distress, responders with higher distress reported greater exposure, greater emotional distress, and greater dissociation at the time of trauma exposure, as well as greater perceived threat and less preparation for the critical incident. After an avalanche on a company of the Norwegian Army, survivors and spontaneous rescuers had higher symptoms than nonexposed participants did. A posttraumatic stress reaction was found among the survivors (9%) and the rescuers (10%), although a reduction of symptoms was seen over a 4-month period. In another study of police officers who were physically handling victims of a major disaster, Alexander and Wells (1991) did not find significant posttraumatic stress disorder (PTSD); the officers' coping styles and good organizational support were credited for the positive results.

A review of a number of studies of disaster workers (Raphael & Wilson, 1994) described several dynamic themes that affect the rescue workers' role and produce symptoms or strain their ability to function. These themes and personal characteristics include the terror of the force and level of destruction of the specific disaster, confrontation with death, helplessness, anger, loss, elation, survivor guilt, and voyeurism. A "counterdisaster syndrome" is described as overinvolvement with the disaster role and a sense that one is indispensable. Stress reduction programs have been popular for emergency personnel, and, although some encouraging results have been seen, the evidence is still sketchy and somewhat controversial (see the review by Mitchell & Dyregrov, 1993).

ETHICAL ISSUES IN TORTURE AND TRAUMA TREATMENT

Because the United Nations (1948) *Universal Declaration of Human Rights* stated that "no one shall be subjected to torture, cruel, inhumane or degrading treatment, or punishment," a series of international laws has attempted to prevent torture and inhumane treatment (Sorensen, 1992). Furthermore, these laws compare with the medical ethics of the World Medical Association (1975), which clearly state a prohibition against physicians participating in torture in any manner and physicians' need for complete clinical independence in determining the health of persons, including prisoners, for whom they are medically responsible. One area of ethical disagreement is in the management of hunger strikes. The complex ethical dilemmas surrounding hunger strikers have been reviewed by Silove, Curtis, Manson, and Becker (1996). Suggested approaches include the appointment of external physicians of confidence, an advance directive about the striker's wishes in the event of a collapse, and the appointment of an ad hoc ethics committee to give advice.

Refugees are often of a different culture from the therapist and as such present unique ethical challenges in treatment. Eth (1992) emphasized the problems of informed consent, conflicting cultural values, and the survivor's search for the meaning of the trauma. Eth pointed out that the search for meaning in the trauma should not be subverted for political purposes.

The principles that should govern ethical practice to avoid therapeutic pitfalls and countertransference reactions have been outlined by Kinzie and Boehnlein (1993). The principles are derived from biomedical ethics and reflect a deontological position, that is, that there are features of human acts other than their consequences that make them right or wrong (Beauchamp & Childress, 1979). These principles applied to PTSD are hierarchical and are as follows:

- **Fidelity:** In this model, the most important ethical principle is the doctor–patient relationship, one that includes trust, honesty, confidentiality, predictability, and consistency.

- **Nonmaleficence (do no harm):** Traumatized patients have already been harmed, deceived, and brutalized, often in unpredictable and arbitrary ways. Acting insensitively, minimizing patients' problems, pushing patients into therapy, pushing patients in life to do more than they can, and overidentifying can all have harmful effects.
- **Beneficence:** The therapist is obliged to provide competent treatment, reduce suffering, and promote health, based on a sound scientific foundation.
- **Autonomy:** The therapist should respect and encourage the survivor as an active partner in the treatment program.
- **Justice:** Justified indignation against wrongs the survivor endured may be encouraged, including a survivor's decision to protest injustice with specific actions.
- **Self-interest:** During the intense treatment of the traumatized patient, the therapist must be able to meet his or her own needs in a healthy manner. To manage stress levels, therapists may need to limit the number of patients or limit their involvement in other stressful professional or community activities. Some, however, may choose to become involved with various advocacy groups to protest unjust acts. Developing a supportive network of colleagues and friends can be extraordinarily valuable for this kind of work.

Therapist countertransference reactions, although widely reported by those who treat survivors of trauma, rarely have been subjected to systematic research. A typology of objective and subjective reactions, such as described by Wilson and Lindy (1994), is a first step. Next, systematic studies of experienced therapists would document the frequency of reactions. Also needed are studies of the outcome of such reactions, such as harm to patients, exacerbation of symptoms, or premature termination of therapy. Equally important is the effect of treatment programs within disaster management organizations, where staff burnout or serious conflict may result. The ethics of treatment need to be further explored; intense interactions improperly handled can lead to exploitation, violation of boundaries, or illegal activities.

REFERENCES

Agger, I., & Jensen, S. B. (1994). Determinant factors for countertransference reactions under state terrorism. In J. P. Wilson & J. Lindy (Eds.), *Countertransference in the treatment of PTSD* (pp. 263–287). New York: Guilford Press.

Alexander, D. A., & Wells, A. (1991). Reaction of police officers to body handling after a major disaster. *British Journal of Psychiatry, 159,* 547–555.

Atshul, V. A., & Sledge, W. H. (1989). Countertransference problems. In A. Tasman, R. E. Hale, & A. J. Frances (Eds.), *Review of psychiatry* (Vol. 8). Washington, DC: American Psychiatric Press.

Beaton, R., Murphy, S., Johnson, C., Pike, K., & Corneil, W. (1998). Exposure to duty-related incident stressors in urban firefighters and paramedics. *Journal of Traumatic Stress, 11,* 821–828.

Beauchamp, T. L., & Childress, J. F. (1979). *Principles of biomedical ethics.* New York: Oxford University Press.

Chodoff, P. (1975). Psychiatric aspects of Nazi persecution. In S. Arieti (Ed.), *American handbook of psychiatry* (2nd ed., Vol. 5). New York: Basic Books.

Comas-Diaz, L., & Padilla, A. M. (1990). Countertransference in working with victims of political repression. *American Journal of Orthopsychiatry, 60*, 125–134.

De Wind, E. (1971). Psychotherapy after traumatization caused by persecution. *International Psychiatric Clinics, 8*, 93–114.

Eth, S. (1992). Ethical challenges in the treatment of traumatized refugees. *Journal of Traumatic Stress, 5*, 103–109.

Figley, C. (1981). Working on a theory of what it takes to survive. *APA Monitor, 9.*

Halifax, J. (1981). *Shaman: The wounded healer.* New York: Crossroad.

Jaranson, J. (1995). Government-sanctioned torture: Status of the rehabilitation movement. *Transcultural Research Review, 32*(3), 253–286.

Jones, D. R. (1985). Secondary disaster victims: The emotional effects of recovering and identifying human remains. *American Journal of Psychiatry, 142*, 303–307.

Kinzie, J. D. (1994). Countertransference in treatment of Southeast Asian refugees. In J. P. Wilson & J. Lindy (Eds.), *Countertransference in the treatment of PTSD* (pp. 249–262). New York: Guilford Press.

Kinzie, J. D., & Boehnlein, J. K. (1993). Psychotherapy of the victims of massive violence: Countertransference and ethical issues. *American Journal of Psychotherapy, 47*, 90–102.

Lundin, T., & Bodegard, M. (1993). The psychological impact of an earthquake on rescue workers: A follow-up study of the Swedish group of rescue workers in Armenia, 1988. *Journal of Traumatic Stress, 6*, 129–139.

Marmar, C. R., Weiss, D. S., Metzler, T. J., Ronfeldt, H. M., & Foreman, C. (1996). Stress responses of emergency services personnel to the Loma Prieta earthquake, Interstate 880 freeway collapse and control traumatic incidents. *Journal of Traumatic Stress, 9*, 63–85.

McCann, L., & Pearlman, L. A. (1990). Vicarious traumatization: A framework for understanding the psychological effects of working with victims. *Journal of Traumatic Stress, 3*(1), 131–149.

Mitchell, J. T., & Dyregrov, A. (1993). Traumatic stress in disaster workers and emergency personnel: Prevention and intervention. In J. P. Wilson & B. Raphael (Eds.), *International handbook of traumatic stress syndromes.* New York: Plenum Press.

Raphael, B. (1986). *When disaster strikes.* New York: Basic Books.

Raphael, B., & Wilson, J. P. (1994). When disaster strikes: Managing emotional reactions in rescue workers. In J. P. Wilson & J. Lindy (Eds.), *Countertransference in the treatment of PTSD* (pp. 333–350). New York: Guilford Press.

Silove, D., Curtis, J., Manson, C., & Becker, R. (1996). Ethical considerations in the management of asylum-seekers on hunger strike. *Journal of the American Medical Association, 276*, 410–415.

Sorensen, B. (1992). Modern ethics and international law. In M. Basoglu (Ed.), *Torture and its consequences.* Cambridge: Cambridge University Press.

United Nations. (1948). *The Universal Declaration of Human Rights.* GA Res. 217 A (III); U.N. Document A/810.

Wilson, J. P. (1997, November). *Countertransference in the treatment of PTSD.* Presented at the annual meeting of the International Society for Traumatic Stress Studies, Montreal, Quebec, Canada.

Wilson, J. P., & Lindy, J. D. (1994). Empathic strain and countertransference. In J. P. Wilson & J. D. Lindy (Eds.), *Countertransference in the treatment of PTSD* (pp. 31–61). New York: Guilford Press.

World Medical Association. (1975). *The Declaration of Tokyo.* Ferney-Voltaire, France.

20

Torture and Human Rights Violations
Public Policy and the Law

DEAN G. KILPATRICK and MARGARET E. ROSS

A chapter on public policy and the law may be unusual in a research document addressing the mental health consequences of torture and related violence and trauma, but in fact these topics are directly relevant for survivors of torture and necessary for those who provide services to survivors or conduct research in this area. How public policy and the law affect the lives of survivors and those who attempt to serve them is reviewed here, along with empirical research findings that suggest that each has important consequences in the treatment of survivors of traumatic events. This chapter concludes with a discussion of public policy approaches toward reparations and restorative justice for survivors of trauma and torture.

DEFINITIONS

In any society, governmental bodies enact laws, make policies, and allocate resources at the local, state, national, and international level. Public policy can be generally defined as a system of laws, regulatory measures, courses of action, and funding priorities concerning a given topic that is promulgated by a governmental

DEAN G. KILPATRICK • National Crime Victims Research and Treatment Center, Department of Psychiatry and Behavioral Sciences, Medical University of South Carolina, Charleston, South Carolina 29425.   MARGARET E. ROSS • Cambridge Business Development Center and International Criminal Defense Attorneys Association, Cambridge, Massachusetts 02139.

The Mental Health Consequences of Torture, edited by Ellen Gerrity, Terence M. Keane, and Farris Tuma. Kluwer Academic/Plenum Publishers, New York, 2001.

entity or its representatives. Public policy is accomplished through enactment of legislation, regulations, and funding priorities. Individuals and groups often shape public policy through education, advocacy, or mobilization of interest groups. The process of shaping public policy is different in western-style democracies than in other forms of government, but it is reasonable to assume that the public policy process generally involves efforts by competing interest groups to influence public policymakers along lines that are favorable to the individual groups.

A major aspect of public policy is the law. In a general sense, the law includes specific legislation and more broadly defined provisions of constitutional or international legal systems. As will be described later, there are many ways that the law can affect the treatment of survivors of torture and can determine the types of services they receive. Likewise, legislation often determines priorities for research and the amount of funding that is allocated. Thus, it is not surprising that a major area of public policy debate is about proposed legislation and funding.

In this context, advocacy can be defined as the process of attempting to influence public policy through education, lobbying, or political pressure. Advocacy groups often attempt to educate the general public as well as public policymakers about the nature of the problems, the legislation needed to address the problem, and the funding required to provide services or conduct research. Although advocacy is sometimes viewed as lacking objectivity or even as unseemly by some in the professional and research community, advocacy clearly plays an important role in setting public policy priorities for service and research funding. Additionally, advocates can use scientific research data in the educational process of both the public and public policymakers, and thereby greatly improve the public policy process.

THE LAW AND TREATMENT AND SERVICES
FOR TRAUMA SURVIVORS

The law can directly or indirectly influence the lives of survivors of torture and other traumatic events in six important ways:

1. State, national, and international law provides a framework for identifying basic human rights and for defining violations of these rights.
2. The law defines behaviors that are proscribed by criminal and civil statutes and provides sanctions for such behaviors in the form of criminal and civil penalties.
3. The law establishes eligibility criteria for legal immigration, asylum, and citizenship—all of which are relevant for many survivors of torture who leave their native lands and seek refugee status in another nation.
4. The law establishes eligibility criteria for a host of services, including veterans' benefits, crime victims' compensation, and disaster relief services.

5. The law has a major effect on the level of funding for mental health and other services that can be provided to survivors of torture and other traumatic events. Public policymakers allocate funding for services through the appropriations process and authorize spending through the enactment of laws that establish special service programs for trauma survivors. For example, the Torture Victims Relief Act, enacted in 1998, authorizes continued and expanded U.S. contributions to treatment centers, both in the United States and around the world, for persons who suffer from the effects of torture. The U.S. Congress authorized special programs for combat veterans and appropriated funds in the legislation that established the National Center for Posttraumatic Stress Disorder (NCPTSD). Also, the Victims of Crime Act of 1984 established funding for crime victim services and compensation.

6. Laws and the governmental appropriations process authorize, set priorities for, and provide funding for research efforts in the area of traumatic stress.

AN OVERVIEW OF INTERNATIONAL HUMAN RIGHTS LAW CONCERNING SURVIVORS OF TORTURE

A comprehensive review of international law is beyond the scope of this chapter. What may be of benefit, however, is a brief discussion of the basic assumptions of human rights law and a description of key documents in international law that are relevant to torture survivors and their treatment.

The concept of human rights developed out of 17th-century philosophical discussions about natural rights or the rights of man. As described by John Locke, Thomas Jefferson, and others, individuals have certain rights by virtue of their status as human beings. The U.S. Declaration of Independence states that "all men are created with certain inalienable rights" and makes the case that a people can reject the authority of a government that violates those rights. From this human rights perspective, if the violation of basic human rights justifies a people severing their ties with their government, it follows that violation of rights by a government is a very serious matter. Therefore, governments play vital roles in defining human rights and in providing legal protection for them. However, Donnelly (1996) notes that the government itself has the potential to be a major threat to the rights of individuals. Thus, a major focus of human rights law is not only to describe rights that are legally protected but also to prohibit actions by governments that violate such rights. Amendments 1 to 10 of the U.S. Constitution, which outline basic rights of individuals and prohibitions against their violation by the government, are an example of human rights law at the national level.

Much of the following discussion of human rights and international law draws heavily on a recent review by Ross (1997). Several fundamental human rights documents have been established at the international level. The United Nations (U.N.) Universal Declaration of Human Rights was enacted by the U.N. General Assembly in 1948. Although the U.N. declaration did not establish enforceable rights, two treaty documents have been adopted that provide some enforcement mechanisms for the rights identified in it. The International Covenant on Civil and Political Rights and the International Covenant on Economic, Social, and Cultural Rights include some enforcement mechanisms for the rights identified in the U.N. declaration for those nations that have signed the treaties. In her evaluation of these documents and related efforts, Ross described five practices that have been used to promote and protect human rights: (a) complaint procedures for those alleging rights violations; (b) reports of impartial experts, including fact-finding efforts; (c) bodies that receive reports on specific measures that nations have taken to comply with human rights; (d) procedures for complaints between nations; and (e) technical assistance to nations to help them meet human rights standards.

Another very relevant international law is the U.N. Convention Against Torture and Other Cruel, Inhuman, and Degrading Treatment or Punishment (1984). Through this law, torture survivors from nations that have ratified this convention are authorized to submit a complaint to the U.N. Committee Against Torture if their country does not provide financial compensation to them.

The U.N. Convention Relating to the Status of Refugees (1951), as updated by the 1967 Protocol Relating to the Status of Refugees, defines the legal status of refugees under international law. Specifically, a refugee is defined as a person who is outside his or her country of nationality because of a well-founded fear of persecution, which must be proven. A major difficulty for some survivors of torture who have fled their country and are seeking asylum in another country is the difficulty in proving that they have a well-founded fear of persecution; such a fear is subjective in nature and hard to document. Moreover, their torture-related psychological trauma often makes them reluctant to discuss painful material, and they may suffer from a torture-conditioned fear and distrust of government officials who are asking them about their experiences. Unless they can demonstrate this well-founded fear, survivors may be returned to their country of nationality.

In summary, a body of international law exists that sets ambitious standards about human rights and, to a lesser extent, provides enforcement mechanisms against nations and governments that violate the rights of citizens. Enforcement is limited because not all governments are signatories to key treaties and conventions. Moreover, governments must agree to relinquish their sovereignty to permit enforcement of sanctions for human rights violations.

ADDRESSING WAR CRIMES AND OTHER MASSIVE HUMAN RIGHTS VIOLATIONS

In the 20th century, there have been numerous instances of massive violations of human rights perpetrated by governments either in the form of war crimes or in the context of suppressing political opposition within nations. Such violations include war crimes perpetrated during World Wars I and II; conflicts in the former Yugoslavia, Rwanda, and Kosovo; government-sanctioned suppression of political opposition in Argentina, Chile, and El Salvador; and the government-sponsored apartheid in South Africa.

In general, two major approaches have been used to address massive human rights violations (Ross, 1997). The first is through international criminal tribunals. Examples of these tribunals include the International Military Tribunal, which tried Germans accused of war crimes after World War II; the International Military Tribunal for the Far East, which tried alleged Japanese war criminals; the International Criminal Tribunal for the Former Yugoslavia; and the International Criminal Tribunal for Rwanda. The tribunal approach uses criminal trial proceedings to ascertain whether given defendants can be convicted of war crimes or criminal civil rights violations.

The second approach, which typically occurs within nations after a change in governmental leadership, is the national truth commission model. This model places less emphasis on locating and punishing perpetrators of violence, torture, and human rights abuses and more emphasis on the importance of the victims. As Ross (1998a) notes, this model is based on the assumption that official acknowledgment of severe abuses by a government-sanctioned body will aid survivor healing, will be less traumatic to the nation than an adversarial tribunal approach, and will deter future abuses. Examples of this approach include the National Commission on Disappeared Persons in Argentina, the National Commission for Truth and Reconciliation in Chile, the Commission on the Truth for El Salvador, and the Truth and Reconciliation Commission for South Africa.

For example, the South Africa Truth and Reconciliation Commission has the overall task of developing a comprehensive picture of the nature, causes, and extent of human rights violations. The Truth and Reconciliation Commission has three committees. The first committee interviews witnesses and takes testimony from survivors and perpetrators; the second committee makes recommendations regarding reparations for survivors; the third committee reviews petitions from perpetrators asking for amnesty.

THE CRIME VICTIMS' RIGHTS LAWS AND THEIR IMPLEMENTATION

There is limited research-based information about the effect of law on the treatment of survivors of torture or other human rights abuses or on how such treatment might have affected their abuse-related mental health problems or well-being. However, research on related topics, particularly on the experiences of crime victims, provides some valuable data that might be applied to survivors of torture and other human rights abuses.

One category of laws in the United States and many other nations focuses specifically on crime victims' rights. At this time, such rights have no protection in the U.S. Constitution, a fact that led the President's Task Force on Victims of Crime (1982) to propose a constitutional amendment that would give crime victims the right to be present and to be heard at all critical stages of judicial proceedings.

Such a constitutional amendment has not been enacted but has been debated in the U.S. Congress (see Barajas & Nelson, 1997, for a recent discussion). However, all 50 states have enacted statutory crime victims' bills of rights, and 29 states protect victims' rights in their state constitutions. The Victims Rights and Restitution Act of 1990 provides victims of federal crimes with many of the rights held by victims of state crimes.

Maguire and Shapland (1997) describe some important differences between the approach used to improve the treatment of crime victims in the United States and the approaches used in other parts of the world, particularly in Europe. For example, victims groups in the United States place considerable emphasis on political advocacy to pass legislation that provides more rights for victims and increased penalties for convicted criminals. In contrast, efforts in Europe are described as focusing on improving services for crime victims rather than on victims' rights per se. Maguire and Shapland note that voluntary groups established to assist victims of crime have multiplied in the United States and most European countries, as well as in other countries such as Australia and New Zealand.

In general, four major kinds of rights are included in victims' rights legislation:

1. The right to notification about case progress and key proceedings in the criminal justice system process,
2. The right to be present at such proceedings,
3. The right to be heard at such proceedings, and
4. The right to receive restitution from a convicted defendant.

The rights to notification, participation, and input are rights held by all defendants in criminal cases, and these rights are protected in the U.S. Constitution. For example, defendants must be notified about their rights (e.g., Miranda warnings). They have the right to be notified about bond hearings and trials. They also have the right to be present at all key hearings and have the right to input, which is generally provided by their defense attorney.

Crime victims' rights advocates have generally sought the same notification, participation, and input rights that defendants have. Thus, crime victims' bills of rights and constitutional amendments typically require the four types of rights listed above. Most victims' rights legislation states that judges must order the convicted defendant to repay the victims for costs they incurred because of the crime (e.g., costs for treatment of crime-related injuries or for destroyed or stolen property).

There is considerable evidence that these victims' rights are important to the general public as well as to crime victims. In a national survey of 1,000 adults in the United States (Kilpatrick, Seymour, & Boyle, 1991), most Americans said it was very important to provide victims and their families with the rights to (a) receive notifications about the times and places of trials (84%), (b) attend trials (82%), (c) discuss the case with the prosecutor during plea negotiations (72%), (d) make a victim impact statement at sentencing (72%), and (e) be informed about the defendant's release from prison (84%). Americans also favored restitution, with 81% stating that it was very important. Of those interviewed, 81% said they would pressure the government to pass laws to improve victims' rights, and 89% said they would support an amendment to their state constitution to improve victims' rights.

A similar study conducted with a household probability sample of 500 adults in South Carolina replicated these national findings of strong public support for victims' rights (Kilpatrick, Best, & Falsetti, 1993). This report also included information from a representative sample of 251 crime victims in South Carolina who had considerable exposure to the criminal justice system (Kilpatrick et al., 1989). As might be expected, an even higher percentage of crime victims than members of the general public thought victims' rights were very important. For example, 84% of South Carolinians, but 93% of crime victims, thought it was important to notify victims about defendants' release on bond.

In another large study funded by the National Institute of Justice, more than 1,300 crime victims were interviewed in four states (Beatty, Howley, Kilpatrick, & Byrne, 1996). The overwhelming majority of these victims said that the following victims' rights were "very important": (a) to be informed about an arrest (97%), (b) to be involved in the decision to drop a case (91%), (c) to be informed about defendant's release on bond (90%), (d) to be heard in decisions about bond (98%), and (e) to make a victim impact statement during parole hearings (85%) and sentencing hearings (82%). In summary, there is considerable evidence that the general public in the United States, and crime victims in particular, express strong support for victims' rights.

With respect to victims' rights in the context of this chapter, three questions should be addressed:

- To what extent are victims' rights provisions actually honored?
- Is there any relationship between the strength of legal protections for crime victims' rights and the way victims are actually treated by the criminal justice system?
- Is there any evidence that treatment of victims has any measurable effect on victims' perception of the criminal justice system?

There is substantial evidence that many crime victims' rights are not honored by the criminal justice system. For example, Kilpatrick et al. (1989) examined the implementation of crime victims' rights legislation in South Carolina. The right to notification and the right to restitution are included in the South Carolina Crime Victims Bill of Rights. This study included a survey of 251 crime victims and a review of court files from a representative sample of 984 recently adjudicated criminal court cases. Only 9% of the court files included documentation that victims were given the opportunity to make a victim impact statement at sentencing, and only 24% of victims said they had been notified about the sentencing hearing. Only 22% of case files with guilty verdicts or pleas included orders to pay restitution, while only 10% of victims said they ever received any restitution. These findings indicate that there was widespread failure to implement key aspects of South Carolina victims' rights legislation.

The extent to which victims' statutory rights appear to have influenced victim participation in the criminal justice system is provided in an excellent review by Kelly and Erez (1997). They conclude that most reforms in statutory rights have only minimal effects on victims because victims are unaware of these rights and do not exercise them. Kelly and Erez (1997) also identified another problem in that statutory bills of rights generally provide no remedy to victims whose rights are violated. Kelly (1990) concluded that victims' rights often remain privileges, which are granted or denied based on the whim of police, prosecutors, or judges.

Attribution and other theories attempt to explain how victimization and treatment by the criminal justice system might be expected to influence or mediate victims' crime-related mental health problems. Kilpatrick and Otto (1987) identified several theories that would predict that providing victims with more information, more opportunities to participate, and more services would improve their satisfaction with the criminal justice system and their psychological functioning. For example, learned helplessness theory (Abramson, Seligman, & Teasdale, 1978) predicts that crime victims who perceive themselves to have the least control and feel most helpless, vulnerable, and passive would be more likely to have more psychological distress than crime victims who perceive greater control and less helplessness. In that regard, Wortman (1983) argued that the "perception of control" variable is particularly important in understanding the effect of victimization. Kilpatrick and Otto (1987) hypothesized that giving victims input into criminal justice system proceedings should increase perceptions of control, decrease feelings of helplessness, and reduce crime-related psychological distress.

Equity theory hypothesizes that crime places the victim in an inequitable, or "one down," position vis-à-vis the criminal and that this position of inequity is what drives victims' psychological distress (Frieze, Hymer, & Greenberg, 1987). Victims can reduce feelings of inequity by either increasing their own outcomes or reducing the criminals' outcomes. For example, the victims' outcomes can be increased by good treatment and provision of needed services. The criminals' outcome can be reduced by timely punishment by the criminal justice system. Kilpatrick and Otto (1987) argued that actual outcome would be less important than how the victims perceive the outcome. Thus, victims who perceive themselves to have been treated less well than criminals should have higher distress than victims who feel that they have been treated as well as or better than the criminal.

After considering all these factors, Kilpatrick and Otto (1987) concluded,

> It appears that victims' treatment by the criminal justice system also plays an important role in their subsequent adjustment and satisfaction. Accordingly, any legislation that provides crime victims with the opportunity to have greater participation in the process could remedy some of the problems noted. Legislators should be careful, however, to insure that any rights conferred are real, that is, the victim has an avenue of redress should these rights be denied. Providing rights without remedies would result in the worst of consequences, such as feelings of helplessness, lack of control, and further victimization. (pp. 26–27).

The aforementioned research project funded by the National Institute of Justice was designed to test the hypothesis that the strength of legal protection for crime victims' rights would have a measurable effect on how victims are treated and victims' perceptions of the criminal justice system (Beatty et al., 1996). The research design involved conducting a legal analysis of the statutory and constitutional protection of crime victims' rights, rank ordering states on the basis of the strength of their legal protection of victims' rights, and selecting states with strong and weak protections for further study. Within each of two strong and two weak protection states, 1,312 adult crime victims were identified from criminal justice system records and interviewed. The sample consisted of victims of physical assault (25%), robbery (24%), sexual assault (11%), relatives of homicide victims (30%), and relatives of other crimes (10%). As had been hypothesized, victims from strong protection states were significantly more likely than victims from weak protection states to have been notified about a number of victims' rights, including bond hearings, victim services, the right to discuss the case with the prosecutor, and the right to make an impact statement. Victims from strong protection states were more likely than victims from weak protection states to participate in several criminal justice system activities, including attending bond hearings, testifying in court, making recommendations about sentences, and making impact statements at parole hearings.

Also, as hypothesized, crime victims from strong protection states were significantly more likely than those from weak protection states to rate several aspects of the criminal justice system process as "more than adequate," including (a) efforts to apprehend the perpetrator and to inform the family about case progress, (b) the fairness of the trial, and (c) the fairness of the verdict or plea. Victims from strong protection states were significantly more likely than victims from weak protection states to state that they were satisfied with police, prosecutors, victims' witness staff, judges, and the criminal justice system as a whole.

To examine potential mechanisms that might explain under what circumstances victims feel supported by the system, Beatty et al. (1996) constructed a 22-item "victim satisfaction scale" that allowed crime victims to rate their experiences with the criminal justice system, a 23-item scale that measured the extent to which victims thought that they had been informed of their rights, and a 5-item scale that measured the extent to which victims thought their victim impact statement was effective. Victim ratings of "satisfaction" were higher among female than among male victims, among White than among African-American victims, and among high-income than among low-income victims. Higher satisfaction ratings were unrelated to age. As expected, victim scores were significantly higher in strong than in weak protection states, and this difference remained after analysis of covariance that controlled for the effects of gender, race, and income. As hypothesized, there was a positive correlation between the extent to which victims were informed about the process and their higher ratings ($r = 0.59$) as well as between the extent to which victims thought their input had an effect on the case and their scores ($r = 0.38$). These findings provided strong support for the hypothesis that increasing notification of victims and providing them with opportunities for input would increase their overall sense of how they had been treated within the system.

In summary, there is substantial evidence from studies conducted in the United States that crime victims' rights are important to the general public and to crime victims, that the strength of legal protection of victims' rights appears to be related to the probability that rights provisions are implemented, and that victims who are informed and provided with opportunities for input are more satisfied with the criminal justice system.

REPARATIONS, RESTITUTION, AND COMPENSATION

The term reparation is defined by *Webster's* dictionary (1995) as (1) "restoration to a good condition, (2) a making of amends, or (3) compensation, as for war damages." In the context of victims of crime, torture, or war crimes, all three of these definitions are relevant. The state or nation has a public policy interest in restoring survivors to a good condition and in providing compensation for damages that the victimization produced. By attempting to compensate survivors for their economic losses and to ameliorate the victimization-related harm they have experienced, the state or nation also is at least partially making amends for the injustice survivors have experienced. Reparation is also consistent with the human capital approach described by Rupp and Sorel in chapter 6 in this volume.

Smith and Hillenbrand (1997) described three basic reparation approaches that have been used in the crime victim field: civil litigation, restitution, and victim compensation. Civil litigation against the perpetrator has potential in some cases, but civil litigation is expensive as well as time consuming, and either side may lack the necessary financial resources. In the United States, the Torture Protection Act allows survivors tortured in other nations to sue their torturer for civil damages in U.S. courts. Although some torture survivors have collected from damage judgments in such cases, the general feasibility of this approach is still unknown.

The second type of reparation approach, restitution, occurs when a judge orders a defendant who has been adjudicated guilty to repay victims for their crime-related economic losses. A clear limitation of restitution approaches is that victims cannot receive restitution unless they report the crime to police; the perpetrator is arrested, indicted, and convicted; the judge orders restitution; and the perpetrator can and does actually pay the restitution. Several studies have found that only a small percentage of eligible crime victims ever collect any restitution (e.g., Beatty et al., 1996; Kilpatrick, Tidwell, Cornelison, & Byrne, 1997; Kilpatrick et al., 1989; Tobolowsky, 1993), either because judges do not order it or because perpetrators cannot pay it. Restitution would appear to offer limited prospects for survivors of torture who are seeking reparations.

The third reparation approach, victim compensation, has considerable applicability, particularly to crime victims. According to the *International Crime Victim Compensation Program Directory* (Office for Victims of Crime, U.S. Department of Justice, 1997), all 50 states in the United States and at least 30 other nations provide some financial assistance to victims of crime or terrorism. This directory provides a list of nations that have compensation programs and describes eligibility criteria, application procedures, benefit and award limits, compensable costs, and funding sources. Unlike civil litigation or restitution, crime victim compensation is paid by a state or national agency. Victims are not eligible to receive compensation unless they report crimes to police within a specified length of time after the crime occurs. Compensable costs for eligible victims vary across jurisdictions but generally include medical expenses for treatment of crime-related injuries, mental health counseling, lost wages, and funeral expenses for homicide victims. Generally, there are maximum limits for compensation. In the

United States, most states pay a maximum of between $15,000 and $25,000. Maximum benefit levels are considerably higher in some nations (e.g., £500,000 in the United Kingdom). Funding in the United States is provided at the state level by fees or charges assessed against offenders. This funding is supplemented by the Federal Office for Victims of Crime Act Fund.

As noted by Smith and Hillenbrand (1997), crime victims' compensation is based on the assumption that the state has an obligation to crime victims. In civil litigation and restitution, the assumption is that the perpetrator has the obligation to repay victims' crime-related financial losses. A clear advantage of this approach for victims is that receiving compensation is not dependent on the arrest and conviction of the perpetrator or on obtaining a judgment in a civil suit. Disadvantages are that financial losses of property crime victims are generally not covered and that only a small percentage of eligible victims know about compensation programs or seek compensation (Elias, 1986; Friedman, Bischoff, Davis, & Person, 1982; Kilpatrick et al., 1989).

Although not labeled as compensation per se, compensation-like reparations are sometimes provided to other types of trauma survivors. For example, combat veterans with service-related disabilities in the United States and other nations are often compensated or provided with free health care services. In the United States, the Department of Veterans Affairs provides legally mandated payments to veterans with service-connected disabilities. Additionally, the Department of Veterans Affairs provides specialized health and mental health care to veterans with service-connected disabilities, including PTSD.

RESTORATIVE JUSTICE

Another important concept in the criminal justice area with implications for survivors of torture and human rights abuses is the concept of restorative justice (Umbreit, 1994). Traditional criminal justice system approaches in the United States view crimes as transgressions against the state, which makes the state the primary victim and the victimized individual the secondary victim. In contrast, restorative justice approaches view the individual crime victim as the primary victim and the state as only a secondary victim. The major focus of restorative justice is to hold offenders accountable for the crime by making them repay victims for their actions (Zehr, 1990). Thus, restorative justice approaches place greater emphasis on making offenders apologize to victims and making good regarding victims' losses rather than on punishing offenders.

In a recent review of research on victim–offender reconciliation programs, Smith and Hillenbrand (1997) note that most of the programs that have been evaluated are those involving minor property crime cases and offenders who are strangers. Typically, these programs are mediated by trained professionals and provide victims with the chance to face their offenders. The victims explain how the crime has affected their lives. Offenders then work out agreements with the victims as to how the offenders will pay back the victims for their crime-related losses.

Coates and Gehm (1989) found that the majority of victims who had participated in victim–offender reconciliation programs were satisfied. Among satisfied victims, factors related to satisfaction included having a chance to learn from
perpetrators why the crime was committed, receiving restitution, and hearing
perpetrators say they were sorry. Umbreit (1994) compared three groups of victims and offenders who participated in victim–offender mediation programs: (a) a
mediation group, (b) a comparison group that was referred but did not participate, and (c) a comparison group that was not referred but was matched on key
variables. Most victims and offenders who participated in mediation expressed
satisfaction with the program; offenders in the program were more likely to pay
restitution, and victims in the program expressed less fear of being revictimized
by the offender after the program than before the program. Thus, the findings
suggest that mediation programs produce promising results that warrant additional research.

Victim–offender mediation programs are not without their problems or crit-
ics, however, and the extent to which such programs are applicable to serious violent crimes is an open question. For example, it is unclear whether victims or family
members of victims of violent crimes such as rape or homicide would be more
interested in mediation programs than in seeing offenders receive appropriate
punishment. Likewise, it could be argued that the state has an interest in violent
crime perpetrators receiving substantial punishment. The state's interest is to
(a) attempt to deter other criminals from committing similar acts by punishing
perpetrators, (b) protect the public from future acts of violence by incarcerating
perpetrators, and (c) provide justice by providing punishment that is commensu-
rate with the crime.

IMPLICATIONS AND POLICY RECOMMENDATIONS

Lessons learned from studies of crime victims and the law in the United States
are not necessarily applicable to other cultures. However, the research findings
from this literature may provide relevant scientific information for those public
policymakers addressing the problems of survivors of torture and serious human
rights violations. These research recommendations and potential implications are
offered with the knowledge that they may not be applicable in all situations.

- Human rights and crime victims' rights are important largely because of
  the resulting substantial harm that is often sustained by victims.
- How crime victims are treated by the system that is processing their case
  has an effect on their satisfaction with the criminal justice system and appears to influence their psychological well-being. Crime victims who have
  enforceable rights within the criminal justice system are more likely to feel
  that they have been treated better if they have been informed about case
  status and proceedings. They are also more satisfied with the criminal justice system than victims without enforceable rights. Victims who think their

input had an effect on the case are more satisfied than victims who lacked input or thought their input had no effect. This finding suggests that survivors of torture and human rights violations also may benefit by having enforceable rights, including the rights to be informed and to provide input.

- Many victims of crime have a powerful need to tell their story, to tell how the crime affected their lives, and to have some vehicle for the state to officially acknowledge the magnitude of what happened to them. As with victims of crime, survivors of torture may benefit from having the opportunity to voluntarily describe the effect of the atrocities they have experienced.

  In most cases, truth commissions provide a voluntary opportunity for survivors to provide this type of testimony, which may have beneficial effects for most survivors who testify because it gives them an opportunity to be heard. By providing this opportunity, such commissions are validating that what happened to victims was important.

- Reparations are important to most crime victims. Moreover, nations have a substantial public policy interest in restoring crime victims to a productive life. Although obtaining and allocating resources can often be very difficult, particularly in developing nations, failing to allocate sufficient resources to help victims recover from the effects of crime, torture, and other human rights abuses can have a major negative effect on a nation's human capital and its ability to be economically productive.

- Several potential funding mechanisms may be appropriate for expanding compensation programs to provide additional services to survivors of torture and human rights abuses: One example is the U.S. Victim of Crime Fund, a compensation fund supported by fines and forfeitures from convicted criminals. Alternatively, governments with existing crime victim compensation programs can expand these funds to include survivors of torture. Additional funding would be required to ensure that sufficient funding is available, but this approach has additional value because such crime victims' compensation programs already exist. In addition, governments could appropriate new funds directly to support compensation programs.

- Based on what has been learned from crime victim research, it appears that restorative justice principles may be expected to benefit survivors of torture and human rights abuses. These principles suggest that it is important to (a) provide the opportunity for public testimony, (b) deliver a clear governmental statement that what happened was wrong, (c) make apologies and offer restitution from perpetrators, and (d) give reparations to survivors. The latter is a significant factor in restorative justice approaches.

REFERENCES

Abramson, L. Y., Seligman, M. E., & Teasdale, J. D. (1978). Learned helplessness in humans: Critique and reformation. *Journal of Abnormal Psychology, 87,* 49–74.

Barajas, R., & Nelson, S. A. (1997). The proposed crime victims' federal constitutional amendment: Working toward a proper balance. *Baylor Law Review, 49*(1), 1–31.

Beatty, D., Howley, S., Kilpatrick, D. G., & Byrne, C. (1996). *Statutory and constitutional protection of victims' rights: Implementation and impact on crime victims.* Final Report submitted to the U.S. Department of Justice, Cooperative Agreement 93-IJ-CX-K003.

Coates, R., & Gehm, J. (1989). An empirical assessment. In M. Wright & B. Galaway (Eds.), *Mediation and criminal justice.* Newbury Park, CA: Sage.

Donnelly, J. (1996). Rethinking human rights. *Current History, 95,* 387–391.

Elias, R. (1986). *The politics of victimization: Victims, victimology, and human rights.* New York: Oxford University Press.

Friedman, K., Bischoff, H., Davis, R., & Person, A. (1982). *Samaritan blues: Victims' and helpers' reactions to crime.* National Institute of Justice, Grant No. 79 NIAX 0059, Summary of Grant Report.

Frieze, I. H., Hymer, S., & Greenberg, M. S. (1987). Describing the crime victim: Psychological reactions to victimization. *Professional Psychology: Research and Practice, 18*(4), 299–315.

Kelly, D. P. (1990). Victim participation in the criminal justice system. In A. J. Lurigio, W. A. Skogan, & R. C. Davis (Eds.), *Victims of crime: Problems, policies, and programs* (pp. 172–187). Newberry Park, CA: Sage.

Kelly, D. P., & Erez, E. (1997). Victim participation in the criminal justice system. In R. C. Davis, A. J. Lurigio, & W. G. Skogan (Eds.), *Victims of crime* (2nd ed., pp. 231–244). Thousand Oaks, CA: Sage.

Kilpatrick, D. G., Best, C. L., & Falsetti, S. A. (1993). *South Carolina speaks out: Attitudes about crime and victims' rights.* Charleston, SC: Medical University of South Carolina.

Kilpatrick, D. G., & Otto, R. K. (1987). Constitutionally guaranteed participation in criminal proceedings for victims: Potential effects on psychological functioning. *Wayne State Law Review, 34*(1), 7–28.

Kilpatrick, D. G., Seymour, A. K., & Boyle, J. (1991). *America speaks out: Citizens' attitudes about victims' rights and violence.* Arlington, VA: National Center for Victims of Crime.

Kilpatrick, D. G., Tidwell, R., Cornelison, V., & Byrne, C. (1997). *Balancing the scales: A master plan for crime victim services in South Carolina.* Final Report submitted to the Bureau of Justice Statistics (#1F94079) through the South Carolina Department of Public Safety.

Kilpatrick, D. G., Tidwell, R. P., Walker, E., Resnick, H. S., Saunders, B. E., Paduhovich, J., & Lipovsky, J. A. (1989). *Victims rights and services in South Carolina: The dream, the law, the reality.* Final Report for Justice Assistance Act Grant No. 86-024, submitted to the Division of Public Safety Programs, Office of the Governor of the State of South Carolina, March 1989.

Maguire, M., & Shapland, J. (1997). Provision for victims in an international context. In R. C. Davis, A. J. Lurigio, & W. G. Skogan (Eds.), *Victims of crime* (2nd ed., pp. 211–228). Thousand Oaks, CA: Sage.

Office for Victims of Crime, U.S. Department of Justice. (1997). *International crime victim compensation program directory.* Washington, DC: Author.

President's Task Force on Victims of Crime. (1982). *President's Task Force on Victims of Crime final report.* Washington, DC: U.S. Government Printing Office.

Ross, M. (1997). *Understanding forced migration through a collective human rights paradigm.* Unpublished manuscript.

Ross, M. (1998a). *National truth commission model for justice after mass violence.* Unpublished manuscript.

Ross, M. (1998b). *Overview of the history of international criminal tribunals.* Unpublished manuscript.

Smith, B. E., & Hillenbrand, S. (1997). Making victims whole again: Restitution, victim–offender reconciliation programs, and compensation. In R. C. Davis, A. J. Lurigio, & W. G. Skogan (Eds.), *Victims of crime* (2nd ed., pp. 245–256). Thousand Oaks, CA: Sage.

Tobolowsky, P. M. (1993). Restitution in the federal criminal justice system. *Judicature, 77,* 90–95.

Torture Victims Relief Act. 28 U.S.C.A. § 1350 (1998). Pub. L. No. 105–320.

Umbreit, M. (1994). *Victim meets offender: The impact of restorative justice and mediation.* Monsey, NY: Criminal Justice Press.

United Nations. (1951). *U.N. convention relating to the status of refugees.* Adopted on July 28, 1951, by the U.N. Conference of Plenipotentiaries on the Status of Refugees and Stateless Persons convened under General Assembly resolution 429 (V) of December 14, 1950, entry into force April 22, 1954, in accordance with article 43. [U.N. publications may be ordered from United Nations Publications, Room DC2-0853, New York, New York 10017, USA Telephone: (212) 963-8302, (800) 253-9646, Fax: (212) 963-3489, e-mail <publications@un.org>, Web site <http://www.un.org/Pubs/Sales>.]

United Nations. (1984). *Article 1, United Nations convention against torture and other cruel, inhuman, and degrading treatment or punishment.* New York: U.N. Department of Public Information.

United Nations. (1985). *Declaration on basic principles of justice for victims of crime and abuses of power.* New York: U.N. Department of Public Information.

The Victims' Rights and Restitution Act of 1990. 22 U.S.C.A. § 2151 (1990). Pub. L. No. 101-647.

Victims of Crime Act, 42 U.S.C.: 10601 et seq. (1984).

Webster's II new riverside university dictionary. (1995). Boston: Houghton Mifflin.

Wortman, C. B. (1983). Coping with victimization: Conclusions and implications for future research. *Journal of Societal Issues, 39,* 195–221.

Zehr, H. (1990). *Changing lenses: A new focus for crime and justice.* Scottsdale, PA: Herald.

VI

Discussion

21

Future Directions

ELLEN GERRITY, TERENCE M. KEANE, FARRIS TUMA, AND SISTER DIANNA ORTIZ

The heart of this book is a summary of what is known about the mental health consequences of torture and other violent and traumatic events. Central to this review are the research recommendations and their implications for treatment, research, and policy. The contributors made a concerted effort to gather and present this information within a scientific context that included the experiences of survivors, clinicians, policymakers, and researchers.

In this final chapter, selected research findings from each section of this book are used to point to a direction for the future. The intention is to help shape research that will provide a greater understanding of the mental health consequences of this most horrific experience and to develop effective services, treatment programs, and relevant policies for survivors of torture. Each contributor summarized the strongest scientific or clinical findings of relevance to research, service delivery, treatment, or policy. The reader is referred to the individual chapters for further information on the specific issues highlighted here.

ELLEN GERRITY • National Institute of Mental Health, Neuroscience Center Building, Bethesda, Maryland 20892.   TERENCE M. KEANE • Department of Psychiatry, Boston University School of Medicine, Boston, Massachusetts 02130.   FARRIS TUMA • National Institute of Mental Health, Neuroscience Center Building, Bethesda, Maryland 20892.   SISTER DIANNA ORTIZ • Guatemalan Human Rights Commission, Washington, D.C. 20017.

The Mental Health Consequences of Torture, edited by Ellen Gerrity, Terence M. Keane, and Farris Tuma. Kluwer Academic/Plenum Publishers, New York, 2001.

335

SUMMARY OF SELECTED RESEARCH FINDINGS

- Precise estimates of the extent of torture are not available at present, and epidemiological studies specifically focused on torture experiences are greatly needed to enhance this knowledge base. Estimates of torture among refugees alone range from 5% to 35% of the world's 14 million refugees, although millions more internally displaced persons and asylees are also at risk. A report from Amnesty International in 1999 stated that systematic use of torture and severe ill treatment was ongoing in 121 of the world's 204 countries. Thus, the experience of torture—how widespread it is, how to help survivors, and how to prevent it—represents a severely understudied area that deserves greater attention from policymakers, researchers, and clinicians.

- Torture survivors can be found in virtually all countries that receive refugees and asylees, but these survivors represent only a small proportion of the number of torture survivors worldwide. Epidemiological studies that focus on the prevalence of torture in various countries need to look beyond at-risk populations (i.e., refugees) to the general population to obtain the most accurate estimates. For example, population surveys or key informant studies with health clinics or treatment providers could be conducted to determine the size of the population of torture survivors in a particular region.

- The experience of torture can result in the development of a wide range of psychological, behavioral, and medical problems, including specific psychiatric conditions, such as posttraumatic stress disorder (PTSD), depression, anxiety disorders, and psychotic conditions. Torture also can lead to sleep disorders, sexual dysfunction, chronic irritability, physical illness, and a disruption of interpersonal relations as well as occupational, family, and social functioning. Often torture occurs in the context of many other life stressors, such as war, terrorism, loss of family and community, and financial setbacks, all of which can be extremely severe stressors. Research suggests that torture exerts an independent effect separate from the effects of the stressful context within which it usually occurs.

- Survivors of torture can recover to the point where they resume functioning at home and at work, but many have severe difficulties. An inability to resume normal functioning exacts a long-standing toll on personal and economic viability. Risk-factor studies have not yet demonstrated specific factors associated with difficulties in recovery, but there is some suggestion that situations that are more unexpected and less controllable are potentially much more likely to result in long-term impairments for individuals. Additional studies of risk factors and resilience are needed to further address these questions.

- Torture can have persistent and lifelong effects. Data from several research programs in the United States, Europe, and the Middle East indicate that the effects of torture can extend throughout the life of the survivor, affecting his or her psychological, familial, and economic functioning. Studies of former prisoners of war and Holocaust survivors confirm that without appropriate intervention, the negative effects of systematic torture can persist throughout the life of the individual.

- Studies conducted over the past 10 years strongly suggest that people who develop PTSD may also experience serious neurobiological changes, including (a) changes in the body's ability to respond to stress (through alterations in stress hormones); (b) changes in attention and arousal (through changes in neurotransmitter systems); (c) changes in the body's response to infection and disease (through changes in the immune system); (d) the development of an imbalance in the noradrenergic system; (e) heightened psychophysiologic arousal and reactivity; and (f) possible changes in the hippocampus, an area in the brain related to contextual memory. Thus, the development of PTSD has direct implications for the functioning of numerous biological systems essential to human functioning. These neurobiological abnormalities may be responsible for the chronic physical health problems often associated with PTSD and depression.

- Over the past several years, assessment instruments have been developed and refined that attempt to measure the extent of exposure to torture and related traumatic events. Other well-established diagnostic instruments that measure PTSD, depression, and other psychiatric conditions are valuable clinical and research tools. Though difficult to develop, sensitive and scientifically based screening instruments are critically important to advance this field and to more accurately assess the mental health consequences of torture.

- As a form of torture, rape and sexual assault have severely negative outcomes. Most commonly used against women, rape may also be systematically used against both men and women and is frequently used to terrorize communities in which there is political unrest and war. The effects of rape are felt by the survivor herself, her spouse or partner, her children, and others in the surrounding community. Research has shown that rape can lead to the development of PTSD, depression, substance abuse, panic disorder, and other psychiatric conditions. Rape can also lead to higher rates of somatic problems and utilization of scarce and expensive health care services. For some survivors, the effect of rape is lifelong and recovery can be slow and, in some cases, negligible. Treatment studies with survivors of acute rape experiences have shown promising outcomes, particularly when professional and paraprofessional staff are available and cognitive–behavioral methods are employed. Research is needed on treatment for adults and children exposed to multiple or long-term rape or sexual assault and on the value of pharmacologic treatment with survivors of rape.

- Treatments specifically focused on torture recovery are in an early stage of development. Most treatments for torture survivors were developed within clinical settings, often under extremely challenging conditions, and many have yet to be fully tested and evaluated. Most psychiatric treatment was provided as part of other health care for refugees. Therefore, multiple methods and treatments were used and involved behavioral, psychopharmacological, psychodynamic, and cognitive methods. Individual, family, and group therapies have also been employed. More recently, treatment programs were developed in neuropsychiatric settings in which empirical tests of treatment efficacy were possible. Initial studies supporting the use of behavioral and cognitive–behavioral interventions appear encouraging. Much more work is needed on the psychiatric treatment of torture survivors and their psychosocial problems and associated impairments.

• Few studies have directly investigated the effectiveness of psychopharmacological interventions for torture survivors. An accurate clinical diagnosis is critical to determine the best medication regimen for the particular pattern of symptoms experienced by each torture survivor. Antidepressant medications, such as selective serotonin reuptake inhibitors, antianxiety agents, and antipsychotic medications, may play a role in the appropriate treatment of a torture survivor. The psychopharmacologist also needs to be aware of potential gender, racial, and cultural differences in response to medications. Pharmacokinetic differences in the metabolism of medications among racial and ethnic groups are well known and need to be considered when prescribing. Finally, the torture survivor's views about medication have been known to be an integral part of the treatment decision-making process. Torture survivors may be open to accepting psychotropic medication, for example, to lessen depression, while also exploring traditional medicines, such as natural remedies prepared by folk healers. Others favor alternative forms of therapy, such as bodywork, massage, aroma or sound therapy, special breathing, and relaxation exercises.

• The cost of disabilities that result from torture and related traumatic events is now being quantified using contemporary econometric methods. As these methods become widely accepted, the exact economic toll of torture on the individual, the family, the community, and the society can be more accurately calculated. The concept of disability adjusted life years, when applied to torture and its aftereffects, may prove to be an important contribution to the measurement of broad-based economic costs associated with torture. The use of these kinds of methods has also begun to show evidence, as it has done with depression, of the economic value of providing treatment and rehabilitation for torture survivors as an important part of broader discussions of the need for care.

• Children and adolescents have experienced torture directly or indirectly (through witnessing the torture of others, especially parents and loved ones). Research has shown that children and adolescents who have been exposed to torture can be identified through sensitive case-finding methods using standardized assessment instruments. These screening methods can also help determine the severity of distress (e.g., PTSD, depression, conduct disorder) among such children and adolescents. A comprehensive approach is needed to help shape developmentally appropriate interventions for optimal healing and recovery of children.

- A family can be severely disrupted by the torture of one or more of its members. In some instances, the parents of traumatized children may also have been tortured or otherwise traumatized, and problems in the parent–child relationships and the family interaction patterns may result. Changes in the course of the child's development are frequently observed in families that have been traumatized and are often an ongoing and serious concern for such families. Interventions geared to remediating developmental changes may prove to be the most effective for the resumption of stable family functioning. In many cases, working with the entire family may be the most beneficial approach, for both the child's recovery and the recovery of the family.

- Research suggests that in relatively stable social contexts, school-based interventions for children and adolescents are among the most enduring because of the involvement of teachers, counselors, and peers in the behavior change process. School-based programs may be most valuable when the parents and siblings are also traumatized, and their daily home functioning is disorganized. Working with the school may result in the most favorable outcomes; however, the conditions in the society must be stable enough to support such interventions. Further research is needed on effective interventions for children and adolescents in refugee camps or in situations in which conflicts are ongoing.

- In settings where few mental health professionals are available, alternative approaches are needed to assist torture survivors with their mental health needs. These alternative approaches may involve (a) using primary care providers (including indigenous providers), (b) training paraprofessionals, (c) involving spiritual or religious leaders, and (d) using whatever media or technology might be available (i.e., radio or television). In some settings, viable mental health programs have been developed by identifying social or political leaders in the communities, training them in methods of education and intervention, and assisting them in providing self-help tools to the communities they serve.

- Timely access to mental health care for torture survivors is an important part of recovery. Programs that are integrated into a well-functioning primary care system that is accessible may optimize effectiveness and improve overall outcomes for the survivors. However, such care needs to be delivered by well-trained providers who are informed of the issues associated with the treatment of torture survivors. It is also important that they possess knowledge not only of the country in which the person was tortured but also of the survivor's culture.

- Many torture survivors are refugees who live in limbo, housed in camps until decisions are made regarding their future. Such uncertain and often uncomfortable circumstances put these populations at high risk for further exposure to trauma, while leaving untreated the consequences of their earlier experiences. Mental health services for torture survivors in these camps should be a standard part of the primary health care services that are made available in the camps.

- The establishment of specialized mental health care for torture survivors in more developed countries has special advantages. Well-trained staff and focused services can be made available locally, and consultants can be made available worldwide. Specialists with backgrounds and experience in PTSD, depression, and other related conditions and providers who are trained in the culture of the targeted population are particularly needed to ensure that the most effective interventions can be offered.

- Conclusions drawn from research on crime victims suggest that the processes associated with restitution, reparation, and restoration may be expected to improve survivors' satisfaction with the system that has been created to promote justice. Timely communication regarding the disposition of cases involving perpetrators and allowing survivors to have input into the decision-making processes regarding restitution, reparation, and restoration may be expected to enhance the recovery process. This research also suggests that efforts to bring together the survivor and the perpetrator may prove of value in the recovery process. In such a meeting, the perpetrator would be obligated to hear directly what the effects of his or her violent actions have been on the survivor, the survivor's family, the community, and the whole society. The principles of restorative justice appear to be applicable to survivors of torture and other human rights abuses. These include the opportunity for public testimony, governmental apology, and reparations to survivors.

- Cultural and language differences often appear when providing care to torture survivors and refugees, and they must be addressed for services to be effective. It is likely that with each situation professionals will need to explore the cultural nuances and the meaning of the experiences of the survivors. Whether survivors are African, Asian, Southeast Asian, Latin American, North American, or European, they will interpret their experiences with a unique worldview. Interventions that incorporate relevant language and cultural factors into treatment will optimize outcomes. A powerful issue for the torture survivor could be the role that governments and health care professionals might have played in the torture experience itself. Understanding and dealing with this issue in a sensitive manner may be critical to the delivery of effective treatments that can be accepted by the survivors.

- Research priorities should include studies of the mechanisms associated with traumatization, risk factors for the development of persistent psychiatric disorders, factors related to resilience and posttorture recovery, the interaction of torture and related stressors such as refugee status and acculturation, the effects of impunity for those responsible for torture, and psychosocial and psychopharmacological interventions. The direct involvement of survivors in the development of research priorities and implementation of research studies is an integral part of conducting meaningful research in this area of science, research that will lead toward improved treatment, service delivery, and human rights policies.

CONCLUSION

Torture has existed throughout history and in diverse forms, including imprisonment, crucifixion, beatings, solitary confinement, and genocidal rape. It has left a permanent legacy on every continent and culture, past and present. History has recorded at least some of the faces and names of those who have borne witness to torture with their bodies and their lives—the early Christians, slaves, the indigenous of many countries, and victims and survivors of the Holocaust, to name only a few.

The diversity of victims throughout the centuries suggests what is obvious: No one is immune to torture. People of any time, ethnicity, age, religion, gender, and social class can be touched by it. Those affected include not only those directly victimized, but also their families, communities, and societies. The swath torture cuts through humanity today is wide and deep. The governments of more than 120 countries engage in torture or similar ill treatment. While the enormity of this crime has led so often to despair and apathy, even its most horrifying effects have failed to completely destroy hope and responsive action to confront it.

Mental health professionals have begun to show that substantial recovery from the effects of torture is possible. In recent years, they have conducted wide-ranging research into torture and its crippling effects and investigated the effects of many forms of severe trauma. They have acknowledged the importance of the issue and the need to understand it. Research into torture has increased, and a new important development has occurred: Torture survivors are not simply, as in the past, subjects to be observed and evaluated. Many mental health professionals now understand that survivors must be among the evaluators and are central to the development of meaningful research and treatment.

In an effort to better understand torture and its effects, the National Institute of Mental Health brought together researchers, clinicians, and policymakers with torture survivors. Mental health professionals listened to the views and experiences of torture survivors from Asia, Africa, North and South America, and Europe. This exchange provided a wide window for the nontortured to receive a glimpse into the survivors' world. Survivors viewed these meetings as a ray of hope in what is often the dark midnight of their own despair; the mental health professionals viewed these meetings as a rare and generous gift, one that seared the soul but also opened the mind and vision to what is needed to shape a better profession and practice. Survivors had the opportunity to reclaim their voice, to define themselves and their own behavior, and to exercise their right to speak for themselves. The mental health professionals had the opportunity to review their own preconceived beliefs, to accept the gift of the reality of the survivor, and to engage in a dialogue that was painful, gratifying, and educational.

Torture has the ability to reduce one to silence. At times, its sole purpose is to punish those who express their views and to send a message to those who otherwise might dare to speak. During the torture, answers are criticized as "wrong" and therefore punishable. After the torture, survivors emerge from that experience of ultimate cruelty with the feeling that no one cares about them and that no one will believe them. To be asked to share their views and to be listened to, cared about, and believed can be a powerful healing experience in itself for survivors. While survivors and mental health professionals certainly do not always agree on every point, they have been able to come together, listen, converse, and learn from one another.

This volume is a public testament to the reality of torture and its consequences. This subject deserves the most serious consideration by those in many professions to reduce the silence that has too often surrounded it. Torture can challenge our most basic concepts about the nature of human beings and reduce people to feelings of helplessness, despair, guilt, and denial.

This work has been an effort to break through the wall of silence and to bring the scientific and decision-making communities together with the general public to share this information. Much of what these diverse communities know of torture is included in these pages and is accompanied by recommendations for future research. These conclusions are drawn not only by academicians and other professionals but also by survivors themselves.

Finally, we conclude with the hope that many who work in this field will find the information in this book of value in their work. All who read this work will recognize that increasing our knowledge of the effects of torture and providing appropriate services for survivors and their families are only two of the issues that challenge us. Research and treatment for torture survivors would not be necessary if torture could be prevented from ever occurring, and thus it is prevention—the abolishment of torture in our world—that would be the ultimate cure.

As noted at the opening of this book, this work is dedicated to those who experience the horror of torture—past, present, and future—and to those who work to end it.

Index

Contributors
Biographical Information

EDITORS

Ellen Gerrity has worked in the field of traumatic stress for more than 20 years as a researcher, clinician, teacher, and research administrator. As the Associate Director for Aggression and Trauma Research at the National Institute of Mental Health (NIMH), Dr. Gerrity headed the NIMH Working Group on the Mental Health Consequences of Torture and Related Violence and chaired the 1997 Interagency Conference on Survivors of Torture: Improving Our Understanding. In 1997, Dr. Gerrity received the National Institutes of Health Director's Award for her work in support of traumatic stress research. Most recently, Dr. Gerrity has worked as a Congressional Legislative Assistant for mental health issues in the office of Senator Paul Wellstone (D-Minnesota). Dr. Gerrity is the coeditor of *Ethnocultural Aspects of Post-Traumatic Stress Disorder* (1996, American Psychological Association Press) and serves on the editorial board of the *Journal of Traumatic Stress.*

Terence M. Keane is Professor and Vice Chairman of Psychiatry at the Boston University School of Medicine. He is also the Chief of Psychology and the Director of the National Center for Posttraumatic Stress Disorder (PTSD) at the Boston Veterans Affairs (VA) Medical Center. Dr. Keane is a Fellow of the American Psychological Association and the American Psychological Society and has published extensively on the assessment and treatment of PTSD. His international contributions to the field of PTSD have been recognized by many honors and awards. During much of the preparation of this book, Dr. Keane was the immediate past President of the International Society for Traumatic Stress Studies.

Farris Tuma is Program Chief of the Traumatic Stress Research Program and the Disruptive Behavior and Attention Deficit Disorder Research Program in the Division of Mental Disorders, Behavioral Research, and AIDS at the National Institute of Mental Health. Dr. Tuma manages an extramural program of research concerning child and adult trauma and victimization, including the behavioral, clinical, neurobiological, epidemiological, and social science aspects of violence and traumatic stress as they relate to mental health and illness.

CONTRIBUTORS

Metin Basoglu is Head of the Section on Traumatic Studies at the Institute of Psychiatry, King's College, University of London, and the Director of the Istanbul Centre for Behaviour Research and Therapy in Turkey. Dr. Basoglu has published extensively on the phenomenology of behavioral and drug treatment of anxiety disorders, including obsessive-compulsive disorder, panic disorder and agoraphobia, and PTSD. He has conducted research into the psychological effects of political violence and torture and effective methods of treating torture survivors. He also has written numerous publications on human rights and psychological effects of torture. Currently, he is coordinating a multisite collaborative study of the psychological and cognitive effects of wars, political violence, and torture.

Brian Engdahl is a consulting psychologist at the U.S. Department of Veterans Affairs Medical Center in Minneapolis, Minnesota, and Clinical Associate Professor at the University of Minnesota (Minneapolis). He has received awards for service to former prisoners of war (POWs) and victims of torture. Clinically, he serves combat veterans, POWs, and veterans with spinal cord and brain injuries. His research focuses on sleep disturbances, brain function, and the diagnosis of PTSD among trauma survivors.

John A. Fairbank is Associate Professor of Medical Psychology in the Department of Psychiatry at Duke University Medical School and Research Scholar in the Department of Psychology, Social, and Health Sciences. His research interests include traumatic stress, PTSD, and mental health treatment. He serves on the editorial board of the *Journal of Traumatic Stress* and serves on the Board of Directors for the International Society for Traumatic Stress Studies. Dr. Fairbank also currently serves on scientific advisory panels for the Institute of Medicine at the National Academy of Sciences and for the Department of Veterans Affairs.

Matthew J. Friedman is Executive Director of the U.S. Department of Veterans Affairs National Center for Post-Traumatic Stress Disorder and Professor of Psychiatry and of Pharmacology at Dartmouth Medical School. He has worked with PTSD patients as a clinician and researcher for 25 years and has published extensively on stress and PTSD. Throughout his professional career, Dr. Friedman has combined his strong concerns about the quality of psychiatric care with a scientific commitment to understanding the etiology, diagnosis, and treatment of clinical phenomena. As a result, his publications span a variety of psychiatric issues, including PTSD, biological psychiatry, psychopharmacology, and clinical outcome studies on depression, anxiety, schizophrenia, and chemical dependency. Dr. Friedman is listed in *The Best Doctors in America*, is a former president of the International Society for Traumatic Stress Studies, and has served on many VA and NIMH research, education, and policy committees, including the NIMH Biobehavioral and Behavioral Processes (BBBP-5) Study Section and the VA's Persian Gulf Expert Scientific Committee. He has received many honors including the International Society for Traumatic Stress Studies Lifetime Achievement Award in 1999.

Merle Friedman is a clinical psychologist and Certified Trauma Specialist. She is Founder/Director of Psych-Action, a management consultancy, and part-time member of the faculty of the Psychology Department, University of the Witwatersrand, Johannesburg, South Africa. She was one of the founders of the Wits Trauma Clinic and is a member of the Board of Directors of Business Against Crime, Gauteng. She is involved in training professional and nonprofessional trauma workers and in research with the South African Police Service. Her primary academic involvement is with issues of reconciliation and violence in postapartheid South Africa.

Malcolm Gordon is a psychologist in the Adult Psychopathology and Prevention Research Branch at NIMH. Dr. Gordon has served as an extramural science research administrator in the areas of child and adult trauma and victimization and adult psychopathology for more than 20 years. He has conducted research in the areas of child abuse, psychobiological development, and adjustment of immigrant children and has a particular interest in behavioral research methodology. Dr. Gordon is a recognized expert in the field of child trauma and has served as an adviser on child and adult trauma research for many federal agencies.

James M. Jaranson is Director of Medical Services at the Center for Victims of Torture in Minneapolis, Minnesota, and Director of the Cultural Psychiatry Training Program at the University of Minnesota, where he holds faculty appointments in the Department of Psychiatry in the Medical School and in the Division of Epidemiology in the School of Public Health. Dr. Jaranson founded the International Mental Health Program in the Psychiatry Department of St. Paul-Ramsey Medical Center (Regions Hospital) in St. Paul, Minnesota. He represents North America on the International Council for Torture Victims, cochairs the section on the Psychological Consequences of Torture and Persecution of the World Psychiatric Association, and is a steering committee member of the Society for the Study of Psychiatry and Culture. Dr. Jaranson has studied, written, and lectured on many aspects of the care of refugee patients and torture survivors and has worked clinically in crosscultural mental health settings since medical school.

Boaz Kahana is Professor of Psychology at Cleveland State University and Fellow of the American Psychological Society and the Gerontological Society of America. His research encompasses both normal aging and the long-term effects of trauma. Among the populations he has studied are Pearl Harbor survivors and survivors of the Nazi Holocaust in three different countries. His ongoing research includes a study of the effects of cancer trauma on the elderly and an 11-year longitudinal study of physical frailty among the elderly with regard to issues of social support, mental health, and other psychological variables. He was recently given an award for Excellence in Gerontological Research by the Ohio Research Council on Aging and the Ohio Network of Educational Consultants in the Field of Aging. He has been awarded NIMH and National Institute on Aging research grants dealing with stress and extreme stress among the elderly and coping and adaptation among the elderly in community and institutional settings. He has also served as a peer reviewer for NIMH, the former Alcohol, Drug Abuse, and Mental Health Administration, and other federal funding agencies.

Eva Kahana is the Pierce T. and Elizabeth D. Robson Professor of Humanities, Chair of the Department of Sociology, and Director of the Elderly Care Research Center at Case Western Reserve University. She is a Fellow of the Gerontological Society of America and has received the Society's Distinguished Mentorship Award. Her other awards include the Mary E. Switzer Distinguished Fellow of the National Institute of Disability and Rehabilitation, the 1997 Distinguished Scholar Award from the section of Aging and Life Course of the American Sociological Association, the Heller Award from the Menorah Park Center for the Aged, and the Polisher Award of the Gerontological Society of America for her outstanding contribution to applied gerontology. She is currently Chairperson of the American Sociological Association's section on Aging and the Life Course. She has published extensively in the areas of stress, coping, and health among the aged; late-life migration; and environmental influences on older persons. Her most recent formulations focus on the role of preventive and corrective proactivity of older adults in shaping successful aging.

Marianne Kastrup is the Medical Director at the Rehabilitation Center for Torture Victims in Copenhagen, Denmark. She is also the Secretary for Finance and Chairperson of the International Review Committee on the Abuse of Psychiatry for the World Psychiatric Association. Dr. Kastrup is a member of the Advisory Board on Mental Health for the World Health Organization in Geneva, Switzerland, and Vice President of the International Federation for Psychiatric Epidemiology.

Dean G. Kilpatrick is Professor of Clinical Psychology and Director of the National Crime Victims Research and Treatment Center at the Medical University of South Carolina in Charleston, South Carolina. He has been involved in the crime victims' rights field since 1974, when he became a founding member of People Against Rape, a Charleston-based rape crisis center. His primary research interests include measuring the prevalence of rape, other violent crimes, and other types of potentially traumatic events, as well as assessing the mental health impact of such events. He has published widely on these topics, served on the fourth edition of *Diagnostic and Statistical Manual of Mental Disorders* (DSM-IV) Posttraumatic Stress Disorder Advisory Committee, and was Principal Investigator on the PTSD Field Trial conducted as part of the DSM-IV revision process. Dr. Kilpatrick has also served as Editor of the *Journal of Traumatic Stress*. In 1990, President George Bush presented Dr. Kilpatrick with the President's Award for Outstanding Service for Victims of Crime, the nation's highest award in the crime victims' field.

J. David Kinzie is Professor of Psychiatry at Oregon Health Sciences University (OHSU), Portland, Oregon, and Director of the Posttraumatic Stress Clinic. Dr. Kinzie practiced medicine in Vietnam and Malaysia and was on the psychiatry faculty at the University of Malaya and the University of Hawaii. He founded the Indo-Chinese Psychiatric Program (now known as the International Psychiatric

Program) at OHSU in 1978 and continues to treat Cambodian refugees. Dr. Kinzie's publications include papers on crosscultural psychiatry and the diagnosis and treatment of PTSDs.

Mary P. Koss is Professor of Public Health, Family and Community Medicine, Psychiatry and Psychology in the Arizona Prevention Center at the University of Arizona College of Medicine in Tucson, Arizona. She cochairs the American Psychological Association Task Force on Violence Against Women and is the author of several award-winning publications on violence against women, sexual aggression, and victimization. She served on the National Research Council Panel on Violence Against Women, is Associate Editor of *Violence and Victims*, and is a member of the editorial board of several leading scientific journals. Dr. Koss has served as a consultant to the United Nations, the World Bank, and the Population Fund. Dr. Koss has received many honors, including the 2000 American Psychological Association Award for Distinguished Contributions to Public Policy.

Kathryn M. Magruder is Associate Professor of Psychiatry and Behavioral Sciences at the Medical University of South Carolina in Charleston, South Carolina. She is currently working on a research project to improve detection and referral for patients with PTSD. She served as Chief of the Services Research and Clinical Epidemiology Branch as well as Director of the Office of Rural Mental Health Research for NIMH. She has written numerous publications in mental health services research, particularly in the area of detection and treatment of mental disorders in primary care settings. Her current research focuses on PTSD in primary care populations and is funded by the Department of Veterans Affairs.

Anthony J. Marsella is Professor of Psychology, Director of the World Health Organization Psychiatric Research Center in Honolulu, and Associate Director of the Collaborative Disaster Management and Humanitarian Assistance Program at the University of Hawaii. Dr. Marsella has published widely in the areas of crosscultural psychopathology and psychotherapy, PTSD, social stress and coping, and schizophrenia, including 10 books and more than 130 other publications. He serves on numerous journal editorial boards and scientific and professional advisory committees and has been awarded numerous research and training grants and contracts. Dr. Marsella has been nationally and internationally recognized for his extraordinary contributions in research, teaching, and public policy through numerous awards, including the 1994 Master Lecturer Award by the American Psychological Association and the 1996 American Psychological Association Distinguished Contributions to the International Advancement of Psychology Award. His international awards include the Medal of Highest Honor from Soka University in Tokyo for his promotion of international peace and understanding. In 1999, Dr. Marsella was awarded an honorary doctoral degree at a ceremony at the University of Copenhagen, which was presided over by Queen Margarethe II of Denmark, for his contributions to cultural and international studies of psychology and psychiatry.

Richard Mollica is Director of the Harvard Program in Refugee Trauma and an Associate Professor of Psychiatry at Harvard Medical School and Harvard School of Public Health in Cambridge, Massachusetts. Dr. Mollica was awarded a Fulbright Professorship to the United Kingdom from 1979 to 1980, and in 1981 he cofounded the Indo-Chinese Psychiatry Clinic, which is now located at the Beth Israel Deaconess Medical Center in Boston. In 1986, Dr. Mollica and his colleagues founded the Harvard Program in Refugee Trauma, which administers Indo-Chinese Psychiatry Clinic's clinical activities and conducts training, policy, and research activities for traumatized populations worldwide.

Sister Dianna Ortiz, born in the United States, was a teacher of Mayan children when she was abducted and tortured by Guatemalan security forces. Since 1994, she has worked with the Guatemala Human Rights Commission/USA and is cofounder of its Coalition Missing project. A survivor herself, she has carried the message to people around the nation, to congressional committees, and to the White House that torture and impunity must end and that the rights of survivors must be protected. In 1996, in an effort to increase public awareness of U.S. involvement in torture in Guatemala, she held a 5-week silent vigil and fast in front of the White House that gained national and international attention. A recipient of numerous awards, she has been invited to speak to human rights organizations and other groups throughout the United States. She has been a guest on major news programs and has been interviewed by the media of a number of nations.

Robert S. Pynoos is Professor of Psychiatry at the University of California at Los Angeles (UCLA) School of Medicine and Director of the UCLA Trauma Psychiatry Service. He is an international authority on children, adolescents, and families exposed to war, community and interpersonal violence, and disaster. His clinical research has included studies of child and adolescent PTSD and complicated bereavement, the developmental neurobiology of PTSD, developmental psychopathology, and posttrauma treatment efficacy. He is a past President of the International Society for Traumatic Stress Studies. His international consultations have included work with UNICEF psychosocial programs in Kuwait after the Gulf War and in Bosnia-Herzegovina and with the Armenian Relief Society after the 1988 Spitak earthquake. He also served as a consultant to the U.S. Department of Education after the bombing of the federal building in Oklahoma City.

Margaret E. Ross is Associate Director of the Cambridge Business Development Center. She is also Research Associate of the International Criminal Defense Attorneys Association and a founding board member of the U.S. division. From 1995 to 1999, she was Program Coordinator at the Harvard Program in Refugee Trauma.

Agnes Rupp is Senior Research Economist and Chief of the Mental Health Economics Research Program at NIMH. Her research has focused on cost-of-illness studies and economic evaluation of various mental health interventions to improve the financing and delivery of mental health services for people suffering from mental disorders. Dr. Rupp also serves as Coeditor-in-Chief of the *Journal of Mental Health Policy and Economics* and chairs the newly established Mental Health Economics Section of the World Psychiatric Association.

Derrick Silove is a member of the School of Psychiatry and Foundation Professor of Psychiatry in the Southwestern School, University of New South Wales, Sydney, Australia. He is Director of the Psychiatry Research and Teaching Unit of the Southwest Sydney Area Health Service. He and his team are actively involved in research with refugees, particularly with asylum-seekers. He is a past Chair and current member of the Management Committee of the Service for the Treatment and Rehabilitation of Torture and Trauma Survivors, New South Wales. Since its inception, he has provided psychiatric services to that agency. He also cochairs the International Committee for Refugees and Other Migrants of the World Federation for Mental Health. He has undertaken several consultancies on refugee mental health both in Australia and abroad.

Eliot Sorel is Clinical Professor of Psychiatry and a consultant in affective and posttraumatic stress disorders and the integration of behavioral health and primary care in the context of health economics and health policy at the George Washington University School of Medicine in Washington, D.C. Dr. Sorel is currently serving as President of the Washington Psychiatric Society, President of the World Association for Social Psychiatry, Chairman of the World Psychiatric Association Violence Task Force, and a consultant for the World Health Organization.

Steven Southwick is Professor of Psychiatry at the Yale University School of Medicine and Professor of Psychiatry at the Yale University Child Study Center. He is also Director of the PTSD Program at the Connecticut Veterans Hospital and Codirector of the Clinical Neuroscience Division of the National Center for PTSD. He has served on the board of directors of the International Society for Traumatic Stress Studies and on the editorial board of the *Journal of Traumatic Stress*. Dr. Southwick is a leading expert on the neurobiology of PTSD and has published extensively in this area. His research has focused on the relationships among trauma, stress hormones, vigilance, and memory for stressful events.